Immunology for Surgeons

Immunology for Surgeons

Edited by
J. E. Castro

Royal Postgraduate Medical School, London

University Park Press
Baltimore

Published in the USA and Canada by
University Park Press
Chamber of Commerce Building
Baltimore, Maryland 21202

Published in the UK by
MTP Press Ltd
St Leonard's House
Lancaster, England

Library of Congress Cataloging in Publication Data
Main entry under title:
Immunology for surgeons

    Includes index.
      1. Immunology. 2. Immunopathology. 3. Immuno-
therapy.
I. Castro, J. E.
QR181.143   617'.07   76-7399
ISBN 0-8391-0932-6

Printed in Great Britain

Contents

List of Contributors

P. R. F. Bell, M.D., F.R.S.C.
Professor of Surgery, School of Medicine, University of Leicester, Leicester, England

J. P. Bramis, M.D.
Transplantation Unit, Mount Sinai Hospital, New York, N.Y., USA

J. E. Castro, Ph.D., M.S., F.R.C.S.
Department of Surgery, Royal Postgraduate Medical School, Hammersmith Hospital, London, W.12, England

G. Currie, M.D., M.R.C.P.
Ludwig Institute for Cancer Research, Chester Beatty Research Institute, Sutton, Surrey, England

J. W. Fabre, M.B., B.S., B.Med.Sc., Ph.D.
Wellcome Senior Research Fellow, Nuffield Department of Surgery, The Radcliffe Infirmary, Oxford, England

M. J. Hobart, M.A., Ph.D.,Vet. M.B.
Department of Immunology, Royal Postgraduate Medical School, Hammersmith Hospital, London, W.12, England

L. E. Hughes, F.R.C.S., F.R.A.C.S.
Professor of Surgery, University Department of Surgery, Welsh National School of Medicine, Cardiff, Wales

E. M. Lance, M.D.
Suite 403, Orthopaedic Associates of Hawaii, Inc., 1441, Kapiolani Boulevard, Honolulu 96814, Hawaii

D. J. R. Laurence, M.A., Ph.D. Cantab.
Unit of Human Cancer Biology, London Branch, Ludwig Institute for Cancer Research in conjunction with the Royal Marsden Hospital, London, England

A. M. Neville, Ph.D., M.D., M.R.C. Path.
Unit of Human Cancer Biology, London Branch, Ludwig Institute for Cancer Research in conjunction with the Royal Marsden Hospital, London, England

J. J. T. Owen, M.A., M.D., B.Sc.
Professor of Anatomy, Department of Anatomy, The Medical School, University of Newcastle upon Tyne, Newcastle, England

J. A. Sachs, M.B., Ch.B., Ph.D.
Tissue Immunology Unit, The London Hospital Medical College, London, E.1, England

J. R. Salaman, M.A., M.Chir., F.R.C.S.
Transplantation Unit and K.R.U.F. Institute of Renal Disease, Royal Infirmary, Cardiff, Wales

C. J. F. Spry, M.A., M.R.C.P., D.Phil.
Department of Immunology, Royal Postgraduate Medical School, Hammersmith Hospital, London, W.12, England

R. N. Taub, M.D., Ph.D.
Mount Sinai School of Medicine, City University of New York, New York, U.S.A.

R. H. Whitehead, M.Sc.
University Department of Surgery, Welsh National School of Medicine, Cardiff, Wales

R. F. M. Wood, F.R.C.S.
Department of Surgery, University of Leicester, Leicester, England

Preface

Immunology is a rapidly developing subject. The contributors in this book present some components of immunological knowledge which relate to the present and the possible future practice of surgery. Aspects of cellular and humoral immunity necessary for understanding are described and consideration given to the mechanisms underlying immunological diseases. Whilst the original interest in immune response was related to microbial resistance, the recent impetus to surgical immunology has been the resurgence of organ grafting. Separate sections of the book deal with clinical organ transplantation, the allograft reaction, graft rejection and immunogenetics. A pre-requisite of successful organ grafting is suppressive control of immune responses. Approaches to conventional immunosuppression and specific non-reactivity are therefore considered.

One method of cancer therapy is strengthening of the host's immune responses. Both experimental and clinical immunotherapy are discussed and components of tumour immunology necessary for their rational understanding are dealt with separately. Successful immunotherapy requires monitoring of immune responses but another method for improving results of cancer treatment is earlier diagnosis by immunological methods.

The book is aimed at practising surgeons who want to know the relevance of immunology to clinical surgery and laboratory scientists needing to understand the applications of their basic concepts.

I am very grateful both to the authors for their contributions and the editorial staff of MTP Press Limited, for their considerable help.

J. E. Castro
April 1976

CHAPTER 1

Introduction

J. J. T. Owen

Introduction

Immunology is an exciting area of study. At an experimental level, it is possible to formulate hypotheses and to design experiments to test these hypotheses. From the clinical point of view, it is quite clear that immunology has important implications for the practice of medicine in general. Interest in immunology grew out of the attempts to deliberately provoke resistance to microbes. Edward Jenner's use of 'vaccination' with cowpox as an attempt to provoke immunity to smallpox is usually quoted as the first experiment along these lines. Subsequently in the late 19th century, Pasteur and others made a more systematic study of methods of immunization and a variety of powerful techniques for use in microbiology and blood grouping were later developed.

Whilst interest in the immune response as a barrier to microbial infection remains a vital area of study, the ramifications of immunology permeate a much broader span of medical practice. We now realize that selective suppression of the immune response may hold the key to the successful transplantation of tissues. Stimulation of the immune response may provide a means by which we can effect the rejection of cancers. Furthermore, disorders of the immune response are probably responsible for a variety of human diseases. Thus, immune reactions directed against an individual's own tissues (autoimmunity) or exaggerated immune responses (hypersensitivity) to foreign substances may result in distressing and harmful symptoms.

Clearly, it is impossible within the very broad span of immunology for any one individual to be an expert on all aspects. However, there is a body of knowledge upon which there is a reasonable level of general agreement.

This should, perhaps, form a basis for the application of immunology to practical clinical problems. It is the aim of this book to try to provide this body of knowledge in relation to the practice of surgery and in this chapter I will attempt to introduce the general concept of immunity; aspects of ontogeny and phylogeny of the immune response; the roles of cells in immune reactions and the application of this knowledge to disease states.

Definition of the Immune Response

First of all, we need to attempt to define what we mean by the immune response. Basically, we are talking about the reaction of an individual to substances or organisms which are foreign to it. The reaction involves a considerable degree of specificity in that once an immune response to a particular foreign substance has taken place, a second exposure to this substance results in a much enhanced response (the so-called secondary response), whereas a first exposure to any other substance elicits only a lower-level primary response. The enhanced secondary response may be elicited some time after the primary response has taken place. Thus, immunological 'memory' can be added to 'specificity' as a hallmark of the immune response.

Phylogeny of the Immune Response

The immune response as defined above is present within all living vertebrates (reviewed by Marchalonis, 1974). Thus, all vertebrates can form antibodies and reject foreign tissue grafts. Of course, within vertebrates there is a good deal of variation in the structure of the lymphoid system and the level of sophistication of the immune response. In lower vertebrates such as the hagfish and lamprey, foreign grafts are rejected, but over a much prolonged time-course than in higher vertebrates. Again, a limited number of classes of antibody are produced in lower vertebrates, whereas five classes of antibody are produced in mammals. Corresponding to these levels of immunological capability, lower vertebrates have less highly organized lymphoid systems than higher vertebrates. Thus, whilst all vertebrate species probably possess a thymus, spleens are present only in species more advanced than cyclostomes and lymph nodes are found only in mammals. However, aggregates of lymphocytes, probably representing a primitive type of lymph node, are found throughout the tissues of amphibians and birds. Organized gastrointestinal lymphoid tissue such as Peyer's patches, etc., is mainly restricted to mammals although birds possess lymphoid aggregates in the intestine and, in addition, they possess a so-called primary lymphoid organ, the bursa of Fabricius, which develops from the cloaca.

The bursa is unique to birds and plays an important role in the development of the antibody response (see below).

When the question is raised as to whether immune responses are present in invertebrates a number of difficulties arise. Certainly, invertebrates do not possess the immunological apparatus, i.e. lymphocytes and antibodies, which we believe are crucial in the vertebrate immune response. Certain invertebrates do possess circulating phagocytic cells, known as celomocytes, which function in the removal of invading bacteria and in the destruction of grafted tissue, and bacteriocidal substances have been observed in some invertebrates although these do not bear any clear structural relationship to the antibodies of vertebrates. In most instances, the responses seen in invertebrates would not fall within the definition of the vertebrate immune response as above. However, recently skin graft rejection reactions have been reported in annelid worms which resemble in a number of respects the transplantation reaction of vertebrates. Thus grafting of skin from one worm to another results in a rejection process, and if a second portion of skin is transplanted from the original donor to the same host, there is an accelerated rejection which is not seen when skin is transferred from an unrelated donor. Celomocytes are seen at the site of graft rejection and they can be used to transfer immunity to non-immune animals. However, elucidation of the molecular mechanisms involved in these rejection processes is crucial to the question of whether rejection responses of annelids are directly homologous to vertebrate immunity.

In summary, it is clear that recognition of foreignness developed at an early stage of evolution, but it is doubtful if many of the mechanisms seen in non-vertebrate species operate by the same molecular mechanisms as the vertebrate immune response. Of course, it is quite possible that the vertebrate immune response evolved out of these primitive mechanisms.

Antigens and Antibodies

Before discussing the types of immune response of vertebrates and their cellular basis, it is necessary to discuss briefly the concepts of antigen and antibody. Antigens are the chemical groupings present upon foreign substances against which the immune response is directed. Generally speaking, for a substance to elicit an immune response it must have a fairly high molecular weight (> 10000). The antibody molecules which are elicited by the antigen bind to specific structures, so-called antigen determinants, on the surface of the molecule. Whilst an antibody molecule is specific for one antigenic determinant there may be several determinants on a single large molecule eliciting the synthesis of many different antibodies.

Chemical groupings which bind with antibody (i.e. which act as antigens) may not be able necessarily to elicit the formation of antibody (i.e. they may not act as immunogens). However, many years ago Landsteiner pioneered work in which he showed that comparatively small molecules (< 10000 molecular weight) could, if they were covalently linked to larger molecules, elicit an immune response. The small molecules which were usually chemically defined groupings of known structure are called haptens and the larger molecules to which they are linked are called carriers. This work is of considerable importance because it suggests ways in which small molecules can act as immunogens and indeed there are reasons for believing that this may be one way by which certain individuals become immunized to drugs.

Antibodies belong to the group of proteins called immunoglobulins. The structure of the immunoglobulin molecule, the types of immunoglobulin class, etc., will be dealt with in Chapter 2. It is only necessary to say here that every immunoglobulin molecule has a fundamentally similar structure consisting of two light chains (about 220 amino acids long) and two heavy chains (about 430 amino acids long). Amino acid sequence studies have shown that the N-terminal half of the light chains and the N-terminal quarter of the heavy chains are extremely variable at a number of amino acid sites, while the rest of the chains conform to a limited number of constant patterns. Since secondary and tertiary protein structure follows from amino acid sequence, a great number of differently shaped combining sites directed at the various determinants of antigens are possible in the variable region of the immunoglobulin molecule. The combination of antigen with antibody is at the heart of the immune reaction. It is usual and useful to think of this in terms of the analogy of the fit of a key to a lock. The structure of the antigen (the key) must be compatible with that of the antibody (the lock) for binding to occur.

Types of Immune Response

Quite early in the study of immunity there was controversy with regard to the relative roles of cells as opposed to soluble factors (antibodies) in the immune response. At that time, Metchnikov proposed that phagocytes (or, as we would now call them, macrophages) were the most important cell type in the immune response. Others believed that antibodies were of crucial importance. Although we now know that both cells and antibodies are necessary in most immune responses, the basic notion of cellular as opposed to humoral (antibody) immunity has persisted and is still valuable today. However, we now look upon lymphocytes as being the specific cells of the immune response (i.e. immunocompetent cells) rather than macrophages.

How do we define these two types of response? Firstly, in an experimental situation, cellular (cell-mediated) immunity can be defined as that immunity which can be transferred from one animal to another by cells. In broader terms, it is that immunity which necessitates the direct participation of cells at the site of the reaction. Examples of this type of immunity are the so-called delayed hypersensitivity responses which are seen, for instance, in the tuberculin reaction and the rejection of foreign skin grafts. Humoral immunity, on the other hand, is defined as the type of immune response that can be transferred by serum. In other words immunity is dependent on soluble factors alone. This type of immunity is probably very important in a variety of infections, but is seen, classically, in the immediate hypersensitivity which takes place in allergic individuals suffering from such conditions as asthma and hay fever.

A recent major advance has been the discovery that there are two major lymphocyte classes corresponding to these two types of immune response. One class of lymphocyte, the T lymphocyte, is generally equated with cell-mediated responses, whereas the other major class of lymphocyte, the B lymphocyte, is equated with humoral immunity. Whilst we know now that these statements are an oversimplification of the true situation and humoral immunity, for example, is dependent upon the co-operation of T cells, nonetheless it is generally accepted that the two types of immunity are primarily dependent on separate types of lymphocyte.

Lymphocytes and the Immune Response

It is remarkable in view of the current interest in lymphocytes how recent has been the acceptance that lymphocytes play a central role in immune responses. Indeed, conclusive evidence for the role of lymphocytes in immune responses has been available only since the late 1950s. Until this time it was generally believed that lymphocytes were end cells and therefore of little functional importance. However, in 1959 it was shown that lymphocytes could be activated to undergo proliferation in tissue culture by a variety of substances, the best known of which is phytohaemagglutinin. These substances, or mitogens as they are now called, usually activate a majority of lymphocytes and do so in a non-specific or non-immunological way (Ling and Kay, 1975). However, subsequently it was shown that similar activation of lymphocytes *in vitro* could be achieved by specific antigens. In this case only a proportion of lymphocytes underwent activation.

In the early 1960s, the importance of lymphocytes in immune responses was further demonstrated by a number of important *in vivo* experiments (reviewed by Gowans and McGregor, 1965). Thus, depletion of animals' lymphocytes by chronic drainage of lymphocytes from the thoracic duct severely impairs the immune response of these animals to various antigens, e.g. tetanus toxoid, sheep red blood cells and skin grafts. If lymphocytes are injected into these depleted animals, their immune responsiveness is restored. Furthermore, if lymphocytes are transferred from an animal already primed to a particular antigen, the depleted recipient will respond to this antigen as though it also had been primed (i.e. it will show a secondary type of response). Thus, lymphocytes can transfer not only immunocompetence but also immunological memory.

Subsequently it has been shown that lymphocytes can transfer immuno-logical tolerance. That is, if lymphocytes are transferred from an animal which has been made tolerant to an antigen to a depleted host, the immune responsiveness of the host will be restored except for reactivity to the antigen to which the donor was tolerant. All of these experiments have indicated the importance of lymphocytes in immune responses and have led to their recognition as 'immunologically competent' cells.

Origins of Lymphocyte Populations: Primary Lymphoid Organs

Most of the evidence for the notion of two major classes of lymphocyte and their importance in the two major types of immune response came from studies on what might be called the ontogeny of immunity. For example, in the early 1960s it was shown that removal of the thymus gland of newborn rodents resulted in a state of immunological deficiency in which the animals were unable to perform cell-mediated immune reactions such as the rejection of foreign skin grafts. Subsequently, it was shown that these animals suffered from a profound deficiency of T lymphocytes in their lymphoid organs; an observation which supported the idea that the thymus was a crucial organ for the production of T lymphocytes (reviewed by Miller and Osoba, 1967).

At about the same time, studies in birds pointed to the importance of a separate lymphoid organ, the bursa of Fabricius, in the production of B lymphocytes. Thus, removal of the bursa of Fabricius at the time of hatching, or ideally before hatching, resulted in an impairment of humoral immunity and a depletion of lymphocytes which were characterized subsequently as B cells (Cooper et al., 1969). The site/s of origin of mammalian B lympho-cytes has remained more controversial, but new information has recently become available and this will be discussed later. Organs in which lympho-cytes are produced from more primitive stem cells are called primary lymphoid organs. This distinguishes them from secondary lymphoid organs which receive lymphocytes from the primary sites.

ORIGIN OF T LYMPHOCYTES: ROLE OF THE THYMUS

It is widely recognized that the thymus is one of the first lymphoid organs to appear during embryogenesis. The framework of the thymus is derived from the downgrowth of epithelial cells of the 3rd pharyngeal pouch of the embryo. This epithelial primordium migrates downwards through the neck to eventually take up its position under the upper part of the sternum. In the past, considerable controversy has centred upon the question of the origins of the lymphocytes which appear within the thymus. Some workers believed that they are derived from the epithelial cells of the primordium, others that they are derived from mesenchymal cells which migrate into the epithelial primordium from some other site.

In recent years, techniques have been introduced which allow cellular migration to be followed. These techniques utilize either isotopic labelling of cells for short-term studies, or chromosome markers for longer-term investigations. The latter technique has found most application in tracing the origins of lymphoid cells. For example, using the T6 chromosome marker in mice, it has been shown that the lymphoid compartment of thymus grafts or the cell-depleted thymus of the irradiated animal are re-populated by stem cells of bone marrow origin (Ford, 1966). The T6 chromosome is a minute chromosome resulting from a chromosomal trans-location and its presence in some mice but not others of the same strain allows experiments of the type above to be performed. Furthermore, it has been shown that there is a natural interchange of stem cells between mice joined in parabiosis, one of which has the T6 marker chromosome, and as a result each thymus contains lymphocytes derived from both animals. Comparable experiments in which chick embryos were joined in parabiotic union via a chorioallantoic membrane vascular anastomosis showed that when embryos were of opposite sex, the thymus of male embryos contained many dividing cells with a female sex chromosome constitution and *vice versa*. These and other experiments have demonstrated the fact that the lymphocytes of the thymus arise by differentiation of cells which enter the thymic primordium from without, namely from the bloodstream. Whilst in the adult, these cells are derived from bone marrow, in the embryo they are probably derived from the major sites of embryonic haemopoiesis, i.e. yolk sac and fetal liver (Owen, 1971).

Once migrant stem cells have entered the epithelial primordium of the thymus they proliferate and mature to small lymphocytes. At least some of these lymphocytes migrate from the thymus to secondary (or peripheral) lymphoid organs such as lymph nodes, Peyer's patches and spleen, where as T lymphocytes they perform a number of important immunological functions (Figure 1.1). Whilst this basic scheme is correct in outline, a number of unresolved problems remain. For instance, controversy surrounds the question of the nature of the intrathymic influence which is responsible for

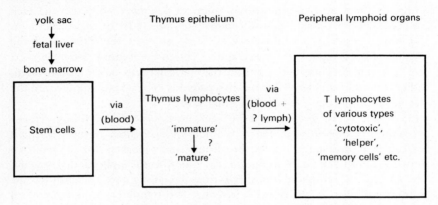

Figure 1.1 Pathways of T lymphocyte maturation

lymphocyte maturation. Is a diffusible substance, a thymic hormone, involved, or is cell contact and interaction within the thymic environment the crucial factor? Furthermore, it is known that, functionally, the majority of lymphocytes within the thymus are inactive and cannot simply be equated with T lymphocytes in peripheral organs. Indeed, the extent of cell migration from the thymus is largely unknown and many cells may die either within the thymus or shortly after migration from the thymus. Another complexity is that there is now evidence for subpopulations of T lymphocytes in peripheral organs. We are unsure as to whether these represent separate lines of T-cell development or whether they are stages in a single differentiation pathway. In either case, it is difficult to see how this peripheral T-cell heterogeneity relates to the heterogeneity of lymphocytes within the thymus.

Thymus hormones

Of the questions posed above, perhaps most interest has been shown recently in the question of thymus hormone/s (reviewed by Trainin and Small, 1973). Although there is a considerable literature on the supposed effects of thymus extracts on a variety of biological functions, work in the last decade has concentrated on the possible effects of thymus preparations on immunological responsiveness, especially on T-cell function. A number of groups have been able to isolate molecules which influence the reactivity of lymphoid cells. These molecules are mostly protein in nature with molecular weights of 10000 to 12000 and represent either separate hormones or sub-units of a single hormone. They have been shown to increase the immune reactivity of animals whose immune responses have been depressed by thymectomy and/or irradiation or animals born with a genetically determined thymic deficiency, such as the 'nude' mouse. Various *in vitro* tests have also been developed to assay the activity of thymus hormone/s. Nonetheless, a major problem in the evaluation of these hormones has been the lack of reproducible assays to measure their effect.

A further problem is the uncertainty as to whether these hormones act upon stem cells which have yet to enter the thymus and/or upon cells which have already migrated from the thymus to peripheral lymphoid organs. This question is of considerable practical importance since in conditions of complete thymic agenesis, a thymic hormone would be effective only if it acted on pre-thymic stem cells whereas a thymic graft would be expected to influence both pre- and post-thymic cell maturation.

Perhaps most information is available on a preparation known as thymosin. It is already undergoing trials for use in immune deficiency of the T-cell type and, more speculatively, it has been suggested that it might be of value in potentiating T-cell responses in neoplasia. In summary, caution is required in the use and evaluation of thymus hormones. At a basic level, we are still ignorant of the nature of the interaction between epithelial cells (from which thymus hormones presumably emanate) and lymphoid cells. Certainly, in animal models the effects of thymic extracts never approach quantitatively the influence of a thymus graft on the restoration of immune competence in immunodeficient recipients.

ORIGIN OF B LYMPHOCYTES: ROLE OF THE BURSA OF FABRICIUS

The bursa of Fabricius, like the thymus, is a major lymphoid organ which appears during embryogenesis. However, unlike the thymus, the bursa is found only in birds. Derived from epithelium, the bursa develops as an outgrowth from the wall of the developing cloaca. The organ is pouch-like in structure and its lining epithelium grows down into the underlying mesenchyme to form follicular structures. It is within these epithelial follicles that lymphocytes are first detected. Whilst there has been controversy in the past as to the origin of these lymphocytes (as in the case of thymus— see above) there is now a consensus of opinion based on cell-marker studies that these lymphocytes are derived from developing haemopoietic tissues such as yolk sac. Thus, there is a migration of stem cells from yolk sac to bursa follicles within which they mature to B lymphocytes (Figure 1.2).

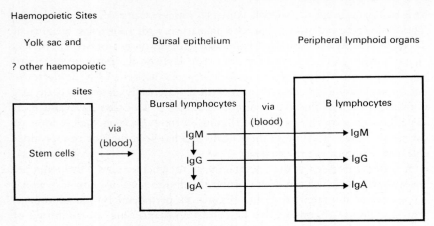

Figure 1.2   Pathways of B lymphocyte maturation

One of the interesting features of the bursa is the fact that it is the first site where immunoglobulin synthesis can be detected in the developing avian embryo using an immunofluorescence technique in which an antibody directed against chicken immunoglobulin and conjugated with a fluorescent marker such as fluorescein is used in fluorescence microscopy (Kincade and Cooper, 1971). Some of the large lymphocytes found within the developing bursal follicles can be shown to have cytoplasmic immunoglobulin at an early stage of embryogenesis. Subsequently, large proportions of bursal lymphocytes can be shown to have membrane-bound immunoglobulin on their surfaces. In a series of elegant studies, it has been shown that the first immunoglobulin class to be synthesized within the bursa is IgM. Later, IgG followed by IgA can be detected. All of these studies have supported the notion that the bursa of Fabricius is an important site of B lymphocyte maturation (the principal distinguishing feature of B lymphocytes as compared with T lymphocytes being the presence of readily detectable surface immunoglobulin). Furthermore, B lymphocytes bearing immunoglobulin of various classes are generated. Interestingly, if IgM synthesis is suppressed by injecting chick embryos with an antibody directed at the μ (heavy) chains of the IgM molecule, IgG and IgA synthesis are suppressed as well. This experiment, together with the fact that a number of 'double' producing lymphocytes are found within the bursa, has led to the suggestion that there is a switch in synthesis of immunoglobulin class in some of the lymphocytes of the bursa such that some lymphocytes which initially synthesize IgM switch to IgG and some of these then switch to IgA. This model of B-cell maturation has the virtue of explaining how generation of heterogeneity of immunoglobulin class may be accomplished within a single cell line without the necessity for repeated generation of heterogeneity of immunoglobulin specificity each time a new class appears.

Following maturation within the bursa, B lymphocytes migrate to other lymphoid organs of the chicken. If the bursa is removed before this migration has taken place, there is a profound depletion in the numbers of lymphocytes bearing membrane-bound immunoglobulin in lymphoid organs and there is an inability on the part of bursectomized chickens to manufacture and secrete the various immunoglobulin classes. As mentioned previously, these results support the notion that the bursa of Fabricius is an essential site of B lymphocyte maturation and that B lymphocytes are precursors of antibody-secreting (plasma) cells. Little is known about the nature of the factors which influence B-cell maturation within the bursa or elsewhere.

MAMMALIAN SITES OF B LYMPHOCYTE PRODUCTION

Following the demonstration of the importance of the bursa of Fabricius in B lymphocyte production, it was suggested by a number of workers that lymphoepithelial organs with comparable functions might exist within the intestinal tract of mammals. A variety of organs, including the tonsils, appendix and Peyer's patches, were postulated to be 'bursa-equivalents'. However, no clear-cut effect on the production of B lymphocytes was found in a series of experiments in which these organs were surgically removed.

Recently, a different experimental approach has been made to this problem. Various embryonic organs have been removed from developing mouse embryos and in the isolated situation provided by tissue culture, their capacity to generate B lymphocytes has been examined (Figure 1.3). In these experiments, a variety of haemopoietic organs have been studied

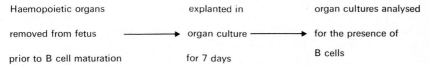

Figure 1.3 Experimental design for determining the origins of B lymphocytes

including fetal yolk sac, fetal liver, fetal spleen and developing bone marrow. It has been shown that with the exception of yolk sac, all of these organs are capable of independently generating lymphocytes synthesizing IgM. These results indicate that there is no distinct lymphoid organ in mammalian development responsible for B lymphocyte maturation, but rather that B lymphocytes are generated along with other blood cells in sites of general haemopoiesis (Owen, 1974). Of course, we are unable to say whether B lymphocytes achieve full maturation within these sites or whether further maturation takes place following their migration to lymph nodes etc.

Secondary (Peripheral) Lymphoid Organs: Migratory Pathways of Lymphocytes

Secondary lymphoid organs are defined as those organs which are dependent upon primary sites for the production and seeding of lymphocyte populations. Possibly, further maturation of lymphocytes may occur within secondary organs but, typically, they are organs within which immune responses take place. Lymph nodes, the various gastrointestinal lymphoid organs and the white pulp of the spleen are regarded as secondary lymphoid organs. If animals are kept in a germ-free environment the development of these organs is seriously affected, which suggests that not only do those organs require lymphocytes from primary sites but that the action of antigens is necessary to stimulate lymphocyte proliferation, thus increasing the overall cellularity of the organs and producing such histological features as lymphoid follicles and germinal centres.

Perhaps one of the most remarkable advances in knowledge of the functional anatomy of the lymphoid system in recent years has been the discovery that a major proportion of lymphocytes are continually recirculating between blood and lymph (reviewed by Ford and Gowans, 1969). Thus, lymphocytes within lymph nodes are not derived from the afferent lymph vessels but, instead, are made up of cells which have passed from blood through the walls of special vessels known as post-capillary venules into the substance of the lymph node. A further remarkable feature is that there is selective migration of T and B lymphocytes to different regions of the node. However, the majority of cells, be they T or B cells, eventually drain from the node through efferent lymphatics into the lymph system and ultimately return to blood via the thoracic duct. A comparable lymphocyte recirculatory pathway has been demonstrated in Peyer's patches.

The significance of this massive recirculation of lymphocytes will be discussed in a following section, but for the moment I will restrict discussion to an account of the anatomical features of peripheral lymphoid organs which are of functional significance to the immune response (Figure 1.4).

It is traditional and useful to divide lymph nodes for descriptive purposes into two regions, cortex and medulla. The outer cortical area contains prominent collections of lymphocytes known as lymphoid follicles. Sometimes these follicles are sites of active lymphocyte proliferation, the cells most active in division being large 'blast'-like cells situated in the centre of each follicle in the region known as the germinal centre. Elsewhere in the outer cortex, lymphocytes are distributed more evenly. The deeper regions of the cortex (the so-called mid and deep regions or paracortex) do not

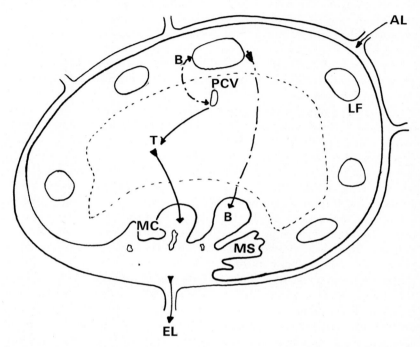

Figure 1.4 Lymphocyte recirculatory pathways in lymph nodes. AL=Afferent Lymphatics; EL=Efferent Lymphatics; LF=Lymphoid Follicles; PCV=Post-capillary Venules; MC=Medullary Cord; MS=Medullary Sinus; —→=T-lymphocyte pathway; ---→ =B-lymphocyte pathway. The region outlined by the broken line is the paracortex.

contain distinct collections of lymphocytes; rather, the lymphocytes are distributed in a random fashion. However, this region is also a site which may be involved in intense cell proliferation, the proliferating cells being large 'pyroninophilic' blast cells. In the medullary region, the two most prominent features are the presence of medullary cords and medullary sinuses. The cords are projections of lymphoid cells radiating from the cortex into the medulla; the sinuses are large drainage areas by which lymphocytes leave the lymph node and enter the efferent lymphatics. Plasma cells (antibody-secreting cells) and macrophages are common cell types in these areas.

It has been shown, using radioactive marker techniques, that when lymphocytes leave blood by migrating through the walls of post-capillary venules which lie in the paracortex, T and B lymphocytes follow separate migratory pathways. B lymphocytes migrate outwards towards the lymphoid follicles; some may actually migrate into follicles. However, from this point onwards the fate of B lymphocytes is less clear. The majority must migrate back through the paracortex into the medulla and so reach the efferent lymph vessels but this pathway has not been demonstrated directly. T lymphocytes follow a separate pathway and mostly migrate into the paracortical zone. Then they continue their migration down through the medullary cords and sinuses into the efferent lymph.

In spleen, lymphoid tissue is organized around the arterioles which radiate through the splenic substance. The lymphoid tissue is usually referred to as 'white pulp' because at a macroscopic level it has a 'whitish' appearance which contrasts with the remainder of the tissue—the 'red pulp'. There is a pathway of lymphocyte migration in the spleen from the marginal sinus which surrounds the white pulp into the white pulp itself. As in lymph nodes, T and B lymphocytes migrate into different regions of the lymphoid tissue; B lymphocytes migrate to lymphoid follicles and T lymphocytes migrate to areas between follicles. Ultimately, both migrate from the white pulp into the red pulp where they enter the vascular system. It should be noted that whereas migration in lymph nodes is from blood to lymph, in spleen it is from the blood of the marginal sinus to the blood of the red pulp.

If T lymphocytes are depleted experimentally by neonatal thymectomy, for example, or naturally as in congenital thymic aplasia, the regions most severely affected in lymph nodes and in spleen are those which are most concerned in T cell migration, i.e. the paracortex of lymph nodes and the diffuse interfollicular area of spleen. These observations have supported the notion that peripheral lymphoid tissues are divisible into T and B regions corresponding to the migratory pathways of these two cell types (Parrott and De Sousa, 1971).

It should be noted that all peripheral lymphoid organs are made up of a sponge-like framework of reticular fibres and cells named in many histology textbooks as 'reticuloendothelial cells'. However, the precise nature of these cells is unclear. In functional terms their most striking activity is that of phagocytosis and it is probably best to regard them as a component of the macrophage system.

The Recognition of Antigen by Lymphocytes

There have been various theories to explain both the diversity and the specificity of the immune response. These can be placed into two broad categories

On the one hand, it has been suggested that an antigen by its structure instructs lymphocytes to produce antibody molecules of a specificity which will combine with the antigen (instruction theory). On the other hand, it has been proposed that all of the information required for the production of a complete range of antibody molecules is already possessed by lymphocytes prior to the entry of antigen and that the role of antigen is simply to select the cell or cells which are producing antibody molecules which 'fit' the antigen (clonal selection theory).

In this brief discussion I hope that it will suffice to say that there is a body of evidence to support the clonal selection view and it is now generally accepted that lymphocytes are heterogeneous in their capacity to recognize and react with antigen. In other words, each antigen will elicit the reaction of one or, at most, a few lymphocytes.

The basis for the restriction of lymphocyte reactivity is another question. It has been argued that somatic mutation may be a frequent event in the organs where lymphocytes are generated and in this way diversity of responsiveness may be generated. On the other hand, the selective expression in individual lymphocytes of genes present within the germ line would result in the heterogeneity of responsiveness which has been observed. Of course, the two views are not mutually exclusive, but the balance of evidence at the moment favours the 'germ line' view. Whatever the origin of diversity, quite clearly there must be considerable heterogeneity in responsiveness between individual lymphocytes to account for the broad repertoire of responsiveness displayed by the immune response as a whole. There is evidence that heterogeneity of responsiveness is not restricted to a particular lymphocyte class, but is present within both T and B lymphocytes. In other words, T and B lymphocytes recognize antigens independently.

An obvious question follows from the preceding discussion; what is the nature of the receptor molecule on the surface of lymphocytes which enables them to bind specifically with one or a few antigens? In the case of B lymphocytes this question can be answered with a fair degree of confidence. B lymphocytes have upon their surface immunoglobulin molecules which are a sample of the type of immunoglobulin (in terms of specificity and, perhaps, class) which the cell can produce in large quantities once activation has taken place. This membrane-bound immunoglobulin can act, therefore, as an antigen-recognition receptor. In the case of T lymphocytes the problem is a more difficult one, because it has proved difficult to demonstrate immunoglobulin on the surfaces of T lymphocytes and, indeed, to show that the immunoglobulin which may be present is the product of T cells rather than absorbed onto the surfaces of cells from the serum. Recently, considerable interest has been shown in the genetic basis of the immune response, i.e. the manner in which individuals react to antigen is determined by the 'immune response' genes they possess. In certain species, these genes are linked to the genes which control the production of histocompatibility factors. It is possible, although not proven, that immune response genes code for a product which is expressed upon the surface of T cells and which is concerned with antigen recognition. This is a matter which will require further investigation.

This is perhaps an appropriate place to point out that the recirculation of lymphocytes described in an earlier section assumes greater functional significance in view of the evidence for the restricted reactivity of individual lymphocytes to antigens. Thus, recirculation greatly increases the chance of lymphocytes contacting antigens with which they will specifically combine and to which they will react.

The Implementation of the Immune Response

The consequences of the activation of lymphocytes by antigen vary according to whether a T lymphocyte or a B lymphocyte is involved. When T lymphocytes respond to antigen they undergo enlargement and enter division. There are many other important changes taking place at a molecular level including increased synthesis of RNA and protein. The enlarged cells are known as 'blast' cells and they are sometimes referred to as 'pyroninophilic' because their cytoplasm contains a considerable quantity of RNA which stains with the dye pyronin. At an ultrastructural level, the cells have a prominent Golgi structure and a large number of ribosomes but they have poorly developed endoplasmic reticulum (cf. activated B cells—see below). Following a series of divisions, the activated cells produced are comparable in morphology to the initial small lymphocyte. However, in functional properties the activated cells are very different and are able to participate in immune reactions as 'cytotoxic' cells, 'helper' cells or perhaps even as 'suppressor' cells. Cytotoxic cells are activated T cells which can lyse cells of foreign grafts bearing incompatible transplantation antigens. Helper and suppressor cells are activated T cells which modulate the reactivity of B cells to antigen and hence participate in the overall control of the humoral antibody response. Activated T cells also liberate factors known as lymphokines which influence the activity of other cells such as macrophages. These various T-cell functions may belong to distinct T-cell subsets and this possibility is discussed in the following section. A further complication is that as well as the generation of effector T cells, so-called 'memory' T cells persist long after the immune response has subsided. They mediate the enhanced immune response seen on secondary stimulation.

When B cells are activated by antigen they also undergo enlargement and mitosis and enter a phase of development which, at least at light microscope level, is very comparable to that seen in T cells. The progeny of the activated B cell is again a large blast cell with pyroninophilic cytoplasm but at an ultrastructural level B 'blasts' possess a much more profuse endoplasmic reticulum than T 'blasts'. The cells which are produced as a result of division of B 'blasts' are antibody-secreting cells (plasma cells). However, some of the progeny of activated B cells are not short-lived (as plasma cells are), but persist as 'memory' cells capable of responding in a 'secondary' fashion to the re-entry of antigen.

The events which follow upon the activation of T and B lymphocytes can also be seen at the whole organ level (Ford, 1973). Thus, antigens which predominantly stimulate cell-mediated immunity and therefore T lymphocyte responsiveness produce changes in the T-dependent region of lymph nodes, i.e. the paracortex. Large numbers of pyroninophilic blast cells appear within this region and we assume that large numbers of effector T cells are produced which migrate from the node to sites of immune reactivity. On the other hand, when humoral antibody is mainly stimulated, the major events are the production of lymphoid follicles, germinal centres and the presence of large numbers of plasma cells in medullary cords and sinuses. The significance of lymphoid follicles and germinal centres has not been fully elucidated. However, there is evidence that germinal centres may be sites where memory B cells are generated. In summary, it is possible to correlate the type of immune response produced by a particular antigen with the anatomical features of the reacting lymphoid organ.

Subsets of T and B Lymphocytes

In previous sections I have dealt with the generation of T cells and their importance in cell-mediated immune responses. At that time, I alluded to the fact that T lymphocytes are also important in many humoral immune responses involving a variety of antigens. T lymphocytes do not themselves produce humoral antibody but they co-operate or help B cells to do so. This helper activity is classically seen in the immune response to haptens. As previously mentioned, haptens alone are unable to elicit an immune response, although they are able to bind antibody once it has been formed. However, if haptens are attached to larger macromolecules (so-called carriers) a humoral antibody response can be elicited. In a series of important experiments it has been shown that when a hapten bound to a carrier molecule is injected into an animal, T lymphocytes recognize and react to determinants upon the carrier molecule, whereas B lymphocytes respond to haptenic determinants. In other words, recognition and responsiveness of T cells to carrier determinants in some way enables B cells to respond to haptens. There is a variety of theories to explain this phenomenon but these are outside the brief of this chapter. However, the phenomenon is an important one and it has been suggested that it may be the mechanism whereby individuals become sensitized to small haptenic molecules such as drugs. The co-operative activity of T and B cells also has a variety of important implications for immunology as a whole. It has been suggested that only T lymphocytes are normally tolerant to the body's own antigens and that B lymphocytes are potentially reactive, but in the absence of helper T cells they do not respond.

Whilst there is substantial evidence for separate categories of functional T lymphocytes such as the 'helper' cells described above and 'cytotoxic' or even 'suppressor' cells mentioned in previous sections, we are still unclear as to whether these categories represent different functional states in a common differentiation pathway or whether quite separate pathways of maturation are involved, perhaps beginning in the thymus. This problem may not be finally resolved until cell markers are available for the identification of the various T cell subsets.

Considerable heterogeneity also exists in B lymphocyte populations. Thus, it can be shown using immunofluorescence tests that not all B lymphocytes have immunoglobulin of the same class on their surfaces and it has been argued that this is the basis for the generation of various immunoglobulin classes during an immune reaction. Previously, I have mentioned the generation of memory T and B lymphocytes during immune responses. As yet, there are no readily available techniques for identifying and separating these cells.

The Role of Ancillary Cells in Immune Responses

Although lymphocytes play a major part in immune responses as immunologically competent cells, it would be a great mistake to ignore the important functions of other cell types. For example, there is a good deal of evidence to suggest that macrophages play a crucial role in a variety of immune responses. They may function at two levels. The first concerns the uptake and 'processing' of antigens by macrophages (reviewed by Nossal and Ada, 1971). When antigen is injected into an animal, it can be shown using radio-isotope labelling techniques that a good deal of it is taken up by macrophages. Macrophages are widely dispersed throughout all lymphoid tissues and, in addition, they are present within the peritoneal cavity, within the sinusoids of liver and as free cells (i.e. monocytes) within the blood. Although a considerable proportion of the antigen taken up by macrophages may be degraded and not utilized for lymphocyte stimulation, there is evidence that some of the antigen which localizes in macrophages is extremely effective in eliciting the reactivity of lymphocytes. It appears that macrophages play an important part both in the 'processing' of antigen and in its presentation to lymphocytes. Relatively little is known about the phenomenon of 'processing' except that antigen recovered from macrophages is often more immunogenic than antigen in its initial state. The presentation of antigen to lymphocytes is another matter which is under active investigation. Certain types of macrophages localized in the lymphoid follicles of lymph nodes (so-called 'dendritic cells') are known to bind antigen to their surfaces probably by means of membrane-bound antibody. It is thought that these cells may play an important part in stimulating lymphocyte proliferation allowing contact between lymphocyte surfaces and antigen.

At a second level, macrophages may operate in the implementation of the immune response. Thus, macrophages have been shown to be potent killers of both normal and cancer cells in tissue culture experiments. It is perhaps significant that they are found in sites of foreign graft rejection as well as in tumours. It is also likely that macrophages play a part in immunity to both bacterial and viral infections. In bacterial infections, macrophages readily ingest organisms which are coated with antibody. In the case of viral infections, the participation of macrophages is less well understood although in experimental models there is evidence that they help in the clearance of virus.

Whilst the reactivity of lymphocytes may depend upon macrophage function, there is data to suggest that macrophages may be influenced by lymphocytes. Thus, a variety of substances liberated from lymphocytes have been demonstrated to influence the activity of macrophages (Dumonde et al., 1969). These substances are known as lymphokines and although they were originally thought to be the exclusive product of T lymphocytes, it is now known that they are liberated from B lymphocytes as well. There is a substance, macrophage inhibition factor (MIF), which slows the migration of macrophages and hence helps to concentrate macrophages in sites of inflammation. Another factor, macrophage activating factor (MAF), stimulates the phagocytic and cytotoxic potentialities of macrophages. Recently it has been suggested that this particular factor is divisible into two components. One component activates macrophages such that they are cytotoxic to foreign cells irrespective of origin, whereas another factor, specific macrophage activating factor (SMAF), activates macrophages selectively against target cells to which the individual is immune (Evans and Alexander, 1972). Much work has yet to be done on the chemical characterizations of these lymphokines as well as upon their role in *in vivo* immune responses. At the moment they are detected by tissue culture techniques, but there is already evidence that they are not simply tissue culture phenomena. They probably play important roles in most types of immune responses, especially those of the cell-mediated type.

Other blood cells, such as polymorphonuclear leucocytes, are important in defence of the body. They are phagocytic cells and can ingest and so remove micro-organisms. Basophil leucocytes and their tissue counterparts, mast cells, are involved in allergy. Thus, the interaction of antigen and antibody with the mast cell surface causes the release of granules which contain a variety of vasoactive amines. In turn, these substances produce the vascular and smooth muscle changes seen in allergic conditions. The role of eosinophil leucocytes is less well understood. It is known that increased numbers of these cells are present during parasitic infections. There is evidence that eosinophilia is dependent on the function of T cells, but the precise role of eosinophils in the resulting immune reaction has not been elucidated.

Changes of Cell-mediated Immunity in Surgical Disease

In recent years considerable interest has been shown in the changes which occur in immune status of individuals who are suffering from a variety of disease states. Attempts have been made to develop assays which will measure the immune status of such individuals (see also Chapter 4). Simple measurements of Ig concentration in serum and the lymphocyte number of blood may help in this respect. However, a variety of more sophisticated measurements of function are now available. These fall into two broad classes. First, there are measurements of non-specific responsiveness. Second, there are specific responses measured to a particular antigen. In the first category, a variety of tests are available, e.g. it is possible to look at the proliferative response of lymphocytes to mitogens. The relative proportions of T and B lymphocytes can be judged by various marker techniques, the best established of which are the sheep red cell rosetting technique for the enumeration of T cells and the detection of surface Ig for the enumeration of B cells. Tests are also available for measuring the cytotoxic potential of lymphocytes, i.e. lymphocytes stimulated by mitogens usually show a capability for the destruction of a variety of target cells in a quite non-specific fashion. Tests are also available for examining the function of macrophages.

In the case of specific tests of immunity, it is possible to measure the degree of sensitization of an individual to a particular antigen by quantitating the reaction of his lymphocytes in mitotic terms to that antigen. On the other hand, a more direct measure of effector function of lymphocytes can be obtained by studying the cytotoxic potential of lymphocytes to a variety of target cells bearing the specific antigen/s in question. The reactivity of lymphocytes to cancer cells is an important example (Currie, 1974).

Studies such as the ones I have mentioned have revealed that there can be a profound depression of immune responsiveness associated with surgical disease. Indeed, surgery alone has been shown to depress the immune response. In the case of cancer, this clearly may have very important implications if, as we believe, the immune response has an important role to play in the control of the neoplastic process. In a more general context, the depression of immune responsiveness may have important implications for resistance to bacterial or viral infection.

We have only begun to understand fully the complex cellular inter-relationships which go to make up the immune response. Until we do understand the inter-relationships of these components we will not be in a position to manipulate the immune response for therapeutic purposes. A major aim of current research in immunology is to achieve this goal.

Acknowledgements

I am grateful to Miss C. Grainger and Mr. B. Layfield for their help with the preparation of this manuscript.

References

Cooper, M. D., Cain, W. A., Van Alten, P. J. and Good, R. A. (1969). Development and function of the immunoglobulin-producing system. *Int. Arch. Allergy*, **35,** 242

Currie, G. A. (1974). Cancer and the immune response. In J. Turk (ed.), *Current Topics in Immunology*, Vol. 2 (London: E. Arnold)

Dumonde, D. C., Wolstencroft, R. A., Panay, G. S., Matthew, M., Morley, J. and Howson, W. T. (1969). 'Lymphokines': non-antibody mediators of cellular immunity generated by lymphocyte activation. *Nature (London)* **224,** 38

Evans, R. and Alexander, P. (1972). Mechanism of immunologically specific killing of tumour cells by macrophages. *Nature (London)* **236,** 168

Ford, C. E. (1966). Traffic of lymphoid cells in the body. In *Ciba Foundation Symposia. Thymus: Experimental and Clinical Studies*, p. 131. (London: Churchill)

Ford, W. L. and Gowans, J. L. (1969). The traffic of lymphocytes. *Semin. Hematol.*, **6,** 67

Ford, W. L. (1973). The cellular basis of immune responses. In R. R. Porter (ed.), *Defence and Recognition*. International Review of Science: Biochemistry Series, Vol. 10, p. 65. (Lancaster: M.T.P.)

Gowans, J. L. and McGregor, D. D. (1965). The immunological activities of lymphocytes. *Prog. Allergy*, **9,** 1

Kincade, P. W. and Cooper, M. D. (1971). Development and distribution of immunoglobulin-containing cells in the chicken. *J. Immunol.*, **106,** 371

Ling, N. R. and Kay, J. E. (1975). *Lymphocyte Stimulation*. Revised Edition. (Amsterdam: North Holland)

Marchalonis, J. J. (1974). Phylogenetic origins of antibodies and immune recognition. In L. Brent and J. Holborow (eds.), *Progress in Immunology II*, Vol. 2, pp. 249–59. (Amsterdam, North Holland)

Miller, J. F. A. P. and Osoba, D. (1967). Current concepts of the immunological function of the thymus. *Physiol. Rev.*, **47,** 437

Nossal, G. J. V. and Ada, G. L. (1971). *Antigens, Lymphoid Cells and the Immune Response*. (New York: Academic Press)

Owen, J. J. T. (1971). The origins and development of lymphocyte populations. In *Ciba Foundation Symposia. Ontogeny of Acquired Immunity*, p. 35. (Amsterdam: Elsevier (A.S.P.))

Owen, J. J. T. (1974). Ontogeny of the immune system. In L. Brent and J. Holborow (eds.), *Progress in Immunology II*, Vol. 5, p. 163. (Amsterdam: North Holland)

Parrott, D. M. V. and De Sousa, M. A. B. (1971). Thymus-dependent and thymus-independent populations: origin, migratory patterns and lifespan. *Clin. Exp. Immunol.*, **8,** 663

Trainin, N. and Small, M. (1973). Thymic humoral factors. In A. J. S. Davies and R. L. Carter (eds.), *Contemp. Topics Immunobiol.*, **2,** 321

Further Reading

Greaves, M. F., Owen, J. J. T. and Raff, M. C. (1974). *T and B lymphocytes* (Amsterdam: Exerpta Medica)

Hobart, M. J. and McConnell, I. (eds.) (1975). Immunobiology. In *The Immune System, A Course on the Molecular and Cellular Basis of Immunity*, p. 91. (Oxford: Blackwell Scientific Publications)

Owen, J. J. T. (1972). *Ciba Foundation Symposium. Ontogeny of Acquired Immunity*. (Amsterdam: Elsevier (A.S.P.))

Owen, J. J. T. (1973). The anatomy of the lymphoid system. In R. R. Porter (ed.), *Defence and Recognition*. (Lancaster: M.T.P.)

CHAPTER 2

Antibodies
and Complement

M. J. Hobart

Introduction

The purpose of this chapter is to present some of the basic facts about antibodies, immunoglobulins and complement which may be needed by
surgeons and also to highlight some of those aspects which he may too
easily take for granted or which seem likely to be of growing importance.

Antibodies serve two functions: that of specific combination with antigens
and that of providing a common 'signal' that an antigen has been encountered so that effector mechanisms may be brought into play to accom-
plish its neutralization or elimination. These two functions have been
brought about by an apparently unique evolutionary process.

One of the best understood effector mechanisms triggered by the combination of antibody and antigen is the complement system. It consists of
at least 16 proteins with complex reaction pathways, and this chapter
attempts to give an understandable, if simplified, account of them and a
little of their biological significance.

Immunoglobulins

Antibodies belong to a family of molecules called immunoglobulins, which
have a common evolutionary history (see below). Their most consistent
characteristic is possession of a common basic anatomy.

BASIC ANATOMY OF IMMUNOGLOBULINS

All immunoglobulins consist of a unit made up of four polypeptide chains
(Fleischmann et al., 1963). These come in two sizes: heavy and light, with

molecular weights of 50000–65000 and 25000 respectively. The polypeptide chains are held together by disulphide bridges formed between cystein
residues (Figure 2.1). These bridges are weak covalent bonds which can be

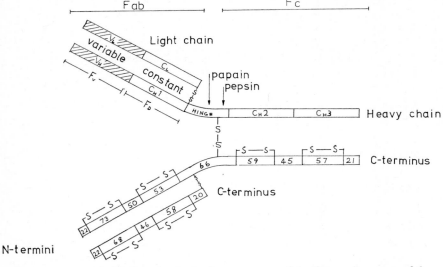

Figure 2.1 A typical IgG molecule. In the upper part of the figure, the names of the
various parts of the molecule are given, while in the lower part, the number of amino
acids in typical domains, and the arrangements of the interchain disulphide bridges are
shown. (Adapted from Milstein and Svasti, 1971)

broken by reducing agents. Although less thermodynamically firm, there
are very important non-covalent forces which hold the chains together and
which influence their folding. By convention, polypeptide chains are shown
in diagrams with their N-terminus (the amino acid with a free α amino
group) to the left. This is appropriate since they are synthesized from the
N-terminus, and in the case of immunoglobulins, the N-termini of both
heavy and light chains are in the same region of the molecule.

Immunoglobulins are rather resistant to attack by proteolytic enzymes,
but certain portions are much more susceptible than others (see below).
Papain attacks a point in the middle of the heavy chain, on the N-terminal
side of the interheavy chain disulphide bridges, dividing the molecule into
three parts of approximately equal size: two identical Fab fragments and an
Fc fragment. The Fab fragments carry the antigen-combining site of the
antibody (Fragment antigen binding: Fab). The Fc fragment of rabbit IgG
crystallizes under mild and undemanding conditions (Fragment crystalliz-
able: Fc). Many of the biological properties of immunoglobulins are mediated

by the Fc part of the molecule. Pepsin degrades the Fc fragment up to near the interheavy chain bridge, leaving a large $F(ab')_2$ fragment.

The most abundant immunoglobulin in serum is IgG, with a concentration of about 10 mg ml^{-1}. IgG is able to activate the complement system and to sensitize particles for uptake by phagocytes (opsonization). It is important in the neutralization of toxin molecules and of viruses, presumably by coating both of them. IgG antibody is usually produced late in an immune response to persisting antigenic exposure (for instance an infection), or as part of the secondary response if the antigenic exposure is short-lived.

By contrast, IgM antibody is made early in the response. It is not present in large quantity, but it does activate the complement system. It can therefore initiate bacteriolysis and complement-dependent opsonization. It has been suggested that the system has evolved in this way to permit a rapid attempt at elimination of pathogenic organisms by IgM and complement, followed by a more sustained attack by IgG, which will neutralize toxic products.

IgE and IgD are both present in very small quantity in the serum. IgD has no clearly identified biological role, but is very abundant on the surfaces of some B lymphocytes, particularly those found in cord blood. IgE, however, has a clearly defined biological role as a reaginic antibody. It attaches passively to mast cells, sensitizing them for subsequent degranulation on exposure to antigen. It therefore plays a central role in immediate-type hypersensitivity reactions (e.g. hay fever).

Some immunoglobulins, especially the macroglobulin, IgM, and IgA, which is the most abundant immunoglobulin in external secretions, are able to form polymers. IgM contains 5 subunits.

In addition to the heavy and light polypeptide chains, two other proteins may be found as parts of immunoglobulins: secretory piece and J chain.

Immunoglobulin Heterogeneity

Since immunoglobulins carry out a greater variety of functions than any other known family of molecules, it is not surprising that they are structurally heterogeneous. This heterogeneity is found at a number of levels.

LIGHT CHAIN TYPES

Light chains are found in two types, κ and λ, which are distinct in their amino acid sequence and their antigenic characteristics. Both are approximately the same size (molecular weight 25 000) and composed of a similar number of amino acids (220). There is a small amount of carbohydrate on

Table 2.1 Physicochemical and biological properties of immunoglobulin classes

Class	Heavy chain		Whole molecule		Carbohydrate content	Placental transfer	Complement fixation	Serum conc. (mg/ml)
	Class	M.W.	Sedimentation coefficient	M.W.				
IgM	μ	70 000	19S	900 000	12%	−	+	0.5–2.0
IgG	γ	50 000	7S	150 000	3%	+	+	8–16
IgA	α	55 000	7S etc.	$(160\ 000)_n$	7.5%	−	−	1.5–4
IgD	δ	65 000?	7	180 000?	12%	−	?	trace
IgE	ε	65 000	8	180 000	12%	−	−	trace

both (about 2%). The ratio of κ to λ is about 2:1 in man, but varies greatly between species. Both types have been recognized in most species which have been examined.

HEAVY CHAIN CLASSES

There are five known classes of heavy chains in humans: α, λ, μ, δ and ε, corresponding to the immunoglobulin classes set out in Table 2.1. These heavy chain classes are distinct both in their amino acid sequence, and in their size, the μ and ε chains having a molecular weight of 65 000 compared with 50 000 for the others. The carbohydrate content of the different classes is shown in Table 2.1.

It is the heavy chains of a specific class which confer class upon an immunoglobulin, with its connotations of the different biological activities which they mediate. Thus, IgG is composed of two γ chains and either two κ chains or two λ chains, IgA of two α chains and two light chains, etc. (see Table 2.1). Most mammalian species seem to have at least 4 out of the 5 classes of heavy chain encountered in humans.

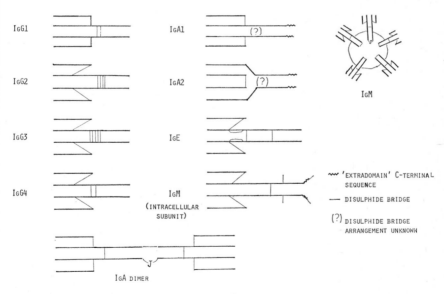

Figure 2.2 Arrangement of chains and interchain disulphide bridges in human immunoglobulins. Note that the IgA2 subclass does not have a heavy–light disulphide bridge and that IgA and IgM have a C-terminal additional sequence including a cystein residue. Note also the additional intrachain disulphide bridge in the Fd region of IgE. (Adapted from Milstein and Pink, 1970)

HEAVY CHAIN SUBCLASSES

Some of the immunoglobulin classes are themselves heterogeneous in the structure of their heavy chains, though these differences do not extend to such fundamental properties as size. They differ, rather, in the amino acid sequences, biological properties, charge and antigenic properties. There are no rules which qualify a group of molecules to belong to one subclass rather than another class, although the distinctions are usually quite clear.

The more important differences between the subclasses of human immunoglobulins are the arrangement of the disulphide bridges between the chains (Figure 2.2). Other properties which distinguish immunoglobulin subclasses are shown in Table 2.2.

ALLOTYPIC DIFFERENCES

Allotypic differences are those not shared by all members of the same species: they are genetically determined differences which are inherited as alternatives in the normal Mendelian fashion, just like blood groups. The differences involved are usually of a single amino acid in the sequence, of the polypeptide chain involved. Human examples include the Gm and Inv grouping systems. Since all genetic concepts are more conveniently dealt with together further consideration will be deferred until later.

THE VARIABLE REGIONS

The ability of antibodies to combine specifically with antigen is due to structural differences in the specialized free ends of the Fab arms. The N-terminal portions of both the heavy and the light polypeptide chains reside in this region, and the N-terminal 110 residues show enormous variability in sequence in both heavy and light chains (the variable regions). Since the sequence of the polypeptide chains determines the way in which they fold and also which groups are presented to the external environment, it is not surprising that specificity is due to effects of this primary structure.

The extreme heterogeneity of immunoglobulins and especially the variable regions would have made investigations of their amino acid sequence almost impossible but for the occurrence of tumours (myelomas) of the cells which make antibodies. All of the cells of such a tumour are derived from a single cell which has completely differentiated before malignant transformation. Such differentiated cells, which derive from a single ancestral cell in which the 'decisions' about the amino acid sequence have been made, belong to the same clone (a term properly used for any asexually derived series of individuals of common ancestry) and therefore produce immunoglobulin with a unique combination of variable region sequences. The monoclonal

Table 2.2 IgG subclasses in man and animals

Species	IgG subclasses	γ chains	Relative electrophoretic mobility pH 8.6	Relative conc. as % serum IgG	Complement activation		Placental transfer	Heterologous skin sensitizing	Other
					Classical	Alternative			
Human	IgG1	γ1	slow	70	++		+	+	binds to macrophages
	IgG2	γ2	slow	20	±		±	–	
	IgG3	γ3	slow	7	+++		+	+	binds to macrophages
	IgG4	γ4	fast	3	–	+?	+	+	
Mouse	IgG1	γ	fast		–			+	
	IgG2a	γ	slow		+			–	
	IgG2b	γ	slow						
Guinea-pig	IgG1	γ1	fast	app. 25	–	+		+	
	IgG2	γ2	slow	app. 75	+++			–	
Cow/Sheep	IgG1	γ1	fast	app. 75	+++	(+)	–	+	in colostrum
	IgG2	γ2	slow	app. 25	–	+	–	–	

immunoglobulin made by the cells of a myeloma, have a uniform structure and are produced in large quantity so they can be purified from the plasma of the patient. Some tumours secrete excess light chains which appear in the urine as Bence–Jones proteins, and these can also be used for sequence studies (Putnam, 1962).

It is clear that the heterogeneity of the variable region is not uniform, nor is it entirely unrestricted. While no two variable regions of identical sequence but from unrelated sources have been discovered, there are sufficient similarities in the sequences of variable regions for them to be classified as belonging to a number of subgroups. There are three or four of these in the human κ chain, three in the heavy chain, but a very large number in the κ chain of mice (Table 2.3). The variability of the variable region is not uniformly distributed along its length. There are a number of parts of the sequence which show much greater variability than others—see Figure 2.3. Recent discoveries of the three-dimensional structure of immunoglobulins show that these hypervariable regions are involved in the formation of the combining site for antigen.

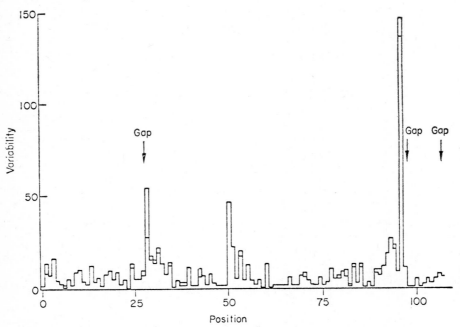

Figure 2.3 Variability within the variable region. Variability at different amino acid positions for the variable region of the light chains. Gap indicates positions at which insertions have been found. (From Wu and Kabat, 1970)

Table 2.3 Sequence data on the N-terminal residue of human κ-chains showing how they can be classified into three subgroups on the basis of sequence homology. Subgroup specific residues are underlined and deletions are shown by dashes

Amino terminal position

	Sequence (positions 1 → ~45, with 10, 20, 30, 40 marked)
Vk₁ Subgroup	
ROY	D I Q M T Q S P S S L S A S V G D R V T I T C Q A S Q D I - - - - - - I F L N W Y Q Q K P
AG	D I Q M T Q S P S S L S A S V G D R V T I T C Q A S Q D I - - - - - - H Y L N W Y Q Q G P
EU	B I B M T Z N P S T L S A S B G D R V S I T C Z A S Z S I - - - - - - T W L A W Y Z Z K P
BJ	D V Q M T Q S P S S L S A S V G D R V T I T C Q A S Q D I - - - - - - K Y - W Y Z (Z K P)
OU	D I Q M T Q S P S S L S A S V G D R V T I T C R A S Z N I - - - - - - S W L B W Y Z (Z K P)
HBJ4	D I Q M T Q S P S T L(S A S V G B R V T I T C R A S Q B V - - - - - - S W L A W Y Q E L P
DAV	D I Q M T Q S P S T L S V S V G D R V T I T C D A S Q Q I - - - - - - S W L I W Y Q Q Y P
FIN	D I Q M T Q S P S S L S A S V G D R V T I T C D A S Q B I - B - - - - S W L I W Y Q Q Y P
KER	D I Q M T Q S P S S L S A S V G D R V T I T C Q A S Q B I - B - - - - D F - W Y - - -
TRA	D I Q M T Q S P S S L S A S V G D R V T I T C Q A S Q B L - K - - - - - - - - - - -
CON	D I Q M T Q S P F S L S A S V G D R V T I T C - - - - - - - - - - - - - - - - - - -
LUX	D I L L T Q S P A I L S V S P G E R V L I T -
BEL	B I N L T Z S P S S L S A S V G D R V T I - - - - - K - - - - - - - - - - - - - - -
PAUL	D I Q M T Q S P S S L S A S V G D R V T I L C Q A S I S - - - - - - K - S L A W Y Z Z K P
Vk₁₁ Subgroup	
Ti	E I V L T Q S P G T L S L S P G E R A T L S C R A S Q S V S - - - N S F L A W Y Q Q K P
FR4	E(I) V V T Q S P(L) T L S L S P G E R A A L S C R A S Q S V R - - - N N Y L A W Y Q Q R P
B6	Z I V L T T S P Z T L S L S P G Z R A A L S C R A S Q S L S - - - G N Y L A W Y Q Q K P
RAD	E I V L T Q S P A T L S L S P G E R A T L S C R A S Q - V S - - - S N S Y L A W Y Q Q K P
CAS	E I V L T Q S P G T L S L S P G D R A T L S C R A S - - - - - - - - - - - - - - - - - -
SMI	E I V L T Q S P A T L S M S P G E R A T L S -
DIL	E I V L T Q S P A T L S L S P G E R A T L S C R A S Q S L S - - - S K S L S W Y Z Z K P
NIG	K I V L T Q S P A T L S L S P G E R A T L S -
GRA	E M V M T Q S P A T L S V S P G E R A T L S -
Vk₁₁₁ Subgroup	
CUM	E D I V M T Q S P L S L P V T P G E P A S I S C R S S Q S L L A S G D G N T Y L N W Y L Q K A
TEW	E D I V M T Q S P L S L P V T P G E P A S I S C R S S Q - H(G B)S - - H(G B)S - -	- - F L N W Y L Q K P
MIL	D I V L T Q S P L S L P V T P G E P A S I S C R S S Q N L L Z S - B G B - - Y L D W Y L Z K P
MAN	D I V M T Q S P L S L P V T P G E P A S I S G R S S Q - B G B - - Y L B - - Y L B ? Y L Z K P
BATES	D I V M T Q S P L S L P V T P G E P A S I S G R S S Q(S) L L H(S) B G B B - Y L B ? Y L Z K P

Key to one-letter amino acid code:

A Ala	G Gly	N Asn	V Val
B Asx	H His	P Pro	W Trp
C Cys	I Ile	Q Gln	Y Tyr
D Asp	K Lys	R Arg	Z Glx
E Glu	L Leu	S Ser	
F Phe	M Met	T Thr	

(From Hood and Prahl, by courtesy of Academic Press)

Each individual antibody molecule has a particular combination of light chain type, heavy chain class and subclass, allotype and sequence of the heavy and light chain variable regions. This detailed composition is shared only by other molecules synthesized by the same cell or by other members of the same clone. With relatively minor reservations, it can be said that each cell in the clone makes only one unique product.

The particular combination of two variable region sequences constitutes the *idiotype* of the antibody: characteristics which are shared with a very small proportion of the other immunoglobulins made by the same individual and very rarely with those made by any other animal, even of the same species. Some of these 'unique' characteristics may make the immunoglobulin antigenic in other members of the same species.

The Structure of Immunoglobulins

The enumeration, classification and sequencing of immunoglobulin chains and the discovery of their chemical linkages was a major preoccupation during the 1960s. These studies have been of immense value both for understanding immunoglobulins and as a stimulus to further work, but it is often easier to grasp structural concepts if they are presented in three dimensions. Recent advances in x-ray crystallographic analysis of immunoglobulin fragments now make this possible.

THE DOMAINS

Both from the evidence of sequence studies and, more recently, from crystallographic studies, it is clear that immunoglobulins are made up of linear arrays of domains (Edelman *et al.*, 1969). A domain is a stretch of about 110 amino acids, with a disulphide bridge linking cystein residues at about positions 23 and 90. A light chain is composed of two domains, α and γ chains of four and the μ and ϵ chains of five domains. The amino acid sequence of successive domains in a chain and of different chains show a small but significant homology, indicating a common evolutionary origin.

A convenient shorthand is used for the identification of domains. A capital V or C indicates whether they are in the variable or constant region of a polypeptide chain. The identity of the chain is indicated by a subscript letter, Greek if specific (e.g. C_γ or V_κ) or Roman if more general (e.g. V_H). The sequential position of a domain in the constant region of a heavy chain is indicated by a number (e.g. $C_\gamma 2$).

The polypeptide chain is thrown into a series of folds so that there are 7 (or 9) 'runs' of the chain in a domain (Poljac *et al.*, 1973; Schiffler *et al.*, 1973; Padlam *et al.*, 1974): '4 there and 3 back', see Figure 2.4. Each 'run'

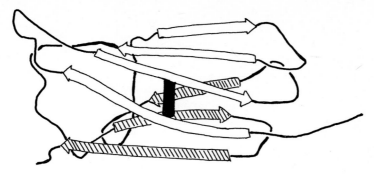

Figure 2.4 Arrangement of polypeptide backbone of a single domain. The polypeptide chain is thrown into a series of folds giving rise to two distinct surfaces involved in interaction: one made up of four chains (white arrows) and one made up of three (hatched arrows). (Adapted from Schiffler *et al.*, 1973)

of the chain is antiparallel to the adjacent one, that is parallel but running in the opposite direction. The folding is such that two distinct surfaces are formed by the runs of the chains, one having three runs and the other four. The two surfaces are held together by the intrachain disulphide bridge described above.

Each domain seems to be a functional unit: thus the variable region is the N-terminal domain of a chain. It interacts with the variable domain of the other chain in the Fab (V_H with V_L). The C-terminal domain of the light chains (C_L) interact with the second domain of the heavy chains (C_H1), and the residual domains of the heavy chains also interact with each other. Some of the biological activities of antibody molecules have been shown to be localized in one or other of these domains: complement fixation in the C_H2 of the γ chain (Utsumi, 1969) ($C_\gamma2$), cytophilic affinity for macrophages and recognition by K cells in the $c_\epsilon3$ (Okafor *et al.*, 1974; MacLennan *et al.*, 1974).

INTERACTIONS BETWEEN DOMAINS

Two kinds of snug-fitting interaction have been observed between domains: those in which they come together with their three chain surfaces apposed and those with the four chain surfaces apposed. The variable domains interact through their three chain surfaces and lie across each other in a cruciform manner, with both the N and C-terminal ends of the polypeptide chains far apart in space. The constant region domains of the Fab pair through their four chain surfaces so that the C-terminal ends of the chains are close together and can form the heavy to light chain disulphide bridge.

The folding of the domain brings only a few residues into the N-terminal end of the C_H1 close to the C-terminus of the light chain, permitting the alternative light to heavy chain bridge which is seen in a number of IgG subclasses, IgA, IgM and IgE.

Feinstein (1974, 1975) has deduced a set of 'rules' from the known structure of a Fab' fragment and from chemical relationships (e.g. the positions of disulphide bridges) which should govern the structure of immunoglobulins. A critical test of these rules is to build a model of IgM, which is structurally the most complex of the immunoglobulins. This model suggests that the domains of a single chain 'zig-zag' down the molecule (Figure 2.5), and the

Diagram of the arrangement of the domains
in the IgM molecule

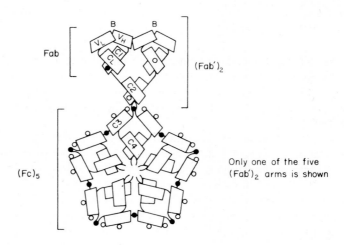

Fab

$(Fab')_2$

$(Fc)_5$

Only one of the five
$(Fab')_2$ arms is shown

●   Interchain disulphide bridge

○   Carbohydrate

B   Antigen – binding site

   Regions of polypeptide chains
   folded into domains

Figure 2.5 Diagram of the arrangement of the domains in the IgM molecule

interaction through the three chain surface is restricted to the variable regions. The final model of the IgM molecule, made accurately to scale on the assumption that all domains are essentially the same as the C_H1 of the γ

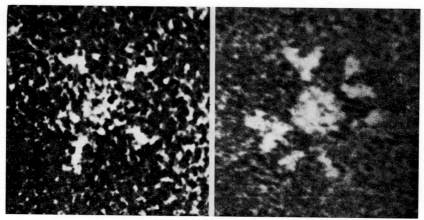

Figure 2.6 Electron micrograph of IgM (from Feinstein *et al.*, 1971)

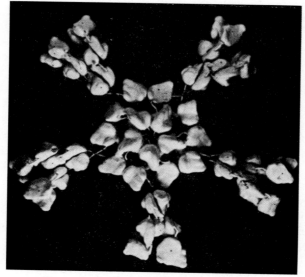

Figure 2.7 IgM model (from Feinstein, 1974)

chain, agrees with electron micrographs of the molecule (Figures 2.6 and 2.7) and is consistent with all of the chemical data. Confirmation of its essential correctness, and for the fact that it is generally true for other classes of immunoglobulins comes from the fact that IgE has a disulphide bridge connecting the $C_\epsilon 2$ domains (Bennich and von Bahr-Lindström, 1974), a feature not found in other immunoglobulins. This disulphide bridge is placed in the sequence at one of the few positions of intimate contact between the $C_\mu 2$s of the IgM model.

THE STRUCTURE OF IMMUNOGLOBULIN CLASSES

The structure of IgM has been refined by use of electron microscopy, protein sequence studies, immunochemical investigations and extrapolation of x-ray diffraction data. Similar methods could probably be used for other immunoglobulin classes.

As described, there are great structural similarities between IgE and one of the subunits of IgM. The difference between these classes lies in an additional polypeptide sequence at the C-terminal end of the μ chain, not possessed by the ϵ chain. This additional sequence contains a cystein residue which is involved in the reactions leading to the formation of disulphide bonds which hold the five subunits of the whole IgM together. Its absence from the ϵ chain makes it impossible for this to polymerize.

There is evidence that IgM is the immunoglobulin class most closely related to the evolutionary archetypal immunoglobulin class and that other classes evolved from it, or a similar common ancestor. The mechanism for IgE would be the loss of the C-terminal additional sequence. However, both IgG and IgA have only four domains in their heavy chains, compared with the five of μ and ϵ. The properties of both IgG and IgA can be readily explained by the loss of a single domain from the heavy chain in the course of their evolution from IgM (Feinstein, 1974). In the case of IgG, the domain lost was the $C_\mu 2$, and in the case of IgA, the $C_\mu 3$. This explains the fact that both IgG and IgM have complement fixing properties, whereas IgA does not. Since the complement fixation site of IgG resides in the $C_\gamma 2$ domain, it seems probable that it is in the $C_\mu 3$ domain of IgM, precisely that which is lost from IgA.

IgA is, however, able to polymerize. It does not do so as extensively as IgM, but it shares with IgM 'the possession of an additional polypeptide sequence at the C-terminal end of the heavy chains which contains a cystein residue involved in the formation of the polymers'.

J CHAIN AND SECRETORY PIECE

One *J chain* per polymer is present in all polymeric immunoglobulins (Koshland, 1975). It is structurally unrelated to the immunoglobulin domains and is rich in cystein residues. It functions by assisting in the formation of the disulphide bridges which hold the subunits of the polymerized immunoglobulins together and is itself incorporated in the polymer by disulphide bridges. It is part of the bridge between IgA polymers but it bridges between two heavy chains of one subunit in the case of IgM (see Figure 2.2).

Secretory piece is also unrelated structurally to immunoglobulins and is attached to IgA *after* it has crossed the basement membrane of a mucous membrane epithelium. It is synthesized by cells other than the plasma cells involved in the production of IgA. Free secretory piece is found in the serum of patients with inflammatory bowel disease, but is not specifically diagnostic. Its function is unknown.

THREE-DIMENSIONAL STRUCTURE, PROTEOLYSIS AND FLEXIBILITY

Consideration of the three-dimensional structure of immunoglobulins indicates the reasons for their resistance to proteolytic digestion. The domains are very compact structures which do not readily permit enzymic attack but certain parts of the chains between the compact areas of the domains are more extended, and hence susceptible. In the case of IgG, there is an extended sequence between the $C_\gamma 1$ and $C_\gamma 2$ domains. This contains the interheavy chain disulphide bridges, a large number of proline residues and it is known as the 'hinge' region. In this region the IgG molecule shows its quite considerable flexibility (Noelkin *et al.*, 1965; Feinstein and Rowe, 1965), for the Fab arms can move through a large arc. However, the importance of this property is much discussed but little understood.

IgM has no hinge region between the $C_\mu 1$ and $C_\mu 2$. The $F(ab')_\mu 2$ arms move as single rigid units, but there is some flexibility where they join the central disc of the IgM molecule made up of the $C_\mu 3$ and $C_\mu 4$ domains. It is possible that the lack of flexibility in the orientation and spacing of the combining sites of the arms of IgM is responsible for the discrepant results found for the valency of its combining sites; some suggest 5, others 10. Clearly, there are ten possible combining sites, but half may be sterically hindered from combination with antigens (Feinstein, 1975).

Biological Activities of Antibodies

Antibodies have two distinct functions: combination with antigens and the provision of a 'signal', recognizable by effector systems.

ANTIGEN BINDING

The immune system allows the generation of a very large number of potential antibody-combining sites. There is a natural selection of those clones of antibody-forming cells which make combining sites with the greatest affinity for a particular antigen. The enormous diversity of the pool from which antibodies are selected and the efficiency of the selection processes result in the production of antibodies which bind very strongly to their antigens.

The strength of binding is a property known as affinity. Since the reaction between an antigen and the combining site of an antibody is reversible, the laws of mass action apply so that the reaction will reach the equilibrium in which there is free antigen, free antibody and antigen:antibody complex,

$$Ab + Ag \rightleftharpoons AbAg$$

If the components of the reaction can be estimated, then it is possible to give an affinity value (k):

$$k = \frac{[AbAg]}{[Ab] \times [Ag]} \qquad [\ ] \quad \text{indicates concentration at equilibrium}$$

This is a formula frequently used by chemists, but perhaps unfamiliar to surgeons. A more comprehensible interpretation is that affinity is the free antigen concentration at which half of the binding sites of the antibodies are occupied (see Taussig, 1975; and Karush, 1970).

The specificity of antibodies may be related to high affinity. The classical experiments of Landsteiner, who showed the abilities of antibodies to distinguish the *ortho-* and *para-*forms of substituted benzene rings should be contrasted with the high incidence of recognizable antibodies in myeloma proteins, often to some unlikely substance, such as DNP (2,4-dinitrophenol). Small molecules like DNP which will combine with antibodies are called haptens. They do not elicit an immune response when injected alone into an animal, but only when attached to a larger molecule which must itself be immunogenic. This is called a carrier, and the mechanisms involved in the responses to hapten–carrier complexes have provided some of the most powerful impetuses for the understanding of the mechanisms of the immune response (Mitchison, 1967). Richards *et al.* (1974) have shown the ability of a crystallized Fab′ fragment from a mouse myeloma to bind a variety of haptens of very different structure with affinities in different *parts* of a single combining site.

Certain methods of detection of antibody which rely on the observation of secondary phenomena, such as precipitation or the initiation of complement activation, may give apparently higher specificities than would be expected from their affinities alone. Usually, more than one part of the antigen to be recognized by antibody before the secondary phenomenon is initiated. For instance, if the antigen has a single reactive site for antibody, precipitation is impossible: at least three are needed. Usually, biological molecules provide three *different* sites, each with their own specific antibody, so that the net specificity of the reagent is that of all three together. Similarly, complement activation depends on the close proximity of a number of IgG molecules on the surface of the antigen. If the antigens are widely separated, no fixation will be initiated. However, if the antiserum contains antibodies to several determinants, each widely separated, but occurring in groups, it will be able to initiate complement activation via antibodies of a number of different specificities acting in concert.

COMPLEMENT ACTIVATION

As described above, complement activation requires the combination with antigen of more than one IgG antibody molecule in close proximity. A single IgM antibody, however, is able to initiate complement activation on combination with antigen.

Not all antibody molecules are able to trigger the complement system, for example IgA and some of the IgG subclasses are unable to do so (Table 2.4). Although recent studies of the complement system suggest that under carefully controlled conditions, IgA, some 'non-complement-fixing' IgG subclasses and even F(ab')$_2$ antibodies are able to activate the alternative pathway.

Two alternative hypotheses are available to explain the difference in complement triggering properties of an antibody molecule which has combined with antigen and one which is still free in the fluid phase. The first suggests that combination with antigen causes a conformational change in

Table 2.4 A comparison of the classical and alternative complement activation sites

	Classical	Alternative (or C3b-feedback pathway)
Activating agents		
Aggregated of human	IgG1 and 3 (and 2), IgM	IgA
rabbit	IgG IgM	F(ab')$_2$
guinea-pig	IgG2	IgG1
ruminant	IgG1	IgG2
		Inulin
	(Lipid A)	Zymosan
		Endotoxin, LPS
Factors required to generate C3	C1	Properdin, factor D
convertase	C4	C3
	C2	Factor B
Total serum requirement	Dilute	Concentrated
Ion requirements	Ca and Mg	Mg
Capacity to produce RBC lysis	High	(Low)
Capacity to generate $\overline{C56}$ in acute phase serum (reactive lysis)	Low	High

(From Lachmann, 1975)

the antibody molecule, exposing a reactive site previously unavailable to C1q, the first of the complement components. Certainly, immunoglobulins do have the required properties of flexibility, but direct proof of this hypothesis is not yet available. Alternatively, it is argued that the requirement for two antibodies close together is evidence for triggering by a difference in the avidity of binding of C1q, due purely to increased 'valency' of available binding sites. The experimental data support this view, but do not exclude a conformation change as well.

REAGINIC ANTIBODY: IgE

IgE antibody has a great affinity for mast cells and basophils, attaching to them by the Fc piece. Its low serum concentration is probably due in part to this affinity. Passively acquired IgE antibody confers the ability of specific activity on the mast cell. If an antigen is bound by the IgE antibodies on its surface, the mast cell is activated to undergo degranulation, releasing its store of pharmacologically active substances, but the molecular mechanics of this process are unknown.

OTHER CELL-BINDING REACTIONS

There are large numbers of reactions which are initiated by IgG antibodies binding to receptors on the surfaces of mononuclear cells, lymphocytes or polymorphs. In some cases, antibodies may be cytophilic for macrophages, giving them a specific receptor for antigen in a similar way to IgE and mast cells. In other cases, the antibody first combines with antigen and is recognized by the cell, sometimes opsonizing the antigen for phagocytosis; for example, IgG1 and IgG3 antibodies do this for macrophages in man. Opsonization for polymorphs is not so demanding and it is not known which subclass of IgG binds to the Fc receptors on the surfaces of B lymphocytes.

TRANSPORT OF IMMUNOGLOBULINS ACROSS MEMBRANES

Like the other biological properties of immunoglobulins, this is also due to the Fc piece of the molecule. Some IgG subclasses are transferred across the human placenta, but IgG2 only very poorly. $F(ab')_2$ antibodies are not transferred across the rabbit placenta.

Immunoglobulin Genetics and Evolution

Immunoglobulins are unusually diverse and the genetic and evolutionary mechanisms involved vary from the conventional through the unique to the unknown!

Natural selection is an exceedingly conservative mechanism. The majority of mutations and other genetic events are, at best, of no survival value, usually disadvantageous, and very rarely advantageous. Immunoglobulins pose a dual challenge to conventional genetics and evolutionary mechanisms: how does a single molecule possess both conserved and diverse regions in its structure; how is the vast diversity of the variable regions generated and how did it arise, when diversity is abhorred by natural selection.

TWO GENES, ONE POLYPEPTIDE CHAIN

The heresy of yesterday's molecular biology is the truth! The problem of molecules which are both diverse and conserved has been solved by the evolution of a mechanism hitherto unique in molecular biology. The variable and constant regions of immunoglobulin polypeptide chains are coded by separate genes. There are three lines of evidence for this:

(a) Rabbits possess a series of heavy chain allotypes which reside in the variable region and which are found on all classes of immunoglobulins (Todd, 1963; Feinstein, 1963).

(b) A few cases of multiple myelomatosis have been found in which the serum contains more than one class of monoclonal immunoglobulin (Wang et al., 1970). The variable regions of the heavy chains in these cases are usually the same, and they use identical light chains. Anti-idiotype antibodies raised against IgG antibacterial antibodies react with IgM antibodies from the same animal (Oudin and Michel, 1970).

(c) All classes of immunoglobulin heavy chains share the same variable region subgroups as determined by sequence studies.

The variable region genes fall into three distinct groups: those for the heavy, the κ and for the λ chains. There is no variable region swapping and the mechanism by which the variable region gene information is welded onto the constant region is not known. It is certainly not at the level of the synthesis of the protein as the chains are each coded by a single messenger RNA (Swan et al., 1972; Stevens and Williamson, 1973). It might be at the level of the transcription of the DNA to RNA, but more probably the event occurs at the DNA level. It is also probable that this unique process is bound up with another unusual phenomenon: that each antibody-forming cell makes a homogeneous product coded by only one of the chromosomes. The antibody-forming cells of animals heterozygous for allotypic markers each only make one or the other allelic product. This phenomenon is called allelic exclusion. The only similar situation known is the Lyon phenomenon, in which the expression of only one of the two X chromosomes occurs in the cells of females, the other being inactivated. In the case of allelic exclusion of immunoglobulins, however, the mechanisms are probably genetic, not chromosomal, as they apply to both the light and the heavy chains which are on different chromosomes. Furthermore, it appears that the variable region gene used is that on the same chromosome as the constant region gene used.

THE ORIGIN OF DIVERSITY

The way in which more than 300 variable region sequences are made available for the synthesis of suitable V regions of each chain is unexplained. On the genetic level, there are two possibilities: the germ line theory or the somatic mutation theory.

The *germ line theory* states that an individual inherits a very large number of V region genes from his parents, enough to satisfy the required number of different antibody molecules. This theory is supported by the following facts:

(a) The discovery of the V region subclasses (Milstein, 1967). This is evidence against the somatic mutation theory, for if there is more than one V region gene in the germ line for each chain, there is no reason why there should not be 100 or 10^5.

(b) The discovery of inheritable antibodies (Krause, 1970; Eichman, 1972). Certain antigens evoke antibody responses of restricted heterogeneity. The characteristics of these restricted antibodies can be shown to be inheritable. It may be that these antigens are truly bizarre in that they can be reacted against by the few variable regions coded in the germ line, but the vast majority of antigens, including threatening ones which should have the most inheritable antibodies, provoke very diverse, non-heritable responses.

(c) A number of experiments provide evidence that the diversity of immunoglobulins might not be so vast as previously supposed (Kreth and Williamson, 1973). The total diversity of the antibody repertoire has been estimated from a few thousand to a few millions. Millions represent uncomfortable burdens on the genome, but a few hundred genes which produce 50000 usable antibodies would take hardly any space. We are quite uncertain as to the extent of immunoglobulin diversity, since the methods used to estimate it produce answers rather close to the potential maxima of the methods, and assumptions are made that any heavy chain V region can get together with any light chain V region to make a potentially useful antibody. The limited evidence available suggests that this is not the case.

The *somatic mutation theory* states that the number of V region genes transmitted in the germ line is rather small (not more than 50) and a process of mutation occurs in the lymphoid cells (but not the germ cells), giving rise to a very large number of cells, each with a different genetic potential.

A number of genetic mechanisms have been proposed for this process, none of them very satisfactory. As an alternative, mechanisms have been proposed which would 'force' the rate of point mutation by increasing the rate of cell division and which incorporate selective pressures which militate against cells which do not mutate. The best arguments in favour of somatic mutation are:

(a) It is philosophically satisfying since it provides a system which is flexible, economical in its demands on the occupation of the genome, avoids the problems of how gene selection occurs, and most important, does not demand the existence of a large number of genes held as a stable cluster. In other cases where multiple copies of genes exist, the situation is highly unstable, with the whole gene set frequently being lost by unequal crossing over.

(b) The *a* heavy chain allotypes in rabbits, mentioned above, which reside in the V regions are inherited as *alleles*. However, it is very difficult to conceive how 300 copies of a gene, all carrying a particular *a* allotype marker, would *never* recombine in a heterozygous animal, giving rise to an offspring which could apparently have three allelic markers. This is best explained by considering the *a* allotype markers as some kind of artefact; for instance all rabbits have all the *a* alleles but they inherit genes which control the set of copies used.

(c) The number of copies of a gene can be estimated by observing the reassociation of copies of the gene to DNA which has been 'unravelled' to a single stranded structure. Studies of this kind are termed annealing studies and, although they are of unique potential, the results require cautious interpretation. A new method involving competition between labelled and unlabelled copies of messenger RNA for light chains strongly suggests that there are a very few copies of the genes for each of the variable region sub-groups (Tonegawa *et al.*, 1974). These recent data are very much more convincing than former annealing studies. On balance, there appears to be a resurgence of belief in somatic mutation.

IMMUNOGLOBULIN GENES

Genetics is a very commonsense subject, even if it has its own jargon and is often translated into mathematical and statistical terms.

The information used to make a polypeptide chain is coded in the DNA. DNA is a linear molecule, organized with other molecules, notably histone proteins, into chromosomes. The DNA code consists of nucleotide triplets which code collinearly for the amino acids. The information for immunoglobulin chains seems to be arranged in three clusters, one for κ, one for λ and one for heavy chains. They seem to be on different chromosomes.

Each gene cluster consists of a segmented linear array of genes (Figure 2.8).

Man		V-genes	C-genes
Light chains	κ	$\overline{\text{Ia}}\ \overline{\text{Ib}}\ \overline{\text{II}}\ \overline{\text{III}}$	—
	λ	$\overline{\text{I}}\ \overline{\text{II}}\ \overline{\text{III}}\ \overline{\text{IV}}$	$\overline{\text{Arg}}\ \overline{\text{Lys}}\ \overline{\text{Gly}}$
Heavy chains		$\overline{\text{I}}\ \overline{\text{II}}\ \overline{\text{III}}$	$\overline{\gamma 4}\ \overline{\gamma 2}\ \overline{\gamma 3}\ \overline{\gamma 1}\ \overline{\alpha 1}\ \overline{\alpha 2}\ \overline{\mu 2}\ \overline{\mu 1}\ \overline{\delta}\ \overline{\epsilon}$

Mouse		V-genes	C-genes
Light chains	κ	$\overline{\text{I}}\ \overline{\text{II}}\ \overline{\text{III}}\ \overline{\text{IV}}\ \overline{\text{V}}\ \overline{\text{VI}}\ \overline{\text{VII}}$ etc.	—
	λ	$\overline{\text{I}}\ \overline{(\text{II})}$	$\overline{\text{I}}\ \overline{\text{II}}$

Figure 2.8 Possible arrangement of the minimum number of genes for human Ig and mouse light chains. The genes on each horizontal line are thought to lie on the same chromosome. In mice the minimum of κ V-genes is probably well above 8 and the existence of a second λ V-gene is uncertain. (From Milstein and Munro, 1973)

There is little information about the 'punctuation' between the genes and we really do not know where the variable region genes are in relation to the constant region genes. We do know that they are not far away, since recombination events between allotypic markers on the variable and constant regions of rabbit heavy chains are not very common (Mage *et al.*, 1971; Kindt and Mandy, 1972). Recombination between genes on the same chromosome (linked genes) occurs by crossing over during meiosis (Figure 2.9). In this way, genes which were separately inherited from mother and father are passed on together to the offspring. Obviously, the closer genes are together, the more infrequent will be crossing-over events between them, and the observed frequency will give a measure of the distance. Genes which are not on the same chromosome will be passed on in recombinant patterns at a rate of 50% just as a matter of chance. When two genes are very far apart on a chromosome, the recombination frequency between them may approach 50% and it would not be possible to be sure that they are on the one chromosome.

The genes which code for the heavy chain constant regions are certainly close together, so much so that recombinants are extremely rare. Sets of similar genes arranged in this fashion are called tandem duplicates.

Humans have a complex series of genetic markers on their immunoglobulins. These allotypes seem mostly to be single amino acid substitutions resulting from mutational events. They are usually detected by the serological

RECOMBINATION

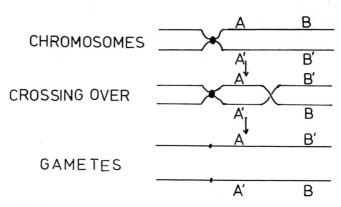

Figure 2.9 Mechanism of recombination between genes on the same chromosome. The chromosome carries two loci (A and B) with alleles A and A′ and B and B′. When crossing over occurs during meiosis, A is inherited with B′ and B with A′

method of haemagglutination inhibition. In this method, erythrocytes are coated with immunoglobulin from an individual of known allotype, usually by one of a number of convenient 'tanning' methods. The cell is then agglutinated with an antiserum to the allotype, and this reaction can be inhibited by prior mixing of the antiserum with test sera from individuals of the same allotype as that on the cells. Owing to an early lack of understanding of the complexities of human immunoglobulins, especially IgG subclasses, and because of the inability of conventional genetic analysis to unscramble this unquestionably complicated series, the system is difficult to understand. The fact that there are or have been at least three systems of nomenclature further complicates the issue.

The most extensively characterized series of markers which occur on IgG are the Gm groups, called after their discoverer Grubb (1970). Markers on IgA are sensibly called Am. Most confusion arises because there are four human IgG subclasses which have all evolved from a common ancestral γ chain (certainly since the primates evolved), and structures which are alleles in one class may be present on others, for instance the non-a (1 −) marker, see Table 2.5. A further source of confusion is that because the genes are very closely linked, recombinants are rare and the arrangement of alleles on each chromosome is usually transmitted as a unit: a haplotype. Certain haplotypes are quite characteristic of different ethnic populations.

Table 2.5 Gm allotypes in man

Chain	γ4	γ2	γ3	γ1
Arrangement of genes (not to scale)			436	214 356, 358
Sequences of homoalleles	N M O		Phe Tyr	Arg AspGluLeu Lys GluGluMet
Old nomenclature	A R K E R S n		c b$^\alpha$ b$^\beta$ b$^\gamma$ b^3 b^4 b s t r^5 – b^2 Rouen 2, 3, SF2 b g	f z a non-a
New nomenclature		23	6 10, 11, 12, 13, 14, 15, 16 7 2 3 18, 19, 20 5 21	4 1 17 1–
Non-allelic markers	non-a or 1– non-g	non-a or 1–	non-a or 1–	1 1–

IMMUNOGLOBULIN EVOLUTION

This section will review very briefly the phenomena which need to be explained and then expand on the genetic, rather than the selective, mechanisms which may have been involved.

All immunoglobulins are made up of subunits (domains) with a common origin, arranged in the molecules in a characteristic way (the four-chain structure). Each chain demonstrates the integration of variable and constant portions, a unique event. The three main groups of chains are on different chromosomes. The heavy chain constant region genes evolved from the μ-like ancestor and are closely arranged as a tandem series.

Since all immunoglobulins are made up of domains, we may assume this as the starting point for their evolution. Clearly, any immunoglobulin is made up of a large number of specialized copies of the domain. The gene of the domain must have been copied many times, to provide a whole series of gene duplicates. Gene duplication can occur in two ways: tandem duplication and polyploid duplication (see Ohno, 1970).

Tandem duplication implies the duplication of a stretch of genetic material on a chromosome, so that the chromosome becomes longer. Probably the most common mechanism is unequal crossing over (Figure 2.10). If the alignment of two chromatids during meiosis is imperfect, then crossovers will have the effect of transferring an 'unfair' amount of genetic material to the daughter chromatids. One will have an additional copy of the overlapped portion, the other will have lost it. This is a rather unstable event for a number of reasons. First, it is often disastrous to be deprived of a given genetic potential and any gamete with such a deletion may give rise to

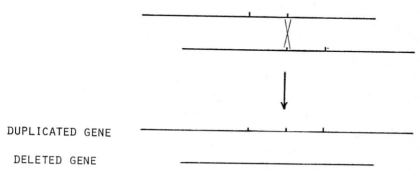

DUPLICATED GENE

DELETED GENE

Figure 2.10 Unequal crossing over. If the chromosomes are misaligned during crossing over, one of them carries two copies of the mismatched section, the other losing its copy

non-viable offspring. Habitual unequal crossing over is, therefore, not encouraged. Even the recipient of the duplicate may have difficulties of gene dosage: for example, too much of an enzyme may be produced, and if the 'controlling' genes for the duplicated gene have not been duplicated at the same time this will be deleterious. A further problem for possessors of duplicated genes is that the greater the number of tandem gene duplications the greater the chances of mismatched synapses and more unequal crossovers.

A 'safer' method of duplicating genes is simply not to undergo a satisfactory meiosis and have extra chromosomes (polyploid duplication). This mechanism has the advantages of retention of control mechanisms but is not available to mammals or any other group which use chromosomal sex determination, since frightful confusion arises as to the sex of anomalies like XXYYs and XXXYs. Nevertheless, gene duplication is essential for evolution. The highly conservative policeman of natural selection will not permit much experimentation with essential genes, so all experiments must be supported by retention of a sufficient genetic potential, and this means that the genes must be duplicated.

In the case of immunoglobulins, it is probable that the primordial domain underwent a (series of?) tandem duplication(s), one duplicate or set becoming specialized as a variable region gene. This arrangement was capable of making a primitive light chain. The division between κ, λ, and heavy chain gene clusters probably now occurred by a process of polyploid duplication, probably undertaken twice. The κ chain set has been relatively stable, but the constant region genes of both the heavy and the λ chains have apparently undergone a series of tandem duplication events. Human λ chains exist in at least four forms, with Lys or Arg at position 191 and Gly or Ser at position 153, and everyone has all four forms. We have already referred to the many duplicated forms of heavy chains but their mechanisms of evolution are of some interest.

It is not difficult to propose a mechanism for the evolution of α and γ chains from the μ chain. The unequal crossovers required are shown in Figure 2.11. Unequal crossover events are probably quite common among immunoglobulin genes in the course of evolution. It seems that the phenomenon of subclasses of heavy chains is transitory. They vary greatly in number between species (from 1 to about 6 or 7 have been reported). There is no functional, antigenic or structural analogy between the different subclasses seen in different species which are not reasonably closely related. Domestic ruminants all seem to have two subclasses of IgG which are antigenically related. There is good evidence from sequence data that the IgG2 of cattle evolved from a precursor which was similar to the IgG1. By the

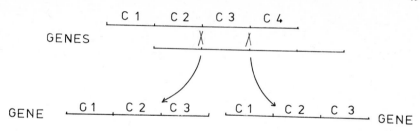

Figure 2.11 Possible origin of γ and α chains from μ chain. Deletion of the $C_\mu 2$ domain could give rise to γ chain, and of $C_\mu 3$ domain to α chain

time that the gene duplication which gave rise to the IgG2 had occurred, the ancestral γ chain was already identifiable as belonging to a ruminant. It seems that immunoglobulin subclasses are merely the current 'experiments' of evolution. Most of them will prove to be of no adaptive value and will be lost by unequal crossing over. What is not permissible is that the ability to make IgG is lost.

Complement

The complement system is the principal humoral effector mechanism of the extracellular fluid and is usually activated by the combination of antibody and antigen. The reaction pathways are complex but not incomprehensible (Figure 2.12). They centre around C3, the most abundant of the complement components and probably the most biologically important, and can be divided into the 'classical', alternative and terminal pathways.

NOMENCLATURE

The components of the classical and terminal pathways are known as Cn, where n is usually a number relating to their position in the reaction sequence. The components of the alternative pathway are known as factors B, D etc., in order of their discovery. Some letters have been abandoned on the identification of alternative pathway factors as numbered complement components, or known complement inhibitors. Of the latter, there are two which are well established: the C1 esterase inhibitor, also known as $\alpha 2$-neuraminoglycoprotein, and C3b-inactivator, also known as KAF (conglutinogen activating factor). When complement components are activated this is indicated by a bar over the abbreviation. Fragmented components are divided into a and b, the larger part usually being designated b. Thus, $\overline{C3bBb}$ is an active complex of the larger fragments of C3 and factor B. Erythrocytes are denoted by E and antibody by A.

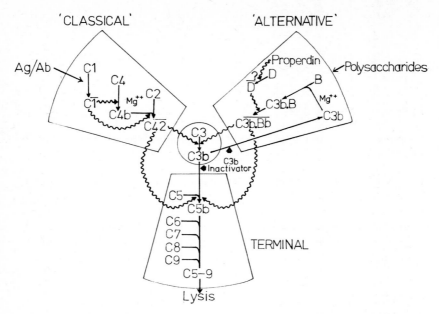

Figure 2.12 General scheme for complement reactions. The central feature of comple-ment action is the splitting of C3. There are two 'complementological' enzymes which do this: the 'classical' convertase, formed by the interaction of antibody and C1, leading to the complex enzyme C42, and the 'alternative pathway' convertase consisting of C3b and factor B. The alternative pathway convertase is readily generated in the presence of C3b, the major split product of C3. Thus, the bulk reaction of the alter-native pathway is a positive feedback cycle. It is under homeostatic control by the C3b inactivator (KAF). In the presence of C3b and a C3 convertase (classical or alter-native), C5 is split, and the terminal complex of C5, C6, C7, C8 and C9 is formed which leads to the generation of the characteristic membrane lesions and lysis of cells

THE 'CLASSICAL' PATHWAY

The 'classical' pathway of complement activation is initiated by the binding of C1 to antigen–antibody complexes. C1 consists of three subcomponents, C1q, C1r and C1s, which are held together by a calcium ion. The C1q has combining sites for antibody. Its interaction with antibody leads to the activation of C1s, a serine–histidine esterase. This attacks the next component, C4, splitting off a small fragment to reveal a short-lived binding site by which the C4b attaches to any local structure. In the presence of magnesium ions, C2 binds to the active C4b and is acted upon by C1 to remove a small fragment. The C4 and C2 form an unstable complex enzyme which attacks C3 and whose half-life at 37 °C is only 7 minutes. At this point, the C1 is no longer required, and nor is antibody. The reaction pathway is a fairly typical 'enzyme cascade' reaction in which an enzyme is activated and produces large quantities of the next enzyme in the series.

THE C3 STEP

C3 can be attacked by a large variety of proteolytic enzymes in addition to $\overline{C42}$. The larger fragment has a short-lived binding site by which the molecule attaches itself to other local structures in much the same way as C4. The quantity of C3 which is fixed in the vicinity of a complement activation site is quite large. It produces a very apparent amorphous coat to the antigen (Figure 2.13). The complement system mediates its most important biological effects via adherence reactions involving C3. A number of cell types including B lymphocytes, polymorphs and macrophages have receptors for fixed C3 on their surfaces. Opsonization of bacteria for phagocytosis by polymorphs is highly dependent on C3 fixation, especially when IgM antibody is involved.

The initial form of fixed C3, C3b, is quite rapidly inactivated by the action of a proteolytic enzyme which is always present in a fully active form in the plasma: the C3b inactivator. Its action prevents the C3 from taking part in subsequent reactions of the complement system, increases its susceptibility to further proteolytic attack, but does not wholly destroy its role as an opsonin.

C3b can take part in at least two more limbs of the complement reaction, the alternative pathway and the terminal pathway.

THE ALTERNATIVE PATHWAY

The term 'alternative pathway' probably conceals at least two reaction mechanisms which are closely related. The best understood of these is the C3b feedback cycle, a remarkable mechanism for the amplification of C3 fixation.

C3b can combine with factor B in the presence of magnesium ions. The factor B is split by factor D in an activated form whose origin is disputed, yielding the complex enzyme $\overline{C3bBb}$. This is a C3 convertase. Note that there are very marked parallels between these reactions and those involved in the formation of the 'classical' C3 convertase $\overline{C42}$, both reactions requiring magnesium and proteolytic attack following the formation of the complex. Furthermore, there is strong evidence for the similarity of C3 and C4 and of C2 and factor B (Table 2.6).

Clearly, any positive feedback cycle of this nature would be explosive in its action if it were under no homeostatic control. This is provided by the

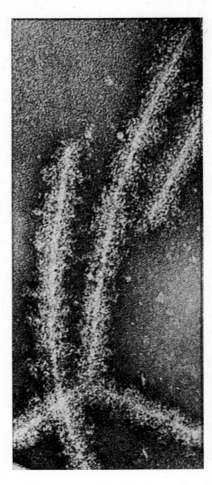

Figure 2.13 Complement sheath on flagella. The action of antibody and complement on flagella and other antigens is the deposition of a thick amorphous coat of complement components, principally C3. (From Feinstein and Munn, 1966)

C3b-inactivator which damps the reaction by inactivating its product and initiator, C3b. The importance of the inactivator both *in vivo* and *in vitro* has been shown by a patient who lacks the enzyme and who has no detectable intact C3 or factor B (Abramson *et al.*, 1971). Experiments involving the removal of the inactivator *in vitro* with F(ab')$_2$ antibody caused spontaneous alternative pathway activation (Nicol and Lachmann, 1973).

As originally described by Pillemer (1954), the alternative pathway was a

Table 2.6 Structurally and functionally related complement components

Groups		Common features
Probable	Possible	
C_{1r} C_{1s}	Factor D	Small proteolytic enzymes, split each other/C2/factor B C_{1r} and C_{1s} have similar subunit structures
C_2 Factor B		I polypeptide chain, same size Heat labile Linked to HLA Bind to C_4b/C_3b in presence of Mg^{++} Then attacked by C_1/factor D Then form part of complex C_3 splitting enzyme
C_3 C_4	C_5	$2(+)_+$ polypeptide chains NH_3^+ sensitive, Hoffmeister salt sensitive ($C_4 > C_3 > C_5$) Activated by proteolytic action to reveal hydrophobic binding site Form complex enzyme with C2/factor B which splits C_3 and C_5 C_3 and C_4 inactivated by further proteolysis, probably by same enzyme
	C_6 C_7	Same size Not readily inactivated by heat, ions, etc. Not (apparently) enzymes Not (apparently) split when incorporated in C_567 complex
	C_{1q} (Collagen) Properdin	C_1 has partially collagen-like sequence Big, asymmetric molecules Resistant to conventional proteolysis (e.g. pepsin) C_{1q} first in reaction sequence, properdin may well be

mechanism for activation of complement by polysaccharides and bacteria in the absence of antibody. The initial reactant was properdin, a substance which fell into disrepute as a consequence of the difficulty of isolating it and its ill-defined properties. Recent work shows that properdin certainly exists and is an exceedingly asymmetric (i.e. probably long and thin) molecule, with a molecular weight of about 180000, a sedimentation coefficient of 3.5s, and a marked resistance to most 'conventional' proteolytic enzymes. It can initiate the conversion of C_3, but how it does this is not known, largely because of the difficulties which result from trying to detect initiating micro-events in the presence of a positive feedback cycle. The simplest hypothesis is that properdin can convert C_3 directly, thus triggering the feedback. There is some experimental evidence to this effect, but the subject is still under discussion.

THE TERMINAL PATHWAY

The terminal pathway of the complement system is that which gives rise to the most dramatic and characteristic reaction of the complement system *in vitro*: lysis. In biological terms, this is probably relatively trivial.

C3b binds C5 which can then be split by either of the C3 convertase enzymes (C42 or C3bBb). The split C5 combines with C6 and then with C7 to form a trimolecular complex which will bind lipid membranes. The C567 complex reacts with C8 and C9 to form the agent which produces the characteristic complement lesion. The exact reaction pathways are not fully characterized, but do not appear to involve further proteolytic reactions, but rather some kind of assembly phenomenon. There is no evidence of an enzymic attack on the lipids and current hypothesis suggests that the C5–9 complex inserts itself into the membrane, giving rise to a functional aperture (Figure 2.14) which cannot be healed and through which ion flux can occur. The cell thus loses its osmotic integrity, swells and bursts.

The efficiency of the terminal components in causing lysis is very much higher in the case of erythrocytes than in the case of nucleated cells. In favourable circumstances, a single complement lesion can cause the lysis of

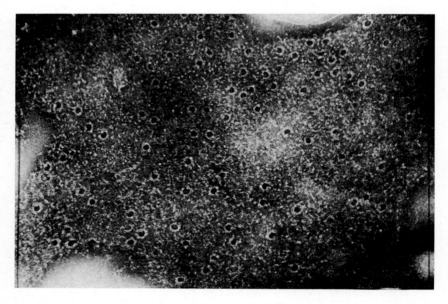

Figure 2.14 Complement lesions in erythrocyte membrane (electron micrograph by Dr. E. A. Munn)

an erythrocyte, but many such lesions are necessary to overcome the repair potentialities of the nucleated cell. This means, of course, that the antibody and complement alone are relatively ineffective in damaging grafts, tumours and virus-infected cells. It also appears to be a general truth that the terminal components of a species are relatively ineffective in lysing its own cells. There is a teleologically obvious adaptive value in this fact: it is less likely that an individual's own tissues will be damaged by the contagious action of complement complexes activated on foreign antigens close by. Nevertheless, it is certainly true that the role of complement in the destruction of cellular antigens *in vivo* has been little studied.

COMPLEMENT-MEDIATED IMMUNOPATHOLOGY

The complement system is not only involved in the defence of the body against invading organisms, but also plays a role in the pathogenesis of a number of diseases. Those afflicting the kidney are particularly important in this respect.

Complement components are involved in both the ultimate form and removal of immune complexes and in the pathogenesis of immune complex diseases. Under favourable circumstances, immune complexes activate the complement system, enclosing the complexes in a coating of fixed C_3, and promoting their removal from the circulation by the reticuloendothelial system. This process occurs predominantly in the liver and the spleen. The complexes are taken up and destroyed by the macrophages and Kuppfer cells.

In certain circumstances, the immune complexes are not adequately dealt with by these mechanisms, for instance when low affinity antibodies are formed or when the antigen load is excessive (e.g. serum sickness). In these circumstances, the complexes may dissociate, leading to the transport of their component parts across basement membranes, particularly in the glomerulus of the kidney. Complement activation may now take place in the extracellular fluid, releasing the anaphylatoxins $C_{3}a$ and $C_{5}a$. These produce an increase in the permeability of capillaries and the filtration of the complexes may be increased. The anaphylatoxins are not adequately neutralized by the plasma carboxypeptidase B, since it is a very large molecule which does not readily traverse the capillary wall. Hence the anaphylatoxins will have a substantially free rein and will produce a florid inflammatory response. Infiltration by polymorphs will occur, whose released lysosomal enzymes contribute greatly to the damage to the basement membrane.

The pathogenesis of membranoproliferative glomerulonephritis is rather less well understood. The disease is characterized by granular C_3 deposition in the glomerulus in the absence of IgG and low plasma C_3 levels. These patients also have raised levels of the mysterious C_3 nephritic factor, which

may be part of the normal complement system, but which defies isolation
free from IgG3. When added to normal serum, this factor leads to C3
breakdown, but the mechanisms by which it causes disease are still poorly
understood (Peters, 1975).

It is important to remember that the kidney disease of these patients
appears to be secondary to a systemic abnormality of the complement
system. It is therefore inappropriate to attempt transplantation unless the
disease process is under control. In the absence of understanding of its true
aetiology and pathogenesis, this is likely to prove rather 'hit and miss'.

COMPLEMENT GENETICS

In early 1974 this subject may have been irrelevant to surgeons, but it seems
that the topic may now be important in the transplant field.

The investigation of complement genetics has progressed along two
separate paths. One is the observation and investigation of infrequent complement deficiency syndromes. This work gives us some clues as to the
biological value of the complement components. Those which have been
recognized in man and animals are shown in Table 2.7. The deficiencies
fall into four classes: the complement inhibitors, the classical pathway, C3,
and the terminal pathway.

Deficiency of complement inhibitors is most serious. Partial deficiency
(heterozygous) of $\overline{C1}$ inhibitor gives rise to the dominantly inherited disease,
hereditary angioedema. Deficiency of the C3b inactivator has already been
referred to, and will be further discussed below.

Deficiencies of the classical pathway components may well lead to a

Table 2.7 Genetic deficiencies of the complement system

Species	Factor deficient	No. of pedigrees	Clinical
Man	C1r	2	Renal and skin disease
	C2	Several	Most healthy, SLE?
	C3	2	Immune deficiency
	C4	1	Skin disease
	C5	1	Skin disease
	C6	1	Healthy
	C7	2	Healthy
	C1-inh.	Many	HAE
	C3b-inactivator (KAF)	1	Immune deficiency
Guinea-pig	C4	1	Healthy
	A component C3-9	1	Healthy but extinct
Mouse	C5	Many inbred	Healthy
Rabbit	C6	Several	Healthy
Hamster	C6	1	Healthy

relatively small increase in susceptibility to viral infections. This may well be the origin of the high incidence of systemic lupus erythematosis which is seen in these patients.

Deficiencies of either C3 or the C3b inactivator, which leads to a secondary C3 deficiency, are extremely serious (Abramson et al., 1971; Alper et al., 1972). None of the patients so far discovered lives outside a relatively wealthy community, and all are under 30 years of age. They suffer repeated systemic pyogenic infections (pneumonias, meningitis, septicaemias). They are probably the products of the antibiotic age.

Deficiencies of the terminal components are probably trivial.

The second line of investigation of complement genetics is the investigation of polymorphisms: allotypes which can be conveniently separated by electrophoretic methods. So far, polymorphisms have been identified in C3, factor B and C6. These investigations are genuinely esoteric but for one fact. One of the preoccupations of geneticists is to locate the genes with which they are dealing. Very great strides are now being made in this direction, partly as a result of new methods involving cell hybridization and partly because the number of genetic markers known is approaching the critical numbers at which linkage relationships can be measured. The great surprise in the mapping field is that two complement components (at least) map close to the HLA system (Allen, 1974; Fu et al., 1974). The two markers concerned are the polymorphism of factor B and the deficiency of C2. The importance of these discoveries are:

(a) The provision of new markers within the region. This might have some ultimate relevance for graft matching.

(b) The possibility that the linkage disequilibrium which apparently exists between C2 deficiency and HLA type may give us a new insight into the origins of linkage disequilibrium and consequently a new understanding of the 'natural history' of the HLA region and of our ancestry.

(c) The fact that genes with functions outside the relatively confined operations of histocompatibility but of obvious immunological relevance lie in the region may lead us to a new functional understanding of cellular interactions.

References

Abramson, N., Alper, C. A., Lachmann, P. J., Rosen, F. S. and Jandl, J. H. (1971). Deficiency of C3 inactivator in man. *J. Immunol.*, **107**, 19

Allen, F. H. (1974). Linkage of HL-A and GBG. *Vox Sang.*, **27**, 382

Alper, C. A., Colten, H. R., Rosen, F. S., Rabson, A. R., Macnab, G. and Gear, J. S. (1972). Homozygous deficiency of C3 in a patient with repeated infections. *Lancet*, **ii**, 1179

Bennich, H. and von Bahr-Lindström, H. (1974). Structure of immunoglobulin E (IgE). In L. Brent and J. Holborow (eds.), *Progress in Immunology II*, vol. 1, p. 49 (Amsterdam: North Holland)

Edelman, G. M., Cunningham, B. A., Gall, W. E., Gottleib, P. D., Rutishauser, U. and Waxdal, M. J. (1969). The covalent structure of an entire γG immunoglobulin molecule. *Proc. Nat. Acad. Sci. U.S.A.*, **70**, 3305

Eichman, K. (1972). Idiotypic identity of antibodies to streptococcal carbohydrate in inbred mice. *Eur. J. Immunol.*, **2**, 301

Feinstein, A. (1963). Character and allotypy of an immune globulin in rabbit colostrum. *Nature (London)*, **199**, 1197

Feinstein, A. (1974). An IgM model. In L. Brent and J. Holborow (eds.), *Progress in Immunology II*, vol. **I**, p. 115 (Amsterdam: North Holland)

Feinstein, A. (1975). The three-dimensional structure of immunoglobulins. In M. J. Hobart and I. McConnell (eds.), *The Immune System* (Oxford: Blackwell Scientific Publications)

Feinstein, A. and Rowe, A. J. (1965). Molecular mechanisms of formation of an antigen–antibody complex. *Nature (London)*, **205**, 147

Fleischmann, J. B., Porter, R. R. and Press, E. M. (1963). The arrangement of the polypeptide chains of γ-globulin. *Biochem. J.*, **88**, 220

Fu, S. M., Kunkel, H. G., Brissman, H. P., Allen, F. H. and Fotino, M. (1974). Evidence for linkage between HL-A histocompatibility genes and those involved in the synthesis of the second component of complement. *J. Exp. Med.*, **140**, 1108

Grubb, R. (1970). *Genetic Markers of Human Immunoglobulins*. (Berlin: Springer-Verlag)

Karush, F. (1970). Affinity and the immune response. *Ann. N.Y. Acad. Sci.*, **169**, 56

Kindt, T. J. and Mandy, W. J. (1972). Recombination of genes coding for constant and variable regions of immunoglobulin heavy chains. *J. Immunol.*, **108**, 1110

Koshland, M. E. (1975). Structure and function of the J chain. *Adv. Immunol.*, **20**, 41

Krause, R. M. (1970). The search for antibodies with molecular uniformity. *Adv. Immunol.*, **12**, 1

Kreth, H. W. and Williamson, A. R. (1973). The extent of diversity of anti-hapten antibodies in inbred mice: anti-NIP antibodies in CBA mice. *Eur. J. Immunol.*, **3**, 141

Landucci-Tosi, S. (1972). Reported in C. Milstein and A. J. Munro: Genetics of immunoglobulins and the immune response. In R. R. Porter (ed.), *Defence and Recognition*, p. 199 (Lancaster: MTP)

MacLennan, I. C. M., Connell, G. E. and Gotch, F. M. (1974). Effector activating determinants on IgG. *Immunology*, **26**, 303

Mage, R. G., Young-Cooper, G. O. and Alexander, C. (1971). Genetic control of variable and constant regions of immunoglobulin heavy chains. *Nature New Biol.* **230**, 63

Milstein, C. (1967). Linked groups of residues in immunoglobulin chains. *Nature (London)*, **216**, 330

Mitchison, N. A. (1967). Antigen recognition responsible for the induction *in vitro* of the secondary response. *Cold Spring Harbor Symp. Quant. Biol.*, **32**, 431

Nicol, P. A. E. and Lachmann, P. J. (1973). The alternate pathway of complement activation: the role of C3 and its inactivator (KAF). *Immunology*, **24**, 259

Noelkin, M. E., Nelson, C. A., Buckley, C. E. and Tanford, C. (1965). Gross conformation of rabbit 7s γ-globulin and its papain-cleaved fragments. *J. Biol. Chem.*, **240**, 218

Ohno, S. (1970). *Evolution by Gene Duplication*. (Berlin: Springer-Verlag)

Okafor, G. O., Turner, M. W. and Hay, F. C. (1974). Localisation of monocyte binding site of human immunoglobulin G. *Nature (London)*, **248**, 228

Oudin, J. and Michel, M. (1970). Idiotypy of rabbit antibodies. II. Comparison of idiotypy of various kinds of antibodies formed in the same rabbits against *Salmonella typhi*. *J. Exp. Med.*, **130**, 619

Padlam, E. A., Segal, D. M., Cohen, G. H. and Davies, E. R. (1974). The three-dimensional structural of the antigen binding site of McPC 603. In E. Sercarz, A. R. Williamson and C. F. Fox (eds.), *The Immune System: Genes, Receptors, Signals* (New York: Academic Press)

Peters, D. K. (1975). The kidney in allergic disease. In P. G. H. Gell, R. R. A. Coombs and P. J. Lachmann (eds.), *Clinical Aspects of Immunology (3rd ed.)*, p. 1127 (Oxford: Blackwell Scientific Publications)

Pillemer, L., Blum, L., Lepow, I. H., Ross, O. A., Todd, E. W. and Wardlae, A. C. (1954). The properdin system and immunity. I. Demonstration and isolation of a new serum protein, properdin, and its role in immune phenomena. *Science*, **120**, 279

Poljac, R. J., Amzel, L. M., Avey, H. P., Chen, B. L., Phizackerly, R. P. and Saul, F. (1973). Three-dimensional structure of the Fab' fragment of a human immunoglobulin at 2.8 Å resolution. *Proc. Nat. Acad. Sci. U.S.A.*, **70**, 3305

Putnam, F. W. (1962). Structural relationships among normal human γ-globulin, myeloma globulins, and Bence–Jones proteins. *Biochim. Biophys. Acta*, **63**, 539

Richards, F. F., Amzel, L. M., Konigsberg, W. H., Manjula, B. N., Poljac, R. J., Rosenstein, R. W., Saul, F. and Varga, J. M. (1974). Polyfunctional antibody combining regions. In E. E. Sercarz, A. R. Williamson and C. F. Fox (eds.), *The Immune System: Genes, Receptors, Signals*, p. 53 (New York: Academic Press)

Schiffler, M., Girling, R. L., Ely, K. R. and Edmondson, A. B. (1973). Structure of a λ-type Bence–Jones protein at 3.5 Å resolution. *Biochemistry*, **12**, 4620

Stevens, R. H. and Williamson, A. R. (1973). Isolation of messenger RNA coding for mouse heavy chain immunoglobulin. *Proc. Nat. Acad. Sci. U.S.A.*, **70**, 1127

Swan, D., Aviv, H. and Leder, P. (1972). Purification and properties of biologically active messenger RNA for a myeloma light chain. *Proc. Nat. Acad. Sci. U.S.A.*, **69**, 1967

Taussig, M. J. (1975). The antibody combining site. In M. J. Hobart and I. McConnell (eds.), *The Immune System* (Oxford: Blackwell Scientific Publications)

Todd, C. W. (1963). Allotypy in rabbit 19s protein. *Biochim. Biophys. Res. Comm.*, **11**, 170

Tonegawa, S., Steinberg, C., Dube, S. and Bernardini, A. (1974). Evidence for somatic generation of antibody diversity. *Proc. Nat. Acad. Sci. U.S.A.*, **71**, 4027

Utsumi, S. (1969). Stepwise cleavage of rabbit immunoglobulin G by papain and isolation of four types of biologically active Fc fragments. *Biochem. J.*, **112**, 343

Wang, A. C., Wilson, S. K., Hopper, J. E., Fudenberg, H. H. and Nisonoff, A. (1970). Evidence for the control of synthesis of the variable regions of the heavy chains of immunoglobulins G and M by the same gene. *Proc. Nat. Acad. Sci. U.S.A.*, **66**, 337

CHAPTER 3

Mechanisms Underlying Immunological Diseases

C. J. F. Spry

Introduction

One of the most important areas of development in immunology is concerned with the ways in which immunological responses are involved in tissue damage. Normally, immunological responses which are directed against bacteria or viruses lead to destruction of the invading organisms. However, in some instances these responses spread to involve and damage non-invaded tissues, and in others the immunological response can also set up a cycle of injury in which the products of damaged tissues initiate further destructive changes. This is a feature of 'autoimmune' diseases where immunological reactions are directed against autoantigens.

Tissue damage which is the result of excessive immunological reactivity should be compared with diseases in which immunological responses are reduced. Here damage results from the uninhibited effects of invading organisms. In the last few years a third category of immunological disease has been proposed in which homeostatic regulation of immunological responses is defective, which results in inappropriate immune responses. In practice these three types of process may occur together in any one patient.

The Inflammatory Response

The inflammatory response is so widespread in nature that it must have evolved at an early stage, even before specific immunological responses arose. The origins of specific immunological responses themselves are still unclear, but it is possible that lymphocytes have an evolutionary origin close to, or involving, cells of the monocyte/macrophage line, but separate from the other main phagocytic cells: polymorphs. In any event, immunological responses *in vivo* cannot be isolated from inflammatory responses, which provide a final common pathway for all types of tissue destruction (Zweifach and McCluskey, 1974).

Phagocytic cells are derived from bone marrow stem cells and they preferentially phagocytise material which has been coated with altered serum proteins. These proteins are of two types: (a) antibodies which have attached to determinants on the surface of the ingested material and (b) complement components. These proteins cover the surface of the foreign material in a way which leaves biologically important regions of the antibody or complement protein exposed. These regions are the Fc portion of immunoglobulin, and the C3b portion of the third component of complement, C3. Phagocytic cells 'recognize' these altered serum proteins through specific Fc and C3b receptors which are present in high density on their surface (Wong and Wilson, 1975). Once attachment has occurred, the coated material is rapidly ingested and digested in phagolysosomes which are formed when lysosomes fuse with the phagocytosed material. Phagocytosed bacteria are killed soon after ingestion (Klebanoff, 1975). The products of digestion may be sufficiently degraded to be non-toxic, but in some instances the material is not degraded, so that when the effector cell dies, the material is released, only to be phagocytosed again by another cell. Recent work has shown that macrophages and neutrophils secrete digestive enzymes into their environment after they have come in contact with foreign material (Weissman, 1975). By this means intrinsically non-toxic but persisting substances can induce chronic inflammatory lesions.

The supply of phagocytic cells and serum proteins to sites of immunological injury is the result of blood flow and its composition, and also of alterations in the vessel walls contiguous to the injury. The supply of cells and proteins involved in inflammatory response is increased when bone marrow and other distant tissues are stimulated by mechanisms which are as yet largely unknown. These stimuli are probably released from the area of tissue damage via draining lymphatics and venules. In sites of chronic inflammation some macrophages can divide locally. Lymphatic drainage from sites of antigen localization determines whether a systemic immunological reaction is initiated. For these reasons it is important to consider the parts played by blood vessels, and the lymphatic connections in areas of tissue damage.

A schematic outline of the various components involved in tissue injury is shown in Figure 3.1.

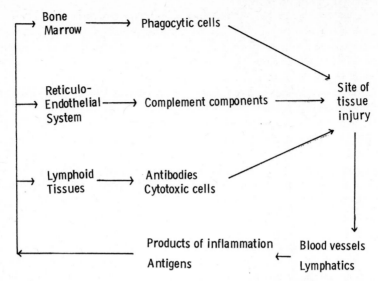

Figure 3.1 Constituents and pathways involved in allergic tissue damage. A large number of components are involved, and their effects are finely balanced in normal individuals

Types of Immunological Tissue Damage

CLASSIFICATION

In most immunological diseases it is possible to classify the response by considering whether the effector mechanism involves predominantly either antibody or lymphocytes. In each case the type of response can be sub-classified by specifying the type of antibody or lymphocyte which mediates the reaction. Other features which may be used in classification are the sites of the response, and the clinical feature of the response.

One of the most widely used classifications of this kind was introduced by Gell and Coombs in 1962 (see Gell, Coombs and Lachmann, 1975). Responses which involve antibody are classed as Type I, II or III, and responses which involve lymphocytes without the interaction of antibodies are Type IV reactions. Type I reactions are anaphylactic reactions, mediated by antibody which is attached to tissue mast cells. Type II reactions are those in which antibody and complement cause damage by attaching to antigens on the surface of tissues or cell membranes. The haemolytic anaemias are the clearest example of this type of reaction. The antigens may be either structural components of the membrane, or they may become attached to the surface as occurs with a number of drugs. Type III reactions involve interactions between soluble antigens and antibodies, and the complexes which are formed initiate immune complex lesions. When these localize in extravascular sites they are termed 'Arthus' reactions. In intravascular sites they produce 'serum sickness'. Type IV reactions are distinguished from all other types in that they can only be transferred by injections containing living lymphocytes and not by antibodies. These include delayed hypersensitivity response, rejection of foreign tissues and graft-versus-host reactions.

In clinical practice it is usually not difficult to distinguish these types of immunological tissue damage, using their main features which are shown in Table 3.1.

Table 3.1 Classification of types of allergic tissue damage (after Gell and Coombs, 1963)

	Type of response			
	I	*II*	*III*	*IV*
Components	Antibody on mast cells	Antibody	Antibody	Lymphocytes and macrophages
Presentation of antigen	Soluble antigens	Antigen on cell surface	Soluble antigen	Antigen on cell surface
Effector cells involved	Tissue mast cell	Neutrophil macrophage lymphocyte	Circulating neutrophil	Macrophage lymphocyte
Effector mechanism	Products of mast cells effect smooth muscle and vessels	Coated cell removed in reticulo-endothelial system (RES) K cell cytotoxicity	Antigen–antibody complex interacts with neutrophils in vessels	Lymphocyte damages cells directly or by activating macrophages
Clinical types	Anaphylaxis	Haemolytic anaemia Haemolysis	Renal disease Vasculitis, arthritis etc.	Delayed hypersensitivity Tissue rejection

ANAPHYLACTIC (TYPE I) REACTIONS

Clinically the commonest anaphylactic reactions encountered are hayfever and allergic asthma. They may also occur when patients are injected with penicillin or with iodine compounds before x-ray studies are done. Invariably these patients have had prior exposure to these antigens, and in a number of cases have known allergy to them.

The mechanism of the response is as follows (see Stanworth, 1973): initially the injected antigen diffuses into perivascular areas rich in mast cells. These cells are found in greatest number surrounding small veins in tissues which are in contact with environmental antigens: skin, respiratory and gastrointestinal tracts. The mast cells have been previously 'sensitized' with IgE (and in some instances IgG).

The nature of the attachment of the IgE to mast cells is not known, but it involves the Fc piece of IgE. When an antigen combines with two IgE molecules on the mast cell surface, a configurational change occurs in the cell membrane which leads to the rapid extrusion of mast cell granule contents into their environment. The granules liberate chemical mediators which include histamine, serotonin, slow-reacting substance of anaphylaxis (SRSA), and vasoactive amines which cause rapid changes in blood vessel permeability. When these substances enter the general circulation they may induce widespread effects, at a distance from the initial localization of antigen. Following the explosive release of their granule contents, mast cells re-synthesize them in about 4–12 hours. The fate of the cell-bound antigen–IgE complexes is not known, and little is known about the steps by which the mast cells become 're-fused' with IgE during the refractory period of about 12 hours before the cell can be triggered again by antigen.

There has been a recent increase in interest in the biological factors which influence the development of IgE antibody responses. This has centred on the finding that normally during early postnatal development environmental antigens in food and air induce the synthesis of the IgA class of antibodies, which have no binding site for mast cells. It is suggested that in individuals who are unable to synthesize IgA normally during first exposure to environmental antigens, the IgE class of antibodies is produced instead. These people would thus produce IgE-mediated (anaphylactic) responses to environmental antigens (Stokes, Soothill and Turner, 1975). If research which is currently under way confirms this interesting idea, 'atopic' individuals could be considered to have a primary IgA deficiency state, or at least a defect in the regulation of the class of antibody which is synthesized.

ANTIBODY-MEDIATED REACTIONS TO CELL SURFACE ANTIGENS
(TYPE II)

Although immunological reactions directed against cell surface antigens have been known for many years, they have proved to be a great deal more complex than was initially suspected. The prototype for this kind of response is seen in the haemolytic anaemias and transfusion reactions where circulating antibodies combine with cell surface antigens (Dacie and Worlledge, 1969). These antibodies are of two main types: the commonest are IgG antibodies which cause red cells to be destroyed by phagocytic cells in the reticulo-endothelial system. The second type is IgM in class, and it induces complement fixation on the erythrocyte membrane which leads to cell lysis with release of free haemoglobin into the circulation.

Less commonly, antigens on cell surfaces are of exogenous origin: drugs or products of bacterial or viral infection. An even rarer type of response in which antibody combines with membrane antigens is seen in Goodpasture's syndrome where antibody combines with glomerular basement membrane (GBM). This type of injury has been studied experimentally in detail using heterologous (e.g. species differing) antisera to GBM (Simpson et al., 1975). The initial reaction involves an immunological response in which heterologous antibody induces injury. A second phase of injury is induced when host antibodies are formed to the injected heterologous serum proteins. These cause further injury by combining with the injected antibody in the kidney. Each of these types of injury is considered in the Gell and Coombs classification to be Type II reaction. A more recently described reaction which can be included with the antibody response to membrane antigens is known as 'antibody-dependent lymphocyte cytotoxicity'. Here antibodies to cell surface antigens initiate a cytotoxic response which involves a class of mononuclear cell now known as a K (killer) cell. Clinical studies have shown that mononuclear cells from patients with Hashimoto's thyroiditis, transitional cell carcinoma of the bladder, and renal transplants, have increased K cell cytotoxicity directed against thyroid, tumour and renal cells respectively. Blood cells have reduced capacity for antibody-dependent cytotoxic reactions in patients with inflammatory bowel diseases, myeloma, macroglobulinaemia, active SLE, and during immunosuppression of acute lymphatic leukaemia.

IMMUNE COMPLEX (TYPE III) DISEASES

The best known immune complex disease is 'serum sickness' which occurs when heterologous serum proteins are injected repeatedly, and it may be induced when patients are treated with antitetanus serum or horse anti-lymphocyte IgG (horse ALG). Circulating antibodies to horse proteins develop and these form immune complexes intravascularly which settle in the walls of blood vessels where they induce a local inflammatory reaction involving neutrophils. This response does not always occur when horse serum proteins are injected into patients, and current research is directed towards making patients tolerant to injected horse serum proteins when they have to be given by using proteins which are freed from aggregates by ultracentrifugation. Aggregate-free serum proteins induce tolerance in animals and this may also be true in man (Jones et al., 1975).

In a number of bacterial and viral diseases in which the production of antibodies does not lead to cure, antigens may be continually released from sites of infection into the bloodstream and these complexes can induce vasculitic lesions which resolve rapidly once antigen shedding has stopped. This type of reaction is seen in patients with active bacterial endocarditis and viral diseases with exanthematous lesions such as measles. Immune complexes are also important in the renal disease of systemic lupus erythematosus, where the complexes are formed with autologous antigens, including DNA (Koffler, Schur and Kunkel, 1967).

CELL-MEDIATED (TYPE IV) REACTIONS

Type IV reactions are defined as immunological reactions which are mediated by lymphocytes directly, as demonstrated by transfer studies in which living lymphocytes (but not serum) from affected donors are able to transfer the reaction to normal individuals. This type of response is evident clinically as:

(i) Delayed hypersensitivity reactions. The biochemical nature of this reaction has been studied in detail. Here thymus-dependent lymphocytes respond to antigenic stimulation by producing a number of proteins (mediators or lymphokines) which induce local lesions characterized by infiltration with macrophages and tissue swelling which is maximal 24 to 48 hours after stimulation (David and David, 1972).

(ii) Graft rejection. This may involve the same mechanisms as delayed hypersensitivity (see Chapter 7).

(iii) Some types of autoimmune disorders, in which recent work has suggested that direct lymphocyte-mediated cytotoxicity is involved (see p. 87).

It should be noted that *in vivo* each of these types of immunological reaction rarely occurs independently of each other, and it is common for a response to progress from one type to another with time. Also *in vivo* there are many factors which affect the final expression of immunological response. This means that the possession of the ability to mount one of these types of immunological reaction to an antigen *in vitro* does not automatically mean that the reaction is playing a significant part in the response to that antigen *in vivo*. In each instance it is necessary to assess the laboratory data in the clinical setting itself.

Immunodeficiency

Immunodeficiency diseases are of two types:

(i) *Primary* immunodeficiency diseases associated with a definable genetic defect. These are rare, and are usually seen only in children or young adults, in whom recurrent infections occur, in combination with other defects.

(ii) *Acquired* immunodeficiency diseases where genetic defects are difficult to define in most instances, and it is usually supposed that some environmental effect has induced the disorder. This type of deficiency state is common, and in some instances may be due to the effects of anaesthetics, surgical procedures, drugs and irradiation on the immune response.

Studies on immunodeficiencies have been done in two ways. The first involves quantitation of cells and proteins involved in immunological responses (see Chapter 4). This method is well suited to routine laboratory work. Deficiencies are then named according to the deficient component. With this approach many clinical syndromes have been studied in which there are deficiencies in the number of stem cells, T lymphocytes, B lymphocytes, immunoglobulins, or complement components, etc. With this background of knowledge about 'constituent deficiencies', it has now begun to be possible to devise a second type of investigation which is designed to look for functional deficiencies in immunological responsiveness. These may occur in the presence of quantitatively normal numbers of cells or proteins. These 'functional deficiencies' are then classified according to whether (i) antigen handling is abnormal (afferent arc abnormalities), (ii) lymphocyte 'triggering' and interactions in lymphoid tissues are defective (central abnormalities), (iii) antibodies, complement, etc., are abnormal in type or quality (efferent arc abnormalities) or (iv) effector lymphocyte, neutrophils or macrophages are functionally defective (effector cell defects). Because knowledge about functional immunological defects is still rudimentary, most classifications emphasize constituent deficiencies. It should be realized, however, that pure constituent deficiencies are rare, and that the majority of immunological diseases are due to functional defects.

PRIMARY IMMUNODEFICIENCIES

There are a number of named immunodeficiency diseases which have distinct clinical features which enabled them to be recognized relatively early (Stiehn and Fulginiti, 1973). The best known ones are listed in Table 3.2.

The correct diagnosis of each of these immunodeficiency diseases at an early stage is important as some of them can be treated with marrow or thymus transplants, immunoglobulin replacement therapy or antibiotics. In children, the main features are a family history of affected siblings, and repeated infections, with failure to thrive. Pyogenic infections occur when maternal antibody is lost at 2–4 months. The absence of pharyngeal tonsilar tissues and the absence of the thymus shadow on chest radiographs are useful initial evidence for B and T lymphocyte deficiencies (see Chapter 4 for details of investigations).

Table 3.2 Classification of primary immunodeficiency diseases

Reticular dysgenesis	Stem cell deficiency
	All lymphocytes and polymorphs deficient
	No immunoglobulins
Severe combined immunodeficiency	Stem cell deficiency
	All lymphocytes deficient
	Tumour incidence increased
Nezelof syndrome★	T lymphocyte deficiency
	Absent secondary antibody response
DiGeorge syndrome★	T lymphocyte deficiency with bronchial arch defects, vascular, endocrine and facial defects
Ataxia telangiectasia	T lymphocyte deficiency with cerebellar abnormalities and telangiectasia, IgA absent in 70%
Wiskott–Aldrich syndrome	Eczema, thrombocytopenia
	No antibody to polysaccharide antigens
X-linked agammaglobulinaemia	B lymphocyte deficiency
	Increased occurrence of atopy, arthritis, dermatomyositis, tumours
Sporadic hypogammaglobulinaemia	Congenital B lymphocyte deficiency with very variable features
Selective immunoglobulin deficiency	B lymphocyte deficiency affecting each antibody class
Chronic granulomatous disease	Phagocyte bacteriocidal defect

★ These types are now considered to be variants of 'congenital thymic dysplasia'

It is especially important to diagnose T lymphocyte deficiencies as these patients should not be immunized with live vaccines (vaccinia, polio, rubella, etc.), and if transfusions are required, blood must be either reconstituted from frozen erythrocytes or given 1000–1500 rads x-rays to destroy donor lymphocytes which could otherwise react to host antigens and induce graft-versus-host disease. These dangers are also present when intrauterine transfusions are given where immunodeficiency is suspected, and in adults who are T lymphocyte deficient (see Chapter 7).

CONGENITAL THYMIC DYSPLASIA

This disease may well have been first described in London in 1849, but it was DiGeorge who brought it to light today. Thymic dysplasia is a sporadic developmental deficiency due to a failure of thymus cell differentiation which leads to T lymphocyte deficiency. Rather surprisingly, the peripheral blood lymphocyte count is only slightly reduced but blood T lymphocytes are absent, and the majority of cells are B lymphocytes. Associated congenital lesions affect the parathyroid glands, ears, mouth, nose and great blood vessels. Infections occur with pyogenic organisms, fungi and large DNA viruses, as might be expected. Following repeated antigenic stimulation, there is only IgM antibody production, e.g. the responses do not mature from primary to secondary type. After thymus transplants, T lymphocytes appear in the blood within several days, but it has been observed on several occasions that T lymphocyte responsiveness recovers in a few hours. This has been cited as evidence suggesting that the thymus produces soluble factors which have a direct effect on peripheral thymus-dependent lymphoid tissues (Businco *et al.*, 1975).

SEVERE COMBINED IMMUNODEFICIENCY

This is an X-linked autosomal recessive disease and is believed to account for about 10% of deaths in children aged 6 weeks to 2 years. The onset is usually at 3–6 months of age with infections due to pyogenic, enteric and fungal organisms. These children often have monilia, with wasting and hyperpigmented skin lesions which may be due to a graft-versus-host reaction induced by maternal lymphocytes. The child's blood lacks lymphocytes and immunoglobulins, but there is often an isolated M component in the serum which is pathognomonic.

These children show no T lymphocyte functions, although the thymus may be enlarged on occasions. Skin grafts are not rejected. Bone marrow transplants have been given on a number of occasions with variable success. When a 'take' occurs, B lymphocytes become activated, and multiple M components are found in the serum. Weight gain is the best sign of improvement.

Recently, a number of children with severe combined immunodeficiency have been found to lack adenosine deaminase in their erythrocytes (Meuwissen, Pollara and Pickering, 1975). This enzyme deficiency has been described in a normal person and on one occasion a successful response took place to bone marrow transplantation from an individual heterozygous for adenosine deaminase deficiency, even though the recipient's erythrocytes remained deficient. In the future it is hoped that further study of purine metabolism in patients with primary immunodeficiency may help elucidate the biochemical basis of these disorders, which may be the result of enzyme deficiency states.

X-LINKED CONGENITAL IMMUNOGLOBULIN DEFICIENCY

This disease was first described by Bruton in 1952, and it is now known to be due to a defective gene on the X chromosome which results in a great reduction in B lymphocyte production, and in rare instances normal B lymphocyte numbers but reduced immunoglobulin synthesis. The affected children present between 9 and 24 months of age with infections due to *Haemophilus*, *Pneumococcus*, *Staphylococcus* and *Streptococcus* organisms. All classes of immunoglobulin are deficient and antibody response to injected antigens is reduced, but cellular immunity is preserved.

A high proportion of affected children who are kept well with immunoglobulin and antibiotics develop a lethal type of dermatomyositis, which affects exterior surfaces initially. Infections with viruses may induce a non-malignant proliferation of lymphocytes, and they have a particular susceptibility to echo virus infections.

ACQUIRED IMMUNODEFICIENCY DISEASES

Acquired immunodeficiency diseases occur where there has been a progressive failure of immunological responsiveness and, by definition, it is assumed that at an earlier period immunological reactivity was normal. Each part of the immune response can be affected non-specifically by drugs, infection, irradiation or tumours, etc. In some cases the induced immunodeficiency state can lead to a worsening of the underlying disease. In many instances the cause of the acquired immunodeficiency remains unknown.

Malnutrition

At the present time, malnutrition in poor areas of the world is probably the most important cause of immunodeficiency, leading to death from infection in early childhood. A similar situation may have occurred in Western countries in the 17th and 18th centuries, and the dramatic increase in population that began then could have been a consequence of improved nutrition, leading to a decline in malnutrition immunodeficiency. (Advances in public health followed this rapid population increase.)

It is only in the last few years that attempts have been made to measure immunological responsiveness in malnourished people, and to look for the way in which deficiency occurs (Neumann *et al.*, 1975). In malnourished children, the principal deficiencies are found in T lymphocytes and their responses (leading article 1975a). By contrast, immunoglobulin levels are high, with all classes raised in concentration, and antibody is produced normally. The clinical features of T lymphocyte deficiency are found: thymic and lymph node atrophy, low blood lymphocyte contents, reduced delayed hypersensitivity reactions and abnormal *in vivo* responses of T lymphocytes. Total haemolytic complement levels are often reduced, and C3 deficiency causes reduced opsonic activity in serum.

Studies on malnourished adults are less clear-cut, but it is to be expected that findings will be similar. Where these defects occur, simple treatment with antibiotics is clearly inadequate, and every attempt should be made to improve nutrition. However this is not without risk, as 'hyperalimentation' with intravenous fluids rich in phosphates can itself induce defective leucocyte bactericidal capacity.

Drugs

Cytotoxic drugs inhibit immunological responses, and some of them are of course used in this role (see Chapter 8). It is often not appreciated that immunological responses are also inhibited by other agents, e.g. anaesthetics including halothane, and a wide variety of commonly used drugs such as diphenylhydantoin, rifampicin and aspirin. These agents also inhibit the proliferation *in vitro* of lymphocytes stimulated with phytohaemagglutinin. This suggests that they may act *in vivo* by a direct action on lymphoid cells (Crout, Hepburn and Ritts, 1975).

Irradiation

Irradiation of lymphoid tissues leads both to direct destruction of lymphocytes and damage to their connective tissue scaffolding. Macrophages and mature plasma cells are resistant to the acute effects of irradiation, and there is also some evidence that memory B lymphocytes are radiation insensitive. Repeated irradiation to one site of the body usually leads to loss of T lymphocytes which are in the recirculating pool (Stjernswärd et al., 1972). This is possibly because these cells are in continual movement along the traffic routes of the lymphoid tissue so that they reoccupy sites which have been irradiated, and are then sited to be irradiated themselves. The effects of irradiation are greater on T than on B lymphocytes, and explanations for this include:

(i) That the rate of replacement of T lymphocyte is less than B lymphocyte.

(ii) That T lymphocytes are more radiosensitive than B lymphocytes.

(iii) That there are more T lymphocytes in the recirculating pool than B lymphocytes.

The effects of irradiation on blood T lymphocytes is evident for periods up to a year (Wara et al., 1975b). Clinically these people are especially prone to sudden overwhelming infections, and this complication is sufficiently common that patients themselves should be made aware of it so that even apparently trivial infections can be treated early.

'EFFECTOR CELL' DEFICIENCIES

When the peripheral blood neutrophil count is less than 2000/ml patients are at risk from infections (Sickles et al., 1975), and special precautions have to be taken. In addition, several diseases have been described in the last few years where the neutrophil counts are normal, but the cells have a decreased capacity to destroy bacteria (Quie, 1975). Some of these can be recognized as part of a definable clinical syndrome, but some are not obvious and require laboratory studies for detection. These studies examine phases of bacterial phagocytosis and killing (Table 3.3).

Table 3.3 Stages in bacterial killing by neutrophils

1. Bacteria coated with antibody, IgG and IgM
2. Complement activation and C3 fixation
3. Membrane contact and adherence by Fc and C3 receptors
4. Ingestion and formation of phagolysosomes
5. Activation of hexosemonophosphate shunt
6. Increased O_2 uptake, H_2O_2, and superoxide production
7. Bacteria killed and digested

Rather surprisingly, neutrophils in patients with acute infections have impaired bactericidal capacity and this can be correlated with the presence of young forms and toxic granulations. Patients with burns show a similar defect, which appears, however, to be absent in victims of trauma.

Defects in chemotaxis have been reported frequently. They may be found as primary defects in children who have recurrent infections, and chemotactic defects may be associated with defective bactericidal capacity. An interesting mechanism underlies the malfunctioning of effector cells in the Chediak–Higashi syndrome. Here lysosomes are large and fusion with phagosomes is defective, so that peroxidase is not delivered to phagolysosomes in the normal way. This disorder may be one of a number of lysosome storage diseases in which there is a secondary defect in effector cell bactericidal capacity.

Secondary defects in chemotaxis are found in patients with diabetes mellitus, cirrhosis, myeloma and rheumatoid arthritis. Malignant neutrophils have reduced bactericidal capacity, but white cells from patients with chronic myeloid leukaemia retain enough function to allow them to be used for granulocyte transfusions in neutropenic patients. In some patients with infections including recurrent staphylococcal abscesses, neutrophil chemotaxis has been found to be low in association with a high level of serum IgE. Neutrophils which lack myeloperoxidase and glucose-6-phosphate dehydrogenase are defective.

A number of drugs induce abnormal bacterial killing *in vitro*. These include morphine and its analogues, steroids, phenylbutazone and sulphonamides. However, it is not known if these agents are associated with defective handling of micro-organisms *in vivo*.

COMPLEMENT DEFICIENCIES

Recently a number of diseases have been described which are associated with deficient production of complement proteins (Brown and Lachmann, 1975). These defects are rare, which may indicate the importance of normal complement function in homeostasis. A list of the diseases associated with complement deficiencies is shown in Table 3.4.

Table 3.4 Complement deficiencies in man, frequencies and disease associations

Deficiency	Pedigrees described	Diseases associated
C1r	2	Skin, joints, nephritis, and infections
C4*	1	Skin
C2*	>24	SLE, nephritis, lipodystrophy
C3	3	Infections, meningitis
C5*	1	SLE
C6*	2	
C7*	2	CRST syndrome
C1 esterase inhibitor*	Many	Hereditary angioedema, SLE, nephritis
C3b inactivator	1	Infections

* Deficiencies occasionally found in normal people

Complement deficiencies fall into four groups:

(i) Deficiencies of the early components (C1, C4, C2), which are associated with clinical syndromes similar to systemic lupus erythematosus (SLE) or glomerulonephritis.

(ii) Deficiencies of the bulk complement component C3. Here the main clinical feature is recurrent pyogenic infections.

(iii) Deficiencies of the late acting complement components C5, C6, C7, which may be symptom free, or associated with SLE or the CRST syndrome. Deficiencies of the alternative pathway components (properdin, factors B and D) have not yet been described.

(iv) Deficiencies of inhibitors of the complement system.

Deficiency of C1 esterase inhibitor is associated with hereditary angio-edema and deficiency of C3b inactivator induces a syndrome indistinguishable from C3 deficiency itself.

Hereditary angioedema

CI esterase inhibitor is a serum inhibitor of the activated form of CI which it neutralizes by combination. When the inhibitor is absent, C2 is activated to a greater extent than normal by the uninhibited activated CI, and this causes increased vascular permeability leading to local edema (Beck *et al.*, 1973). Attacks of angioedema occur unpredictably, and when they involve the airways death can follow rapidly, unless emergency tracheostomy is carried out. Recurrent attacks of abdominal pain are an important feature of this disease, and frank intestinal obstruction can occur due to mucosal wall edema. This is a rare but important disease which should be considered in the differential diagnosis of small bowel obstruction and the acute abdomen. Treatment here should be conservative. Some immediate benefit usually follows injection of hydrocortisone, adrenalin and fresh plasma. The clinical features of the condition which make it stand out distinctly from other settings where angioedema can occur are:

(i) The disease is inherited in most cases.

(ii) There is often a history of death from asphyxia in a relative.

The definitive diagnosis is made by assaying serum for CI esterase inhibitor either by immunodiffusion or by measuring the amount of functioning esterase inhibitor which is present. The latter method is preferred as 20% of patients with the disease have normal antigenic levels of non-functional inhibitor.

TREATMENT OF IMMUNODEFICIENCY DISEASES

It is often not possible to remedy immunodeficiency states, so that treatment is normally aimed at the eradication of each episode of infection as it occurs. The survival of many older people with immunodeficiency is largely due to this approach. However, attempts have been made to replace the deficiency by injections of immunoglobulin or by grafting fetal thymus or bone marrow. (Marrow grafting is discussed further in Chapter 7.)

Patients who are unable to make antibodies to common pathogenic organisms have repeated attacks of infection. They are treated with prophylactic injections of normal pooled gammaglobulin which contains antibodies to these organisms. Initially it was thought that patients with normal amounts of immunoglobulin were not at risk, so that gammaglobulin was reserved for patients with serum IgG levels of less than 200 mg/100 ml. However, the indications for treatment have enlarged as clinical studies have shown that it is effective in preventing infections in patients with higher levels of IgG. Treatment is needed in the following circumstances:

(i) IgG less than 200 mg/100 ml, even if symptomless.

(ii) IgG less than 500 mg/100 ml if repeatedly infected.

(iii) IgG normal, with repeated infections and absence of antibodies to common pathogens.

(iv) IgA low or absent, with repeated respiratory infections.

(v) Immunodeficiencies with known antibody deficiencies, such as the Wiskott–Aldrich syndrome.

IgG is prepared by precipitation of serum with 25% alcohol, and it contains 90% IgG. The preparations for use in Britain contain 150 mg IgG/ml, 4–5 mg IgA/ml and 1–2 mg IgM/ml. Patients are usually given 25 mg/kg per week intramuscularly. Reactions to injections include urticaria and bronchospasm which may be due to histamine release from mast cells by aggregates of IgG. Particular care should be taken in treating patients with pulmonary hypertension, as reactions of this type can be fatal in them.

Thymus grafting has been used to treat children with congenital thymus lymphocyte deficiencies. The grafts can be obtained from fetal tissues and they are usually implanted into the muscle of the abdomen. If the graft is viable, there is usually a dramatic clinical improvement, but it is usual for a graft–versus–host reaction to occur at some later stage and this may be fatal. The long-term survival of these grafts is still not certain. It is also not clear how far the grafted thymus provides a normal environment for host T lymphocyte maturation, or whether it is necessary for a chimera to be produced of donor T lymphocytes and host B lymphocytes. The possibility that the thymus provides a humoral stimulus for normal T lymphocyte development is an area of current research, and it has been claimed that injections of extracts of thymus ('thymosin') restore T lymphocytes to deficient individuals (Wara et al., 1975a). If this is confirmed some T lymphocyte defects may also be treated by regular replacement injections.

In the last decade, a number of enthusiastic reports have suggested that extracts of peripheral blood lymphocytes can restore deficient T lymphocyte responsiveness. Very low molecular weight lysates from normal cells are known as 'transfer factor' and considerable hope was raised about their potential use in patients with immunodeficiency, infections and tumours. Unfortunately these hopes have not yet materialized, although remarkable individual responses have been described. Generally, there seems to be little scope for the use of this material at present except in some patients with T lymphocyte deficiency or persistent infections with intracellular organisms. It can only be provided on an *ad hoc* basis from immunologists who are specially interested in it (Basten et al., 1975).

Deficiencies of effector cells have not proved easy to treat in the past. The introduction of blood cell separators has changed this, and it is now clear that regular infusions of neutrophils from normal individuals or patients with chronic granulocytic leukaemia will reduce the incidence of infection in these patients (Higby and Henderson, 1975). Unfortunately this type of replacement cannot normally be used for more than a short time as donor leucocytes cannot be 'banked' in the same way as erythrocytes, and the effects of the transfused neutrophils probably last for only a few hours. Its main use is in the management of acute infections in granulocytopenic patients.

Allergic Responses in Infections

INTRODUCTION

By the end of the 19th century, immunity to infections was found to occur when antibodies developed, and there were striking successes in preventing some infectious diseases by immunization. However, it was soon apparent that in many infections diseases immunization did not confer protection, and it was also established that antibody was not involved in the eradication of established infectious. At the same time studies with macrophages demonstrated that they destroyed bacteria by phagocytosis, and it was thus held for many years that these two systems were the basis for immunity to micro-organisms. It was only when methods were developed for transferring lymphocytes between animals, that they too were found to induce immunity to intracellular bacteria in recipients, independent of antibody. This distinction between lymphocytes and antibody in immunity is referred to as 'cell-mediated immunity' and 'humoral immunity'. In the last 15 years other mechanisms have been found to be involved in immunity to bacteria. These include the 'activation' of macrophages by soluble products from stimulated lymphocytes, demonstrating that there are links between each of these responses, which were initially considered to be distinct.

Immunity to micro-organisms requires T lymphocytes both to cooperate with B lymphocytes in antibody responses, and to produce soluble factors which activate macrophages. T lymphocytes may also destroy cells which express viral antigens on their surface by a direct cytotoxic reaction (T cell cytotoxicity). B lymphocytes are required to produce antibody which coats infective organisms. These coated organisms may be phagocytosed more easily (e.g. the antibody has 'opsonic' properties) or lysed by complement. Recently K cell cytotoxicity has also been demonstrated in infectious diseases: here antibody-coated fungi were killed directly by lymphocytes of the K cell class.

These responses are normally protective, but in certain cases they lead to further tissue damage.

This distinction between protective and other types of immunological responses to infections was clearly made over 70 years ago by von Pirquet, and the application of this important concept today has led to a reintroduction by Coombs of the term 'allergic' in its originally defined sense: to indicate 'an altered state of host specific reactivity' (which is neither necessarily good nor bad for the host), and to restrict the term 'immune' to situations where the host benefits. The following terms are therefore now widely used by immunologists (Table 3.5).

Table 3.5 Terms used to distinguish protective immuno-logical reactions from other types of response

	Outcome of response	
	Not defined	*Protective*
Antigen	Allergen★	Immunogen
Type of response	Allergic response★	Immune response
State induced	'Allergized'	Immunity

★ Note that the widespread but restricted use of these terms by allergists to describe Type I (anaphylactic) responses is now not recommended

Unfortunately, there is no generally accepted term to cover immunological responses which compromise the host, but the discussion which follows should help at least to show their clinical importance in a wide variety of infectious diseases.

VIRUSES IN IMMUNOLOGICAL DISEASES

Antibody provides one of the main mechanisms of defence against viruses which are present in the blood but cell-mediated responses are more important in the eradication of established viral infections. This has been well established in the case of measles (Ruckdeschel *et al.*, 1975). The role of antibody has been demonstrated experimentally in mice using intravenous injections of Coxsackie B-3 virus where animals were protected by prior injections of antibody. In a similar way in man, antibody to polio virus prevents infective particles from spreading from the gut to susceptible tissues through the blood. Failure of this mechanism is seen in children with severe hypogammaglobulinaemia who are more liable than normal children to develop paralytic poliomyelitis after exposure to natural or vaccine strains of virus. The incidence of paralytic poliomyelitis in adult immunoglobulin-deficient patients is also increased. Occasionally immunodeficient patients fail to eliminate the virus from the intestinal tract so that they become chronic carriers of polio virus. Many viruses have antigenic variants, but they commonly share some determinants. Where this occurs, the antibody response to each variant induces the production of increased amounts of antibody to the first variant encountered, with a corresponding decrease in the response to later variants. This has been named 'original antigenic sin', indicating that responses in older life are dominated by the effects of the initial exposure to antigen. This is an important factor in the development of vaccines. For example, patients immunized against some dead measles vaccine did not become immune to measles infections, but unlike unimmunized individuals, they had pre-existing antibody to some measles antigens, so that when they developed measles they developed immune complex disease in addition.

The role of antibody in the elimination of viruses other than polio and hepatitis A virus, is less clear. Clinical observations of children with various types of immunodeficiency suggest that macrophages and T lymphocytes play the major part in protection from measles, chickenpox, vaccinia, herpes simplex, cytomegalovirus and other viruses. These T lymphocytes are not only required to act as helper cells for B lymphocytes in the production of antiviral antibodies, but they also function as cytotoxic cells, directed specifically against virus-infected cell surface antigens. These cytotoxic T lymphocytes divide after contact with antigen, and migrate from lymphoid tissues into the blood. Some of them enter sites of viral infection where they can damage infected cells by a direct action (T lymphocyte cytotoxicity). 'Activated' macrophages may also play a role in the elimination of virus-infected cells. Other effector cells, including polymorphs, prevent direct cell-to-cell spread of viruses. This has been demonstrated in herpes simplex infections, where neutrophils limit infection by interposing themselves between susceptible and infected cells.

Several viruses cause a lymphopenia in man, including influenza, varicella, measles, herpes simplex, and adenovirus. In rubella severe lymphopenia can occur, which may be due to the development of antibodies to lymphocytes (lymphocytotoxins). This complication is of clinical importance, as the patients are particularly likely to develop fatal superinfection (Huang and Hong, 1973). Recent work on chronic viral infections has led to the possibility that they could be responsible for a number of chronic immunological diseases in animals and man. Attention is especially directed towards diseases which are known to have the features of chronic immune complex and delayed hypersensitivity disease. Considerable research effort has been put into attempts to detect the viruses involved, with striking successes in some instances. For example Australia antigen–antibody complexes have been detected in some patients with polyarteritis, and high titres of antimeasles antibodies often occur in subacute sclerosing panencephalitis, multiple sclerosis and chronic active hepatitis. These persisting viruses are either sequestered in cells where they remain in an inactive state, or they replicate and continue to be released despite the presence of an immunological response. Most of the information about these types of infection has been derived from experiments in mice infected with chronic lymphocytic choriomeningitis, or cytomegalovirus infections (Olding *et al.*, 1975).

It is probable that the majority of viruses which produce persisting infections in man are either budding RNA (or 'negative') viruses, such as measles, or DNA viruses, including herpes, cytomegalovirus and EB virus. Chronic measles infections can occur in children who have been infected *in utero*. Here the measles virus produces optic, auditory and cardiac defects, and the virus can be isolated from many tissues. Older children with persisting measles virus infections develop diffuse neurological damage, which leads to subacute sclerosing panencephalitis. It is a surprising feature of these persisting infections that high titres of antibody are present, and lymphocyte cytotoxicity is usually not decreased.

Bacteria

As in viral infections, immunity depends on humoral and cellular responses (Mudd, 1970). Bacteria which multiply in tissues release antigens into the blood and lymphatics, and these induce antibody formation and cell-mediated responses. For example, in streptococcal infections antibodies are produced to nuclear and cell wall antigens and delayed hypersensitivity response can be demonstrated to constituents of streptococcal culture fluid. Bacteria which only grow on the surface of external epithelia and do not invade tissues do not give rise to immune responses. For example, in uncomplicated *Salmonella* food poisoning or *Shigella* infections, where septicaemia does not occur, antibodies are not produced.

Infective organisms provide the majority of antigens to which people are exposed, and it is probable that most of the 'natural' immunoglobulins in normal serum are produced in response to them. This seems likely in view of the low levels of immunoglobulins present in germ-free animals fed on sterile but otherwise normal diets, and the absence of immunoglobulins in the serum of fetal ruminants in which placental transfer of maternal antibody does not occur.

Bacterial infections give rise to harmful allergic reactions in a number of ways. Bacterial antigens may be suddenly released into the blood, and where antibody is present, antigen–antibody complex formation occurs, which can cause activation of complement. This in turn induces widespread changes in vascular permeability, leading to shock. Gram-negative bacteria produce endotoxins which are able to activate complement directly, via the alternative pathway, to produce the same effect. Here the reaction is called the Schwartzmann reaction. The edema and haemorrhagic necrosis that occurs in this response is a consequence of increased vascular permeability induced by C3a and C5a, and the subsequent localization and degranulation of marginated neutrophils at the sites of increased permeability. A clear-cut example of this type of reaction is seen in haemorrhagic meningococcal septicaemia. Similar but less severe reactions are seen in other septicaemic states due to gram-negative organisms. It follows that in surgical practice, particular care must be taken to prevent these responses when chronic abscesses are drained, by not allowing the abscess contents to spill into serous cavities or disseminate into the blood. Unfortunately once the endothelial damage has been induced, there is little that can be done therapeutically besides replacing lost intravascular fluids, and giving mechanical respiration if the lungs are involved.

Chronic antigen release from persisting bacterial infections also causes immune complex disease. These complexes may cause local damage at the site of antigen liberation. This occurs in lepromatous leprosy where peripheral nerve lesions occur as a consequence of the formation of local complexes, in addition to the direct effects of the bacteria themselves. In other infectious diseases the complexes are intravascular, and settle in glomeruli to produce immune-complex nephritis (which is also seen in leprosy).

Harmful cytotoxic reactions to bacteria are probably less common than to viruses. It has been suggested that the extensive lobar reaction to pneumococci (which do not produce any directly toxic products) is a delayed hypersensitivity response, but this is difficult to prove. The significance of delayed hypersensitivity reactions in the pathogenicity of tubercle bacilli remain unsettled (Youmans, 1975). Here an equally strong case can be made for protective and destructive effects of delayed hypersensitivity reactions. Studies with immunogenic but normally non-pathogenic strains of tubercle bacilli, especially BCG (Bacillus Calmette Guerin) have been particularly interesting. In unsensitized animals intravenously injected killed BCG has little effect, but in tuberculin-positive animals marked lesions are produced, which may be even greater than those produced by viable BCG in tuberculin-positive animals. This clearly shows that delayed hypersensitivity reactions, like immune-complex injury and massive complement activation, can lead to excessive self-induced allergic tissue damage even when the organism is dead.

Fungi

Fungi present a number of special problems, both because they may grow in tissues without a significant local host response, and because hypersensitivity reactions to small amounts of fungal antigen can cause excessive tissue damage. Repeated exposure to fungal antigens in aerosols in a sensitive individual, leads to pulmonary fibrosis as seen in 'farmer's lung'. Here fungi growing in mouldy hay induce formation of antibodies, so that repeated challenge results in antigen–antibody formation in lung tissue. This produces a local Arthus reaction in which neutrophils predominate. Damage is progressive and the end result can be extensive fibrosing alveolitis. A similar process occurs in 'bird fancier's lung' and a number of occupational diseases.

Other organisms

In syphilis, the reaction between organism and host usually causes little tissue damage. This is particularly clearly shown in congenital syphilis where tissue reactions to the presence of the treponeme are minimal. In adults, the early secondary stage of syphilis is also associated with immune suppression, produced by the organism (Friedmann and Turk, 1975). Many other types of infection, including leprosy, show reduced Type IV responses when the organism is present in large numbers (Schwab, 1975). Diagnostic tests for syphilis commonly detect antibodies which are made to three types of antigens:

(i) Lipoidin (Wasserman cardiolipin).

(ii) Group-specific antigens found on different species of treponeme including Reiter's treponeme.

(iii) Species-specific antigens which are usually assayed by *Treponema pallidum* immobilization tests.

In syphilis, the host factors which lead to tissue damage are unknown, but they probably involve allergic reactions which are seen both during the late secondary stage when Type IV reactivity is marked and when large amounts of antigen from dead spirochetes are released when penicillin is injected— the 'Herxheimer reaction'.

Other organisms with extended tissue survival induce allergic tissue damage. Examples of these include allergic reactions to *Filaria bancroftii*, and *Schistosoma haematobium* infections. Many parasites induce IgE antibody formation and eosinophilia and give rise to asthma and urticaria. Diarrhea in ascaris infections has an allergic basis. Anaphylactic reactions are important in hydatid disease where release of cyst contents into serous cavities can induce a fatal reaction identical to that produced by anaphylactic reactions to bee or wasp stings.

From this discussion it is clear that allergic reactions are often of considerable clinical importance in infectious diseases, not only because they provide the basis for specific antimicrobial immunity, but because they can extend and perpetuate tissue damage. Both of these factors have to be considered in assessing the outcome of any infectious disease.

REACTIONS TO DRUGS

Reactions to drugs are very common in clinical practice (Parker, 1975) and they are usually easily dealt with by simply stopping treatment. Surprisingly little research has been done in this important area but several interesting findings have been made. Generally, drugs induce allergic responses only after they have combined with carrier macromolecular substances, but this union is often weak and reversible. Genetic factors also determine degrees of responsiveness to different drugs, and the type of response is variable.

Antibodies are produced to many drugs which are injected, and these may not be pathogenetic. IgE antibodies to the penicillin derivative penicilloyl polylysine are found, for example, in patients who show no reaction to penicillin, and most patients with delayed hypersensitivity reactions in the skin to test doses of penicillin show no systemic effect when it is given intramuscularly. For these reasons it has been suspected that there are un-known factors involved in drug reactions which cannot be assessed at present. In fact the evidence that allergic reactions are responsible for most drug-induced lesions is at best circumstantial. This criticism does not apply to drug-induced blood dyscrasias, where the interaction of drug and target cell can be studied much more easily *in vitro*. Here there are three types of response:

(i) The drug combines with erythrocytes, and a Type II lytic reaction occurs: penicillin is the best example.

(ii) The drug combines with antibody, and the complex attaches to cells giving a Type III reaction.

(iii) The drug induces autoantibody formation, as shown in methyldopa haemolytic anaemia, or sets up a sequence of events which mimic systemic lupus erythematosus (chloroquine, hydralazine, procaine amide) or systemic sclerosis (practolol) (Harpey, 1974).

When a drug reaction is suspected, useful investigations include the Coombs' test, blood counts, serum complement levels and detection of immune complexes in serum. Unfortunately it is usually impossible to incriminate any one drug in a mixture except by reintroducing it, and this may not be acceptable.

AUTOALLERGIC DISEASES

Introduction

These are diseases in which allergic reactions are directed against host antigens, leading to tissue damage. The clearest example is autoallergic haemolytic anaemia, where antibodies induce either erythrocyte lysis with complement, or coat cells so that they are phagocytosed and digested. Many other diseases are associated with the presence of autoantibodies, but where a destructive role for these antibodies has not been demonstrated, they should be considered separately as 'diseases with associated autoallergic phenomena'.

Terminology in autoallergic diseases has been clarified in recent years. The term 'collagen diseases' has been discontinued, as has 'autoimmune', in favour of 'autoallergic' (see page 77). In parallel with the rationalization of terminology, there has grown up a healthy scepticism among clinicians for the suggestion that autoallergic mechanisms underlie most chronic diseases: from rheumatoid arthritis on the one hand to pernicious anaemia on the other (Stiller *et al.*, 1975). This has led some people to the extreme view that autoantibodies are nothing more than opsonins for tissue breakdown products which would otherwise be removed poorly from the blood. Unfortunately it is often not possible to determine whether autoantibodies play an active or passive role. Irrespective of where the truth lies between these extremes, in practice autoallergic responses are important indications of tissue damage and they can be measured and used for diagnosis and management (Glynn and Holborow, 1974).

Experimentally, autoallergic responses can be induced to a very wide range of autoantigens, especially using antigens which are found in the inner layer of membranes, or contained in the cytoplasm. It appears that under appropriate conditions, responses can occur against a wide variety of autoantigen. An important exception to this general rule is that autoallergic reactions cannot be induced against histocompatibility antigens. This is taken as evidence that there are no lymphocytes in adult animals capable of responding to autologous histocompatibility antigens. Burnet has suggested that this is due to the destruction of these lymphocytes in fetal life, by a process known as 'clonal elimination' (Burnet, 1959).

But clonal elimination of autoantigen-sensitive lymphocytes cannot be a general phenomenon, as circulating lymphocytes have been detected which have receptors on their surface for autoantigens including thyroglobulin, and the principal questions in this area are therefore: 'What prevents autoallergic reactions from occurring in all individuals' and 'Which factors lead to that production?'

Unresponsiveness to autoantigens

At present, there are two main types of hypotheses to explain the apparent unresponsiveness of normal individuals to autoantigens. Both rely on experiments which show that autoantigens are T lymphocyte dependent. In the first type of hypothesis it is suggested that autoantigens are normally found in a concentration which is too low to stimulate autoantigen-sensitive T lymphocytes, or that these T lymphocytes are unusual in that they possess a high 'threshold' for stimulation by autoantigens. Autoantibodies would then be formed only when autoantigens are present in excess concentration, or when lymphocytes have a reduced 'threshold'. The second hypothesis proposes that a state of 'low zone' (T lymphocyte) tolerance exists to autoantigens, or that suppressor T lymphocytes specifically inhibit autoantigensensitive T lymphocytes. This hypothesis predicts that autoantigens stimulate antibody production by 'bypassing' the requirement for these tolerant or suppressed T lymphocytes. It should be noted that these two hypotheses are not mutually exclusive.

Support for the second type of hypothesis has come from a variety of experiments in rabbits, guinea-pigs and mice in the last few years. In the best-known studies autoallergic thyroiditis was produced by coupling autologous thyroglobulin to carrier molecules and more simply by using slightly different thyroglobulins from related species. Mechanisms of this type have been used to explain how a variety of different drugs can induce a single type of autoallergic disorder resembling SLE. However, there has been a move away from these artificially induced models of autoallergic diseases with the discovery that autoallergic diseases also occur spontaneously in inbred animals. These include: NZB mice with autoallergic haemolytic anaemia; NZB/NZW, Swan, B/W mice and dogs with 'systemic lupus erythematosus'; 'A' strain mice with 'rheumatic heart disease'; and obese white Leghorn chickens and Buffalo rats with autoimmune thyroiditis. Manipulation of these animal models has already produced some interesting results. The SLE-like syndrome in dogs appears to be related to a C-type virus which can transmit the disease to other dogs and even other species (Schwartz, 1975). The thyroid disease in obese chickens has provided a useful model as it has been shown that autoantibodies are pathogenic and not just a result of tissue damage. In these studies bursectomy of susceptible chickens caused a reduction in the severity of the thyroiditis.

Genetics of autoallergic diseases

Animal studies using inbred strains will also provide insights into genetic factors involved in autoallergic diseases, which have been known to occur with increased frequency in related individuals.

Recently, genetic studies on autoallergic diseases in man have produced the remarkable finding that many of them are linked with the possession of a number of histocompatibility genes (McDevitt and Bodmer, 1974). The situation is clear enough in ankylosing spondylitis where virtually all patients possess the histocompatibility antigen HLA 27. The linkages in other diseases are not as dramatic as this, which shows that possession of certain histocompatibility genes is not a necessary condition for development of an autoallergic disease. Nor can it be the only requirement, as only a small number of people with these HLA antigens actually develop the disease. For example, only about 5% of individuals with HLA 27 develop ankylosing spondylitis. The genetic basis for autoallergic diseases is probably not dependent on the possession of certain histocompatibility genes, but on some closely related genes. Strong candidates are the nearby 'immune response genes' (ir genes) which determine whether individuals are 'high' or 'low' responders to antigens. If it can be shown that ir genes control responses to autoantigens, this would provide support for the hypothesis presented earlier that autoallergic diseases develop in individuals with reduced 'threshold' for T lymphocyte activation.

These important discoveries about the genetics of autoallergic responses have not been matched as yet by studies on the 'triggering' factors which initiate these reactions, although many workers in this area feel that viral infections are the most likely candidates, and interest has centred especially on 'C-type' viruses, as described earlier (Schwartz, 1975).

Autoantibodies

There is an ever-increasing list of diseases in which autoallergic reactions can be detected and used in diagnosis and for following the progress of disease (Table 3.6).

Autoantibodies are commonly detected using fluorescent microscopy. Frozen tissues are cut on a cryostat and then covered with the patient's serum on a glass slide at room temperature. The slides are then washed and reincubated with fluorescent antibodies directed against human immunoglobulin. After washing again, the distribution of fluorescence is studied microscopically. The fluorescent label can be either fluorescein or rhodamine. Where soluble autoantigens are concerned, such as thyroglobulin, DNA, immunoglobulin, C_3 and intrinsic factor, the autoantibody can be measured by precipitation, agglutination or radioactive binding methods. The latter methods provide quantitative measures which are difficult to produce using fluorescent techniques.

Autoantibodies have been a special area of study in Grave's disease and myasthenia gravis. The culmination of a great deal of research has shown that sera from patients with Grave's disease contain two unique types of autoantibodies which combine with the thyroid-stimulating hormone receptor on thyroid cells (leading article, 1975b). They can be detected in at least 90% of patients with diffuse toxic goitre. Blood levels of one type of antibody, the 'human thyroid stimulator' correlate closely with ^{131}I uptake

Table 3.6 Diseases in which autoallergic reactions are present

Endocrine diseases
  Hashimoto's thyroiditis, Grave's disease, myoedema, diabetes mellitus, Addison's
  disease, etc.

Neurological diseases
  Encephalitis, neuropathies, multiple sclerosis, etc.

Liver diseases
  Chronic active hepatitis, cryptogenic cirrhosis, primary biliary cirrhosis, etc.

Gastrointestinal diseases
  Ulcerative colitis, pernicious anaemia, celiac disease, etc.

Diseases affecting the musculoskeletal system
  Myasthenia gravis, dermatomyositis, systemic lupus erythematosus, rheumatoid
  arthritis, rheumatic fever, etc.

Skin diseases
  Pemphigus vulgaris, pemphigoid, etc.

Renal diseases
  Goodpasture's syndrome, etc.

into the thyroid. Serum containing this autoantibody has been shown to increase thyroid activity of volunteers (Smith, 1975). A second type of autoantibody which can be assayed using only mice, called the 'mouse thyroid stimulator', also binds with human thyroid cells, but does not stimulate activity. (These antibodies were formerly known as LATS-P and LATS respectively.) This property of an autoantibody to increase 'target cell' activity is unique. It is of course far more common for autoantibodies to be separated from the antigens with which they could combine, as the majority of autoantigens are intracellular.

In myasthenia gravis, antibodies have been described recently which combine with acetylcholine receptors on muscle (leading article, 1975c). This prevents the transmission of the normal nerve impulse at the endplate. This antibody may be the same autoantibody that binds to smooth muscle and thymic myoid cells. It has been shown experimentally that antibodies to acetylcholine receptor protein from electric eels produce a syndrome analogous to myasthenia, and they cross-react with thymus myoid cell antigens. The success of thymectomy in some patients with myasthenia may be due to the removal of these myoid cell antigens which are presumed to be involved in the development of the disease. It should be noted that each of these developments has stemmed from the introduction of sensitive and quantitative assay systems for autoantibodies. Advances in other areas of autoallergic disease may well depend on similar technical advances.

Type IV reactions to autoantigens

Histologically, most tissues affected by autoallergic responses are infiltrated with lymphocytes, plasma cells and mononuclear cells. These are the hallmarks of 'cell-mediated' or Type IV reactions. It therefore comes as no surprise that *in vitro* assays for reactions of this kind have demonstrated that they are indeed present in many autoallergic diseases (Table 3.7).

Table 3.7 Type IV reactions to autoantigens

Disease	Antigen
Hashimoto's thyroiditis ⎫ Pernicious anaemia ⎬ Primary biliary cirrhosis ⎭	Rat liver mitochondria
Primary biliary cirrhosis	Liver extracts
Hashimoto's thyroiditis	Human mitochondria, thyroid, kidney, liver
Pernicious anaemia	Human mitochondria, liver and stomach
Addison's disease	Human adrenal
Diabetes mellitus	Rat liver mitochondria Nuclear antigens
Systemic lupus erythematosus	Nuclei, DNA, nucleoprotein
Cryptogenic fibrosing alveolitis	DNA
Asbestosis	DNA
Rheumatoid arthritis ⎫ Ankylosing spondylitis ⎬ Reiter's syndrome ⎭	IgG

The principal methods that are used to show this are based on the technique for measuring the area of migration of guinea-pig macrophage out of the open end of glass capillary tubes in culture. When lymphocytes from the patient are incubated with the autoantigen, they produce a number of mediators (or lymphokines) which inhibit the migration of these macrophages. Assays with macrophages detect macrophage 'migration inhibitory factor' (MIF) (David and David, 1972). Assays in man commonly use human peripheral blood cells instead of macrophages as they contain both lymphocytes and neutrophils which are inhibited from migrating in the same way as macrophages. This assay detects 'leukocyte inhibitory factors' which are probably different from MIF.

References

References marked ★ are suggested for further reading

Basten, A., Croft, S., Kenny, F. and Nelson, D. S. (1975). Uses of transfer factor. *Vox Sang. (Basel)*, **28,** 257

Beck, P., Wills, D., Davies, G. T., Lachmann, P. J. and Sussman, M. (1973). A family study of hereditary angioneurotic oedema. *Q. J. Med.*, **42,** 317

Brown, D. L. and Lachmann, P. J. (1975). Inherited complement deficiences and disease. *Curr. Titles Immunol., Transpl. Allergy*, **3,** 121

Burnet, F. M. (1959). *The Clonal Selection Theory of Acquired Immunity*. (London: Cambridge University Press)

Businco, L., Rezza, E., Giunchi, G. and Aitui, F. (1975). Thymus transplantation. Reconstitution of cellular immunity in a four-year-old patient with T-cell deficiency. *Clin. Exp. Immunol.*, **21,** 32

Crout, J. E., Hepburn, B. and Ritts, R. E. (1975). Suppression of lymphocyte transformation after aspirin ingestion. *N. Engl. J. Med.*, **292,** 221

★Dacie, J. V. and Worlledge, S. M. (1969). The autoimmune haemolytica anemias. *Prog. Hematol.*, **6,** 82

★David, J. R. and David, R. A. (1972). Cellular hypersensitivity and immunity. Inhibition of macrophage migration and the lymphocyte mediators. *Prog. Allergy*, **16,** 3co

Friedmann, P. S. and Turk, J. L. (1975). A spectrum of lymphocyte responsiveness in human syphilis. *Clin. Exp. Immunol.*, **21,** 59

★Gell, P. G. H., Coombs, R. R. A. and Lachmann, P. J. (1975). *Clinical Aspects of Immunology*, 3rd Ed. (Oxford: Blackwell Scientific Publications)

★Glynn, L. E. and Holborow, E. J. (1974). *Autoimmunity and Disease*, 2nd Ed. (Oxford: Blackwell Scientific Publications)

Harpey, J.-P. (1974). Lupus-like syndromes induced by drugs. *Ann. Allergy*, **33,** 256

Higby, D. J. and Henderson, E. S. (1975). Granulocyte transfusion therapy. *Ann. Rev. Med.*, **26,** 289

Huang, S. W. and Hong, R. (1973). Lymphopenia and multiple viral infections. *J. Am. Med. Ass.*, **225,** 1120

Jones, V. E., Lance, E. M., Abbosh, J. and Graves, H. E. (1975). Intensive immunosuppression in patients with disseminated sclerosis II. Tolerance to equine IgG and effect on immunoglobulin and complement levels. *Clin. Exp. Immunol.*, **21,** 13

Klebanoff, S. J. (1975). Automicrobial mechanisms in neutrophilic polymorphonuclear leucocytes. *Semin. Haematol.*, **12,** 117

Koffler, D., Schur, P. H. and Kunkel, H. G. (1967). Immunological studies concerning the nephritis of systemic lupus erythematosus. *J. Exp. Med.*, **126,** 607

Leading Article (1975a). Lymphocyte function in malnutrition. *Nutr. Rev.*, **33,** 110

Leading Article (1975b). Hyperthyroidism and Grave's disease. *Br. Med. J.*, **ii,** 457

Leading Article (1975c). Myasthenia gravis. *Lancet*, **i,** 1227

McDevitt, H. O. and Bodmer, W. F. (1974). HL-A, immune-response genes and disease. *Lancet*, **i,** 1269

Meuwissen, H. J., Pollara, B. and Pickering, R. J. (1975). Combined immunodeficiency disease associated with adenosine deaminase deficiency. *J. Pediat.*, **86,** 169

★Mudd, S. (ed.) (1970). *Infectious Agents and Host Reactions* (London: W. B. Saunders)

Neumann, C. G., Lawlor, G. J. Jr., Stiehn, E. R., Swendseid, M. E., Newton, C., Herbert, J., Ammann, A. J. and Jacobs, M. (1975). Immunologic responses in malnourished children. *Am. J. Nutr.*, **28,** 89

Olding, L. B., Jensen, F. C. and Oldstone, M. B. A. (1975). Pathogenesis of cytomegalo virus infection I. Activation of virus from bone marrow-derived lymphocytes by *in vitro* allogeneic reaction. *J. Exp. Med.*, **141,** 561

Parker, C. (1975). Drug therapy: drug allergy. *N. Engl. J. Med.*, **292,** 511, 732 and 957

★Quie, P. G. (1975). Pathology of bacteriocidal power of neutrophils. *Semin. Haematol.*, **12,** 143

Ruckdeschel, J. C., Graziano, K. D. and Mardiney, M. R. Jr. (1975). Additional evidence that the cell-associated immune system is the primary host defence against measles (rubella). *Cell. Immunol.*, **17,** 11

Schwab, J. H. (1975). Suppression of immune response by microorganisms. *Bacteriol. Rev.*, **39,** 121

Schwartz, R. S. (1975). Viruses and systematic lupus erythematosus. *N. Engl. J. Med.*, **293,** 132

Sickles, E. A., Greene, W. H. and Wiernick, P. H. (1975). Clinical presentation of infections in granulocytopenic patients. *Arch. Int. Med.*, **135,** 715

Simpson, I. J., Amos, N., Evans, D. J., Thomson, N. M. and Peters, D. K. (1975). Guinea-pig nephrotoxic nephritis I. The role of complement and polymorphonuclear leucocytes and the effect of antibody subclass and fragments in the heterologous phase. *Clin. Exp. Immunol.*, **19,** 499

★Stanworth, D. R. (1973). Immediate hypersensitivity. The molecular basis of the allergic response. *Frontiers Biol.*, **28**

★Stiehn, E. P. and Fulginiti, A. (eds.) (1973). *Immunologic Disorders in Infants and Children.* (New York: Saunders)

Stiller, C. R., Russell, A. S. and Dossetor, J. B. (1975). Autoimmunity: present concepts. *Ann. Int. Med.*, **82,** 405

Stjernswärd, J., Jondal, M., Vánky, F., Wigzell, H. and Seally, R. (1972). Lymphopenia and change in distribution of human B and T lymphocytes in peripheral blood induced by irradiation for mammary carcinoma. *Lancet*, **i,** 1352

Stokes, C. R., Soothill, J. F. and Turner, M. W. (1975). Immune exclusion is a function of IgA. *Nature (London)*, **255,** 745

Wara, D. W., Goldstein, A. L., Doyce, N. E. and Ammann, A. J. (1975a). Thymosin activity in patients with cellular immunodeficiency. *N. Engl. J. Med.*, **292,** 70

Wara, W. M., Phillips, T. L., Wara, D. W., Ammann, A. J. and Smith, V. (1975b). Immunosuppression following radiation therapy for carcinoma of the nasopharynx. *Am. J. Roentgenol., Radium Ther. and Nucl. Med.*, **123,** 482

★Weissmann, G. (ed.) (1975). *Mediators of Inflammation.* (New York: Plenum Press)

Wong, L. and Wilson, J. D. (1975). The identification of Fc and C3 receptors on human neutrophils. *J. Immunol. Methods*, **7,** 69

Youmans, G. B. (1975). Relation between delayed hypersensitivity and immunity in tuberculosis. *Am. Rev. Resp. Dis.*, **111,** 109

★Zweifach, B. W. and McCluskey, R. J. (1974). *The Inflammatory Process.* (London: Academic Press)

CHAPTER 4

The Assessment of Immune Status

L. E. Hughes and R. H. Whitehead

The Assessment of Immune Status

The term 'immune status' may loosely be considered as synonymous with the older term of 'host resistance', a concept in relation to disease which has been championed by some but ignored by others for many years. There have been attempts to augment host resistance by immunological manipulation since immune processes were first discovered at the beginning of this century. Early attempts were crude and directed towards increasing immunity to specific antigens, usually microbial, such as tuberculin extracts or bacterial vaccines. It was hoped that the increase in immunity to a particular antigen might be reflected in increased general immunity or 'resistance'. It will be seen in this chapter that such concepts and techniques are still widely used today.

However, with the advances in the understanding of immune reactions in the past 25 years, it is becoming possible to dissect the immune response in order to study the different aspects of the immune process and to measure the competence of the individual cellular elements which take part in these processes. In some cases this 'homing down' approach may enable one to determine the precise nature of any deficiency, but in most clinical situations broad tests measuring overall response to a complex antigen still give the best indication of general immune competence.

The measurement of immune status is most important and most exact in relation to certain congenital immunodeficiency disorders. Here an accurate assessment of the different elements of immune response is essential to characterizing the particular deficiency. For example, in the Swiss type of hypogammaglobulinaemia a combined deficiency of both cellular and humoral immunity is present and the disease is usually fatal before the age of 2 years. On the other hand, in the DiGeorge Syndrome, thymic agenesis is associated with defective cellular immunity (deficiency of T cells) while B cell-dependent areas of lymphoid tissue and immunoglobulin levels are normal (suggesting that the B cell line is present and capable of full differentiation). Such clear-cut immune deficiency diseases are rare, and of little interest to surgeons except in relation to possible therapeutic approaches such as thymic transplantation.

In surgical conditions measurement of immune status has many possible applications but in most the role of immunity is much less precise than in those conditions just described. Even though less precise, the indirect evidence that immune competence is an important facet of many surgical conditions is sufficiently established to warrant the very large amount of research which is being carried out in this field at the present time. At the same time, our understanding of the role of immunity is so limited that it is doubtful whether consideration of immune competence has as yet any role in practical management of surgical disease. Enthusiastic application of incompletely understood immune concepts to diseases such as cancer is widespread and may prove to be counterproductive. On the other hand, knowledge in this field is advancing so fast that it may soon be possible to manipulate host resistance to the benefit of the patient.

To understand what we are doing when we study immune status it is helpful to look at the two situations where these studies are of greatest potential importance in surgery, organ transplantation and malignant disease.

TRANSPLANTATION

After transplantation, unless the donor kidney is from an identical twin, the body recognizes foreign histocompatibility antigens within the tissue and this recognition will lead to the development of a variety of immune responses whose purpose is to destroy the grafted tissue. Clearly the aim of therapy is to diminish or suppress this immune response, that is, to produce an 'immune deficiency state'.

Such a deficiency of immune responsiveness may be of two types—it may be specific to a particular antigen, e.g. the particular histocompatibility antigen or antigens present in the donor kidney (this is the situation seen in immunological tolerance), or alternatively, it may be a general inability to recognize or respond to any foreign antigen (including the specific antigen of the donor kidney). Thus a specific defect, as in tolerance, may exist in the presence of normal general immune responses of the host, but a deficiency of general immune competence will be reflected in specific immune deficiencies as well. It is mainly the assessment of general immune competence which is covered in this chapter.

MALIGNANCY

The question of host resistance to cancer is far less clear-cut than in the case of transplantation. The situation is best illustrated in terms of the natural history of cancer, where in one patient a small, apparently early breast cancer without evidence of spread may result in death from widespread metastases in a matter of months, while in another patient an advanced tumour may be associated with long-term survival. These differences in behaviour may be described in terms of 'the host–tumour relationship' and this obviously consists of at least two parts, the aggressiveness of the tumour and the resistance of the host. It has been widely assumed that this host resistance may be defined in immunological terms, although there are almost certainly factors involved other than immunological processes. Any immunological element in host resistance must presuppose the presence of specific tumour antigens in the cancer cells. From the immunological point of view, the therapeutic aim is the antithesis of that in transplantation. Tumour immunology sees cancer as a foreign tissue graft which the body is unable to reject because of a deficiency in its immune mechanisms. Manipulation of immunity then has two important roles. The first is to increase host immune competence (both specific and non-specific) so that it can reject the 'foreign' tumour tissue. The second is to assess all forms of tumour treatment in terms of their effect on host immune competence, so that those types of treatment may be chosen which will have the least depressant effect on immune competence, thus giving maximum benefit to the host and minimal benefit to the tumour.

Whilst there is much indirect evidence to support the concept that host resistance to cancer is an immune function, it must be realized that at present there is little clear-cut evidence in the clinical situation that will stand scientific scrutiny. However, it is to this field that the greater part of surgical research in cancer is directed, and this will form the material for most of this chapter.

As in the case of transplantation, host immune reaction to cancer may be considered in specific or non-specific terms. Whilst specific immune reactions have been well defined in some animal tumours, they remain difficult to investigate in clinical cancer since well-defined cancer antigens have not yet been isolated from human tumours. On the other hand, general immune competence can be evaluated with considerable precision, and this aspect of immunity is at present being widely investigated in the clinical situation.

GENERAL VERSUS LOCAL IMMUNITY

Before discussing the measurement of immune competence in patients, it is important to consider differences in competence in different parts of the body. Most of the tests for general immune competence reflect the immune status of the body as a whole, and in particular the situation in the bloodstream. However, the findings obtained by such general tests may not apply to all regions of the body. Certain sites, known as 'immunologically privileged' sites, show little immune response because of anatomical barriers. This occurs in the anterior chamber of the eye, into which effector mechanisms such as lymphocytes and gammaglobulins cannot penetrate, and the central nervous system, which is deficient in efferent lymphatics, so that antigens within the nervous system do not readily reach immunologically competent tissues.

Because of the tendency of immunologically competent cells to 'home' on certain tissues, such as the gut and lymph nodes, the distribution of such cells in the sites where they accumulate may be very different from that in the bloodstream. Obviously the local immune status of such areas may differ from that of other areas of the body. Likewise, some pathological processes have the effect of attracting lymphocytes and 'sequestrating' them in the local area, so reducing the numbers available for general circulation. Many aspects of this problem remain to be investigated: for instance, there is some evidence that a tumour may exert an inhibitory effect on a local draining lymph node that is not reflected in the general immune competence. Nind et al. (1973) studied patients with colon cancer and melanoma looking at the ability of lymphocytes from several sites to kill tumour cells in tissue culture. They showed no killing of tumour cells by lymphocytes found within the tumour; killing by lymphocytes from a draining regional node could be shown in only 5%, yet killing by circulating blood lymphocytes was found in 50% of patients. Thus circulating lymphocytes were much more active than those in the draining lymph nodes.

An even less well defined, but clinically interesting example of local host resistance is occasionally seen following radiotherapy, where rapid tumour growth may occur in an area corresponding exactly to the area subjected to irradiation (Figure 4.1). Here it is believed that radiotherapy has in some way damaged the local immune status and allowed the tumour side to dominate the host–tumour equation. It is not known what aspect of immunity has been depressed in this area, and the situation has not yet been defined scientifically. It may be that other forms of injury can have a similar effect; for instance it has been suggested, although with little supportive evidence, that the 'resistance' of thinly cut flaps during mastectomy may be

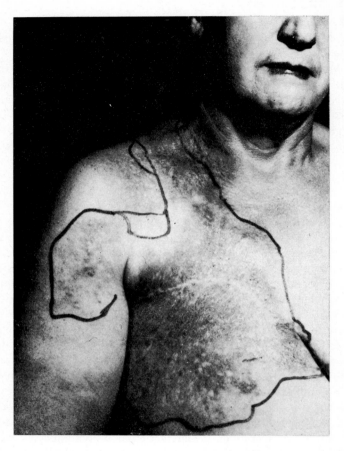

Figure 4.1 Local recurrence of breast cancer developing preferentially in the area receiving postoperative radiotherapy

less than in the case of thickly cut flaps, so leading to a higher incidence of tumour seeding.

This is a whole aspect of tumour immunology which awaits detailed examination. The lesson at present is that while immune competence of the body as a whole is important, the possibility that local immune competence may be quite different should always be considered.

Measurement of Immune Response

THE IMMUNE RESPONSE

The nature of the immune response has been discussed elsewhere, but it is important to recall the main features in order to understand measurement of immune status. The immune response consists basically of three 'limbs', the afferent, the central and the efferent. Through the afferent limb the body recognizes a foreign antigen and sets in motion the immune response. The main elements involved are small (T) lymphocytes and macrophages, the role played by each varying to some extent with the nature of the antigen. Little is known about the central limb of the response, but it is particularly related to storage of immunological information. The efferent limb may be expressed in one of two main groups of responses—the cellular, where immunity is effected by the lymphocytes, either directly or through mediators known as lymphokines, and the humoral, where immunity results from antibody of different classes produced by (B) lymphocytes and plasma cells. However, the situation is in fact much more complex, for humoral and cellular types of response may co-operate to give a more effective response, or interact in antagonistic fashion. Antibodies may also combine with macrophages which then act as a final destructive mechanism. In addition, other substances such as complement play a vital role in these effector mechanisms.

MEASURING GENERAL IMMUNE COMPETENCE

Against this background one may look at the methods available for the assessment of general immune competence. They may be divided into two broad groups. The first group measures, as a whole, the immune response to any convenient test antigen. In the second group, individual elements of the immune mechanism are taken and analysed separately. (In addition to, and quite distinct from these techniques for measuring general immune competence, there is the whole field of measurement of specific immune response to an individual antigen, specific to the condition being studied, for example, tumour specific antigens.)

The first group of tests of immune status (Table 4.1) examine the ability of the host to respond to an individual antigen, and use that response as a general index of the overall ability to produce an immune response. These tests are widely used and are valuable methods of measuring immune competence, and again fall into two main subgroups—response to a new antigen, which has not been encountered before, and response to a previously encountered antigen. The former requires competence of both recognition

Table 4.1 Examples of tests of immune competence using convenient test antigens

	Cellular immunity	Humoral immunity
Primary response	DNCB	Tetanus toxoid
	BCG	Flagellin
Recall response	Mantoux	Diphtheria toxoid
	Streptokinase/dornase	Tetanus toxoid
	Mumps antigen	Proteus

(afferent) and effector (efferent) limbs of the response. It follows that a positive response will reflect competence of all aspects of immunity, but on the other hand, deficiency of either limb of the response will result in failure, so that one cannot determine whether recognition or effector aspects are at fault. With such a test, using a new antigen, it is necessary to sensitize to the antigen, and to challenge with the same antigen 10 to 12 days later, that is after an interval sufficiently long to allow the development of a primary immune response.

Response to a previously encountered antigen (a 'recall' response) measures only the central (memory) and efferent limbs of the response. It depends on the fact that once the body has produced a primary immune response, appropriate memory cells should circulate for the rest of the patient's life. The antigen will mobilize small lymphocytes already sensitized to that antigen, so that immunity will be expressed more rapidly. In this case only a challenge dose (usually much smaller than a sensitizing dose) is used. If no response occurs, one can assume that the efferent limb is then incompetent, provided one is certain that the patient has met the antigen before. With most antigens commonly used, e.g. tuberculin, in the Mantoux test, one does not know this with certainty for an individual patient, although one does know that a certain percentage of a particular population (age group, social class and ethnic origin) can be expected to have met the antigen earlier in life. Thus in an individual non-responder, one does not know whether the patient has previously been sensitized and lost that sensitivity as the result of the disease process (e.g. cancer) or whether he has never met the antigen. It is obvious that when looking at immunity of, for example, cancer patients, one can only compare this group as a whole with a group of appropriate controls, and it is important in this type of test to use an antigen which a high percentage of the population will previously have encountered.

In each of these two situations (primary and recall responses) one may use an antigen which results in a mainly cellular response, or a mainly humoral response. Cellular response is commonly measured by delayed hypersensitivity skin tests. The chemical 1-chloro-2,4-dinitrobenzene (DNCB) is useful in the primary response and tuberculin for the recall response. (It is also possible to study a cellular recall response *in vitro* and this will be discussed later.) Tetanus toxoid or flagellin may be used to measure primary humoral response, and levels of antibody to Proteus have been used as a measure of recall humoral responses.

Instead of measuring the overall response to an antigen, one may take individual elements of the immune mechanism and study them quantitatively or qualitatively. These elements and ways in which they may be studied are shown in Table 4.2.

Table 4.2 Measurement of individual elements of the immune response

Elements	Quantitative response	Qualitative (functional) assessment
Lymphocytes	Total lymphocyte count T & B lymphocyte count K lymphocyte count Null cells	Response to mitogens
Polymorphs	Direct count	Particle ingestion
Macrophages	Not available	Colloidal clearance
Immunoglobulins	Serum levels Immunoassay Local concentration Immunofluorescence	
Complement	Serum levels	

It is essential that testing be carried out prior to any form of treatment since many therapeutic modalities may influence these results. For instance, radiotherapy may cause temporary depression of many aspects of immunity, as may surgery of even moderate degree. Steroid drugs may either decrease or increase the tuberculin reaction, depending on the mode of administration and testing, and anti-mitotic agents may likewise depress the response. For these reasons, studies can only be considered to reflect the untreated state where initial testing is done prior to any form of therapy, or at least 3 months (longer in the case of radiotherapy), subsequent to such therapy.

GENERAL TESTS OF IMMUNE STATUS (see Table 4.1)

Primary cellular immune response

This is tested most conveniently by means of the simple organic chemical 1-chloro-2,4-dinitrobenzene (DNCB) (Aisenberg, 1962) which is used in industrial processes but to which natural sensitivity does not occur. It is a potent allergen which produces a delayed hypersensitivity response, somewhat similar to that induced by tuberculin. As DNCB does not occur naturally, and as most normal individuals can be sensitized to it, it can be used to measure the ability of a patient both to become sensitized and to express a delayed hypersensitivity response.

DNCB is believed to act as a hapten and this means that it needs to be conjugated with a carrier protein in the skin in order to become immunogenic. Various techniques of testing have been used, but differences between the methods are relatively slight. DNCB is dissolved in acetone to give a 2% solution and 0·1 ml of this solution is placed on the skin of the arm (Figure 4.2). The area is covered with a light occlusive dressing for 48 hours. At the same time as sensitization, a challenge dose of 100 μg (0·1 ml

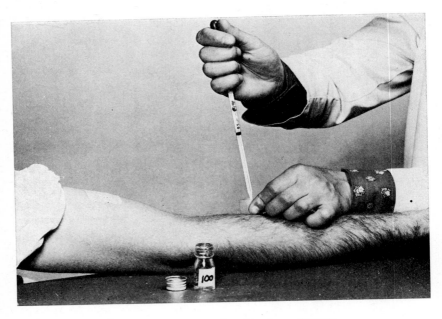

Figure 4.2 Technique of sensitization to DNCB

of the 0·1% solution) is applied in a similar manner to the forearm to confirm the absence of prior sensitization. Fourteen days after sensitization, a challenge dose of 100 μg of DNCB is applied to the forearm in the same manner. Further dilutions (e.g. 50 μg; 5 μg) may also be used to quantify the effect. (It is obviously important that any research worker using this technique should take stringent precautions to ensure that he does not sensitize himself by accidental contact.)

Where the patient has become sensitized, the delayed hypersensitivity reaction consisting of erythema and edema with itching, will be seen in 48–72 hours (Figure 4.3). Various methods of grading responses have been

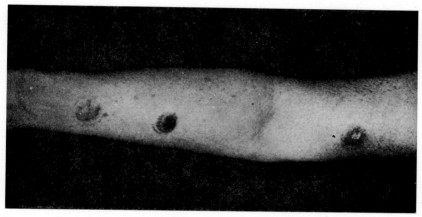

Figure 4.3 Typical delayed hypersensitivity responses to DNCB—sensitizing dose above the elbow, and challenging doses of 100 μg and 50 μg below the elbow

used, one being a simple numerical response as follows:

Response strength 0 = No response.
1 = Erythema alone.
2 = Erythema and induration.
3 = Induration + small vesicles.
4 = Larger or confluent vesicles.

0 and 1 are considered negative and 2, 3 and 4 positive.

Patients with a 4 response or a troublesome reaction should not be retested as further excessive reaction may be expected. The further grading of the response to different doses of DNCB is more helpful in comparing patient groups. This is based on challenge with two dilutions (50 μg and 100 μg).

Grade 0 = Negative to both 50 μg and 100 μg.
1 = Negative to 50 μg but positive to 100 μg.
2 = Positive to 50 μg and 100 μg.
3 = Positive to the initial 100 μg applied at the same time as the sensitizing dose.

This technique based on dosage of DNCB has the advantage of less observer variation, since response is graded as being positive or negative, rather than by degree of response. Using this technique we have found that 5% of healthy patients (patients with benign breast disease) do not become sensitized, while 75% show a Grade 3 response. Many disease processes result in diminution in positive responses and the number of negative responses may be decreased by increasing the sensitizing dose of DNCB— with corresponding increase in morbidity in the form of unpleasant local reactions. A more detailed assessment may be obtained by using a greater range of dilutions, but again this results in an undesirable increase in the number of skin reactions.

A normal DNCB response consists of redness and erythema with itching at the site of application of the doses. The local changes gradually resolve over 2 weeks, but a patch of pigmentation may persist for up to 3 months. We have not seen any systemic complications of DNCB sensitization. While it has been shown that a considerable proportion of DNCB in the guinea-pig is localized in the liver, serial liver function tests in our patients have shown no abnormality. However, it is doubtful that such testing can be justified ethically in normal patients.

Most workers have found that approximately 95% of a normal population will react to DNCB. It is less widely recognized that general non-malignant disease can markedly affect the response. A diminished response is seen in children with protein calorie malnutrition, and in one series only 50% of patients with chronic active tuberculosis were positive. We have found that patients requiring surgery for benign gastrointestinal disease, such as peptic ulcer and diverticulitis, show a 20% negative rate and only 30% show a Grade 3 response (compared with the 5% negative rate and 75% Grade 3 response seen in healthy patients with benign breast disease). The results in malignant disease are discussed later.

A further test which has been used as an index of primary cellular response is the rejection of skin allografts. It has been shown that rejection of such allografts is delayed in patients with advanced skin cancer. The usefulness of this test is limited. Since histocompatibility differences between individual patients vary, it is difficult to determine what a normal value would be. Furthermore, the ethical problems are considerable in anyone other than those with terminal cancer, particularly in relation to possible transfer of hepatitis antigen. It is doubtful if this test should ever be used in the clinical situation.

Recall cellular response

The test most commonly used for measuring this is the tuberculin test, which has the advantage of an immense amount of background data available due to the widespread testing of the population. As only approximately

70% of the normal population will be tuberculin responders, a negative response may indicate either absence of prior exposure or a defect in the ability to express delayed hypersensitivity. For this reason the test cannot be used as an index of general reactivity in the individual patient but only as a comparison between large groups of patients with various disease processes.

The problem of absence of prior exposure may be minimized by using a battery of recall antigens—suitable ones include streptokinase/streptodornase, mumps antigen, trichophytin extract, and *Candida albicans* extract. Of these streptokinase (about 70% of controls positive) and mumps (90% controls positive) are particularly suitable. Results may be expressed in one of three ways. Each test may be considered in isolation, anergy considered to be present only with failure to respond to all the antigens, or an additive score may be used (Anthony *et al.*, 1974). In either case, maximal depression is seen with lymphoreticular malignancies such as Hodgkin's disease and lymphatic leukaemia, less marked depression in advanced solid tumours, and minimal impairment in early cancer. As with the DNCB test, there is considerable evidence that general disease states and malnutrition may affect results. For this reason it is vital that control populations be matched for degree of illness and also for social and racial factors, which may affect the expected incidence of prior contact with antigen.

The recall cellular immune response may also be measured *in vitro*. In this situation the lymphocytes are cultured with the antigens to be tested, such as tuberculin, and their ability to undergo blast transformation measured. Details of this technique are in many ways similar to those described later with mitogens. However, the technique is not as readily controlled as in the case of substances like phytohaemagglutinin and for this reason the technique is not widely used.

Primary humoral response

Attempts to measure humoral immune responses have not been pursued as vigorously as have the cellular responses outlined above. Many early papers are difficult to evaluate because of such factors as failure to give details of treatment schedules and progress at the time of testing, or failure to eliminate the possibility of prior exposure. In the case of tetanus toxoid, patients may have forgotten early immunization, or indeed may have been unaware that it was included among the various assaults suffered during military service or childhood. However, the possibility of prior contact with tetanus toxoid or other similar antigens can be eliminated by appropriate schedules timed to detect an anamnestic response indicating previous exposure. Other workers have used viruses as immunizing antigens.

A further antigen which is suitable for this type of investigation is flagellin, a protein obtained from the flagella of the organism *Salmonella adelaide* (Rowley and Mackay, 1969). As *Salmonella* organisms containing flagella antigens which cross-react with those of *Salm. adelaide* are rare, most people will not have had prior exposure. This antigen has the advantages that it can be produced in a chemically pure form, and a large amount of experimental work has been carried out in accurately defining the mechanisms and the kinetics of the immune response. In the human situation, many data are available in relation to the immune response it evokes in normal patients of various ages, and in a variety of disease states. For instance, there is little alteration with age, but females give a better response than males, and general hospital patients show a decreased response compared with 'normal' people. It has the advantages of standardization held by DNCB in relation to cellular responses and so will probably come to hold the same position for humoral immunity.

Recall humoral responses

These have been measured on a number of occasions by an anamnestic response to a previously encountered antigen—e.g. diphtheria toxoid. Another approach has been to measure serum levels of antibodies which are generally present in the normal population—e.g. agglutinins to Proteus organisms—which are found in 95% of normal adults, or serum antibodies to *Candida albicans*. There have been obvious methodological problems associated with the studies that have been reported in this field, so that it is not possible from the present work to give an assessment of the effects of disease processes and malignancy on secondary humoral immune responses. In future studies it is likely that only primary humoral responses, e.g. to flagellin, will be used to any large extent.

More recently, the whole subject of humoral immune response has been neglected in favour of studies on cellular immunity and this is not surprising when one recalls that the major immunological mechanisms against foreign solid tissues are cellular in nature.

On the other hand, it is becoming increasingly obvious that serum antibodies may play a much greater role in the destruction of foreign tissues than has been previously thought. It will be seen in chapters dealing with tumour immunology and transplantation that antibodies may themselves be cytotoxic to cells, or that they may have a 'blocking' effect and so counteract even strong cellular immunity, or again that by means of 'macrophage arming activity' humoral antibodies may yet prove to be the most potent of all immunological mechanisms. Hence in the future it could be that the most important factors governing immunotherapy regimes against cancer will be related to the ability to produce a satisfactory, desirable cytotoxic humoral antibody response, or to suppress the production of an undesirable (blocking) humoral response to the cancer antigens. Should this prove to be the case, humoral mechanisms will be subjected to the same intense study as cellular immunity.

Tests of Immune Status Related to Individual Elements of the Immune Response (see Table 4.2)

QUANTITATIVE ASSESSMENT OF LYMPHOCYTES

Total lymphocyte count

The total lymphocyte count can readily be determined by differential leucocyte counts, and this simple assessment shows important variations in disease states. For instance, it has been clearly shown that in patients with colon cancer, total lymphocyte count decreases, both in absolute terms and as a percentage of total white cell count, as the disease becomes more advanced, and provides a rough prognostic index in this condition. On the other hand, the opposite situation has been found in gastric cancer where the lymphocyte count rises as the disease becomes more advanced (Bolton et al., 1975). While these changes are of interest, recent work discussed in Chapter 1 has shown that the lymphocyte population is made up of a number of subgroups, e.g. T and B cells, with disparate immunological functions. It is clear that overall immune function will be greatly affected by the relative proportions of the different subgroups and hence it is necessary to repeat most, if not all, previous work to take this into account. Work on lymphocyte subpopulations in humans is in an early phase, and undoubtedly further subclasses will be defined, again calling for re-evaluation. Already a third group of lymphocytes (antibody-dependent cytotoxic cells, known as 'K' or 'killer' cells) has been defined, and in some disease states such as cancer, a proportion of lymphocytes do not show the characteristics of any of these groups and have been called 'null' cells.

The future clinical significance of lymphocyte subpopulations with varying functions is so great that the present situation regarding their assessment will be discussed in some detail.

T and B cell determination

Distinctive cell surface markers for subdividing the lymphocyte population were initially well characterized in rodents and chickens. In recent years, the application of similar techniques to human lymphocytes has shown that two major subpopulations exist, T (or thymus-derived) and B (or bone marrow-derived). Marker systems used to detect T and B lymphocytes (Figure 4.4) have been recently reviewed (Greaves *et al.*, 1973). The percentage of T cells is determined by making use of their ability to form

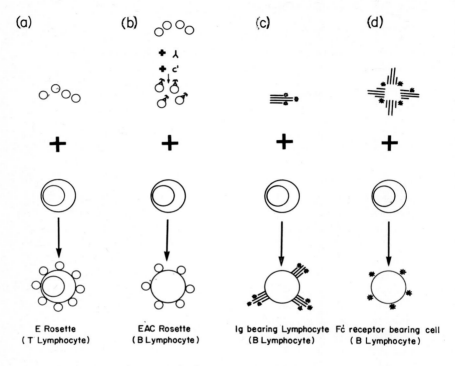

(a) **(b)** **(c)** **(d)**

E Rosette   EAC Rosette   Ig bearing Lymphocyte Fċ receptor bearing cell
(T Lymphocyte)   (B Lymphocyte)   (B Lymphocyte)   (B Lymphocyte)

Figure 4.4 Summary of the method for determining T and B cells

rosettes with sheep red blood cells at 0–4 °C (E rosettes). Rosetting, a technique developed on empirical grounds, rather than on a clear immunological basis, occurs when lymphocytes are mixed with certain red blood cells. When more than three to five red cells are attached to an individual lymphocyte, it is counted as a rosette.

B cells bear three determinants on their surface which may be used in their identification:

(i) They have receptor for C_3 (C_3 is the third component of complement) (see Chapter 2) which can be used to bind complement. Complement is provided already attached to an antigen–antibody complex, which itself acts as a marker. A convenient test is to use sheep red blood cells as the marker, together with antisheep red blood cell antibody (which combines with the sheep red blood cells to form a complex which will bind complement); the bound complement then fixes to the surface of the lymphocyte. In this way the red cells may be made to rosette on the B lymphocytes. (These rosettes are known as EAC rosettes, from erythrocyte, antibody and complement used in their formation.)

(ii) B cells carry immunoglobulin on their surface, which may be detected by immunofluorescence techniques using an antihuman gammaglobulin (anti-IgG) labelled with fluorescein isothiocyanate (FITC).

(iii) B lymphocytes also have receptors for the F_c portion of the immuno-globulin molecule. The F_c portion of the immunoglobulin molecule has been described in an earlier chapter, it does not carry the antibody-reacting sites but does have sites for fixation of complement. It is normally detected by staining the cells with a heat-aggregated human immunoglobulin (AggHIgG) labelled with FITC.

At present it is not known whether all three markers appear on all B lymphocytes. Recently Brown and Greaves (1974) have shown that most, but not all, cells with immunoglobulin on their surface also bind AggHIgG. They also found that a small proportion of T cells also bound AggHIgG. All these cells were lymphoblasts suggesting that activated T cells may synthesize or expose an F_c receptor. Monocytes are also known to have F_c receptors and C_3 receptors on their membranes and therefore could give false-positive results in measurement of T and B cells.

Recently double-labelling techniques have been described which make possible the simultaneous counting of B and T cells. The simplest of these methods uses erythrocytes from two animal species. T cells are detected as usual using sheep erythrocytes, while the B cells are detected by using a pigeon erythrocyte/antipigeon erythrocyte antibody/complement combina-tion. The final result is that the T cells form rosettes with the sheep cells and B cells form rosettes with the pigeon cells. The two types of erythrocytes can be distinguished by shape and by the fact that the avian erythrocytes are nucleated. These double-labelling techniques have revealed the presence of lymphocytes which do not form rosettes on either test and these have been appropriately termed 'null' cells. It has been reported that the percentage of null cells is increased in patients with advanced cancer.

A number of technical factors need to be borne in mind when determining B and T cells. These have been reviewed recently by a WHO/IARC spon-sored workshop (1974). It is essential to check the efficiency of the cell-separation method used to obtain lymphocytes. The most common separa-tion technique is centrifugation of heparinized blood (diluted $\frac{1}{3}$ to $\frac{1}{5}$) over a layer of ficoll/hypaque; the lymphocytes being lightest stay suspended above the heavy ficoll/hypaque solution. The yield of lymphocytes should be checked as should the morphology, as this separation method gives a higher proportion of monocytes than is present in whole blood.

In order to obtain optimal E rosettes, a number of points are important. The sheep red blood cells should be between 1 and 3 weeks old, the lymphocytes should be washed two or three times but not centrifuged too vigorously, and incubation of lymphocytes should be carried out at 0–4 °C for at least 1 hour and can be continued overnight. The final resuspension must be very gentle and tapping of the tube with the finger is sufficient. The treatment of the red blood cells with neuraminadase is claimed to give more stable rosettes. It is obvious that great attention to detail is necessary, and these difficulties of technique may explain many of the variable results reported by different workers. The methods for B cell detection are more stable but again attention should be paid to the details set out in the WHO/IARC Workshop Report.

The normal level of B cells is usually given as 20–30%. Reports of T cell counts have varied greatly but recent papers have agreed on a range of 70–80%. Little is yet known of the fluctuation in T and B cell levels in normal people and in disease. Steel et al. (1974) measured T cell levels (using sheep red blood cell rosetting) in six healthy subjects at four intervals during a morning and found only a small fluctuation—from 5–11%—in different individuals. However, strenuous exercise gave a marked lymphocytosis lasting for 45 minutes although these were mainly non-T cells. In disease states, Stjernswärd et al. (1972) described the decrease in T cells and a relative increase in B cells following irradiation in breast cancer patients, which lasted for at least 12 months in some cases. Anthony et al. (1975) have studied the B and T cell levels in lung cancer patients and report that low T cell levels were associated with a poor prognosis and that T cell levels remained constant until shortly before death, when they dropped sharply.

In a recent study (Niklassen and Williams, 1974) of T and B cells in acute infections, the T cell percentage was depressed in early stages of the disease and the proportion of B cells was increased. The increase in B cells occurred earlier in viral and mycoplasmal infections than in bacterial infections. The decrease in the number of T cells present was concomitant with an increase in the number of null cells.

Antibody-dependent cytotoxic (K) lymphocytes

As well as the two major lymphocyte subpopulations described above, a third subpopulation termed K (or killer) cells has been described. These cells are identified by their ability to kill in non-specific fashion target cells which have been coated with antibody (Perlmann et al., 1972). That is, one has a situation where specific antibody is able to attach to a cell bearing the corresponding antigen without leading to cell destruction. (This may be due to several causes, the most common one being inability of the antibody to fix complement.) If these K cells are then added to the antibody-coated cells they are able to bring about destruction of the cells in a quite non-specific fashion. Although these cells interact with the antibody bound to the target cell through an F_c receptor on their membrane, their nature is unknown. The two possibilities are that they are either a subpopulation of B cells or that they are a non-phagocytic monocyte (macrophage). The major problem with the K cell assay in its present form is that it is qualitative rather than quantitative. All that is measured is the amount of target cell death produced, measured by isotope release from antibody labelled target cells in the presence of varying concentrations of K lymphocytes. Results are normally expressed as a percentage of the known normal levels of the test, as the actual number of K cells cannot be determined by the method used.

There is some experimental evidence in animal tumours that non-specific killing by monocytes or lymphocytes activated by antibody may be an important mechanism in tumour cell destruction, so further work in this field will be awaited with great interest. Little has yet been reported concerning changes in the proportion of these cells in disease states, although Skinner et al. (1974) have reported that azathioprine preferentially suppresses the K cell population. A patient with macroglobulinaemia has been described who was K cell deficient but had apparently normal T and B cell function. Ting and Terasaki (1974) showed that K cell activity is less in cancer patients than in normals or patients with non-malignant diseases.

Null cells

At present null cells can only be quantitated by subtracting the combined B and T cell counts from 100%. As more is learned about the nature of these cells, more direct methods of assessment may become available.

QUALITATIVE MEASUREMENT OF LYMPHOCYTE FUNCTION

Lymphocyte stimulation

When a lymphocyte comes into contact with an antigen for which it is coded, it is transformed into a blast cell and undergoes mitosis. This process yields a clone of cells specifically active against the stimulating antigen. In the process of transformation, many soluble products with specific activities (known as lymphokines) are liberated by the activated lymphocyte. Both the ability to undergo blast transformation and measurement of the production of different types of lymphokines have been used as indices of lymphocyte function.

Non-specific stimulation

It has been known for many years that protein extracts of various bean species are able to induce lymphocytes to proliferate. The term mitogen is used for these substances because of their ability to stimulate mitosis. The most widely used substance in the immunological sphere is phytohaemagglutinin, and its mitogenic activity was noticed during its use as an haemagglutinating agent in haematology. This mitogenic effect is antigenically non-specific but most of the mitogens (phytohaemagglutinin, concavalin A, leucoagglutinin) have been shown to be stimulants of T cells. Pokeweed mitogen is believed to be primarily a stimulant of B cells and specifically so in low concentrations. Higher concentrations probably stimulate T cells as well as B cells. This non-specific stimulation appears to mimic the specific transformation occurring with antigens *in vivo* and has been used by many workers to measure the integrity of the cell-mediated part of the immune response (in the case of T cell mitogens) in many disease states. While the actual nature and significance of the non-specific stimulation is not understood, in general there is a fair degree of correlation between cellular immune competence and non-specific T cell stimulation by mitogens. On the other hand, a PHA response will not necessarily correspond to a tuberculin or DNCB response in a given patient, nor is there good evidence that the same result will be obtained in a given patient with different mitogens. In spite of these reservations, it seems that the general concept has a useful degree of validity. In the study of human disease states, a very large majority of the work has used PHA as the mitogen.

Stimulation is normally assessed by incubating lymphocytes (or whole blood) with phytohaemagglutinin (PHA) or one of the other mitogens for three days, at which time blast transformation should be well established (Figure 4.5). Tritiated thymidine is usually added 4 hours before the incubation is terminated and the amount of radioactive label incorporated into the DNA is measured. This technique gives a measure of the cell growth rate (DNA turnover) and hence the amount of stimulation induced by the mitogen. Figure 4.6 shows the sequence from small lymphocyte to blast cell.

In earlier techniques the actual number of blast cells was counted, either by morphological criteria in a stained blood smear, or by means of autoradiography after incorporation of an isotope label into the DNA of the lymphocyte. Such methods were not only time-consuming but have a low degree of reproducibility and have largely been discarded in favour of techniques using liquid scintillation counting. Most workers have tended to use large doses of PHA in attempts to obtain maximal responses, in spite of reports that suboptimal doses are better for detecting lesser degrees of im-

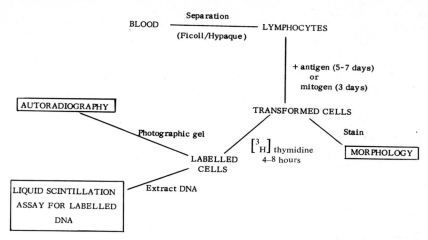

Figure 4.5 Procedure for lymphocyte stimulation. The number of blast cells present or the amount of incorporation of [³H]thymidine into DNA is a measure of the degree of stimulation

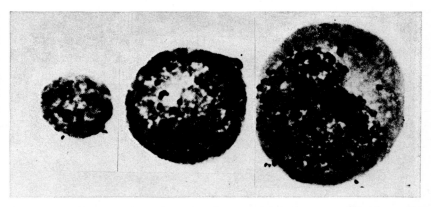

Figure 4.6 Progression of transformation from small lymphocyte to blast form. The newly formed DNA has been labelled by tritiated thymidine

mune stimulation. We have found that suboptimal PHA concentration gives the best discrimination between groups of cancer patients with good and poor immune response, as shown in Figure 4.7, which shows the results of a dose–response curve in a series of breast cancer patients grouped according to expected prognosis (Whitehead et al., 1975). This also shows that maximal doses of PHA do not yield the highest levels of stimulation, especially in normal people. For this reason such a dose–response curve using three doses,

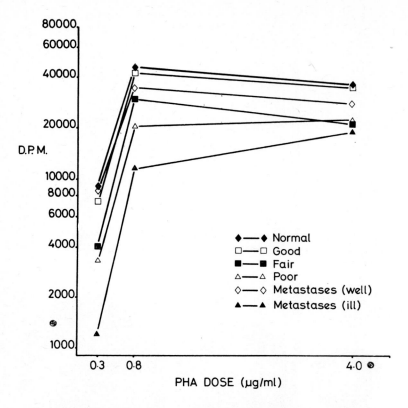

Figure 4.7 Lymphocyte response to PHA in patients with breast cancer, as shown by a dose–response curve

or at least a suboptimal and an optimal dose, will give more useful information than a single dose. In the normal patient group and those with early breast cancer, the amount of stimulation rises until the optimum dose is reached and then falls as this is exceeded. In advanced cancer patients, however, the dose–response curve continues rising with the highest dose but the responses are all at a lower level than in normal control patients.

We have found the following method to be highly satisfactory: lymphocytes are separated from heparinized blood using ficoll/hypaque, washed three times and suspended in McCoy's 5A medium + 15% fetal calf serum, at a concentration of 1.25×10^6 cells/ml; 0.2 ml of this suspension is dispensed into each of 12 wells of a microculture dish. Three concentrations of purified PHA are used, 20 μg/ml, 4 μg/ml and 1·5 μg/ml and 0·05 ml of each of these is added to three wells to give a final PHA concentration of 4 μg/ml, 0·8 μg/ml and 0·3 μg/ml. Saline is added to the final three wells which act as controls. The plate is then incubated at 37 °C in an atmosphere of 5% CO_2 and 100% humidity for 72 hours. Four hours before harvesting the cells, 0·05 ml of 10 μCi/ml of tritiated thymidine is added and the plates reincubated. For harvesting, the plate is chilled, the cells washed from the wells and collected on filter paper. They are then processed for counting in a liquid scintillation counter. Results should be expressed in disintegrations per minute and can be expressed either as a stimulation increment (stimulation in test wells—stimulation in control wells) or as a stimulation ratio (stimulation in test wells/stimulation in control wells).

The 'PHA response' in normal persons varies very widely both between individuals and within the same individual from day to day. This is partly due to the difficulties of standardization of the technique, but probably also due to random variations in lymphatic responsiveness. This means that in general, a tenfold difference is needed between two readings before they should be considered as significantly different. It is obvious that each laboratory should determine its own 'normal variation' before assessing the significance of its findings, and papers reporting small changes in PHA responsiveness should be assessed critically.

Taking these factors into consideration, there is usually a marked depression of responsiveness in patients suffering from immunological disease states associated with impairment of cellular immunity (DiGeorge Syndrome, Swiss-type agammaglobulinaemia, ataxia-telangiectasia). Responsiveness has also been reported as diminished in as varying disease states as kwashiorkor, celiac disease, primary biliary cirrhosis, tuberculosis and Sjögren's disease. Some workers have also found diminished responses in patients with Crohn's disease but other workers have reported normal responses in these patients.

Several drugs including aspirin, have also been reported as reducing lymphocyte stimulation. Lymphocyte responsiveness is depressed for at least 7 days following surgery (Berenbaum et al., 1973). The cause of this depression is not known but has been shown to be related to the extent of operative trauma, but not necessarily to the length of operation. Radiotherapy is known to depress lymphocyte stimulation. This depression has been shown to last for long periods (up to 12 months) and appears to be due to a selective T lymphocyte depletion.

There have been many reports of a depressed lymphocyte responsiveness to phytohaemagglutinin in patients with cancer of varying histological types. The reports are difficult to compare directly because many different techniques have been used, some varying in almost every respect. In spite of these limitations it is evident that a tumour is in some way able to depress the host's immune system.

Other tests of non-specific competence

The ability of peripheral lymphocytes to mount a graft-versus-host reaction has also been used as a means of measuring the competence of lymphocytes from cancer patients. Lymphocytes are injected into the skin of an animal and the size of the inflammatory nodule produced as the patient's lymphocytes react against the animal's histocompatibility antigens gives a measure of the competence of the patient's lymphocytes.

An ingenious variation on this theme also measures the general functional capacity of lymphocytes. Lymphocytes are injected into the footpad of irradiated rats and after a number of days, the draining lymph nodes are removed and weighed. The weight is compared with that of the same nodes from the opposite limb into which formalinized cells have been injected. The increase in weight indicates that the injected lymphocytes have populated the node and are reacting against the host tissues.

The 'non-specific' competence of lymphocytes has also been assessed *in vitro* by using a variety of specific antigens to stimulate blast transformation—the specific antigen being used to measure general immune response in the same way as the Mantoux test has been described earlier. The two antigens used most commonly have been PPD and Varidase, and they may be considered as an *in vitro* analogy to the corresponding skin tests.

The mixed lymphocyte reaction is an extension of this technique. In this test the ability of the patient's lymphocytes to recognize foreign lymphocytes and respond to them is measured. In practice the stimulating lymphocytes are inactivated by irradiation or mitomycin C to prevent them responding also. The incubation period needs to be longer (5–7 days) than for PHA stimulation. It has been claimed that this test gives a more sensitive measure of immune depression in cancer patients than PHA stimulation tests. This would certainly seem to be true for the older PHA techniques using maximal doses, but may not be so for dose–response curves with PHA. The technique is of great relevance in assessing the suitability of donors in transplantation and will be discussed in Chapter 6.

Polymorphonuclear leukocytes

Polymorphs can be quantitated in blood smears and their functional capacity can be measured *in vitro* by allowing them to ingest latex particles or heat-killed yeast. The number of ingested particles per cell can be counted. It has been found that although the number of polymorphs is not diminished in cancer patients, their functional capacity (normally expressed as a phago-cytic index, K) is diminished in patients with disseminated disease. In patients with leukaemia, this phagocytic index was shown to return to normal during drug-induced remissions only to decrease again when the patient relapsed.

The monocyte/macrophage system

This group of cells forms a very significant part of the body's defence system whose importance is becoming more obvious as it is subjected to more intensive study.

It is generally accepted that macrophages process antigen for presentation to the small lymphocyte and it has been shown that the macrophage is essential for initiating a delayed hypersensitivity response if the antigen is larger than a critical size.

Monocytes originate primarily from the bone marrow, whence they enter the bloodstream, circulating for 1-3 days before they randomly leave the circulation to become a 'fixed' tissue macrophage—where they will bear a label dependent on the site in which they settle—Kuppfer cells, fixed splenic histiocytes, pulmonary alveolar macrophages, epithelioid cells, etc. Their survival in these tissues is measured in weeks unless they are called to take part in a local inflammatory reaction. The cells of this system may be studied in vitro by harvesting blood monocytes, or in vivo when the total function of the fixed tissue macrophages (reticuloendothelial system) may be assessed.

Much work is at present in progress to develop techniques for isolation of cells of this system in order to study their function in a manner similar to the in vitro tests for lymphocytes. While this is done quite easily in the case of animals (since macrophages can readily be harvested from the peritoneal cavity after injection of a mild irritant such as paraffin oil), the situation is much more difficult in the case of human studies. Attempts to isolate pure suspensions of human monocytes from peripheral blood use such techniques as passing the blood through columns packed with glass beads to which the macrophages can adhere. Monocyte preparations can be isolated in this way, but require large amounts of blood—100-150 ml to produce useful yields. It can be expected that tests of macrophage function analogous to those of lymphocytes will soon be available.

Immunoglobulins

The levels of the various immunoglobulins IgG, IgA, IgM and IgE can be quantified using standard immunodiffusion techniques. Kits are available commercially for this purpose. Using an immunodiffusion technique Hughes

(1971) measured IgG, IgA and IgM levels in 984 patients with various carcinomas, melanomas and sarcomas. IgG levels were shown to be within normal limits in patients with most cancer types but were raised in male patients with skin cancer and in all patients with lung cancer. IgA levels were raised in patients with cancer of the gastrointestinal tract, respiratory system and skin. These results might be expected as these are the regions in which IgA production is concentrated. IgM levels were within normal limits in most cancer types, but were significantly raised in females with malignant melanoma and males with sarcoma.

Interest in IgE levels has been stimulated by reports that people with a history of allergy have a significantly lower incidence of cancer. Initial reports of IgE levels in cancer patients did suggest that some cancer patients had abnormal IgE levels but more recent reports have highlighted the great technical problems with the very intricate methods used, and the question must still be considered an open one.

While serum immunoglobulins can be conveniently measured, it is possible that immunoglobulin levels in peripheral blood do not reflect the local situation within and around the tumour. Immunoglobulins can be measured in tumour extracts using the same techniques as are used for peripheral blood determinations. These studies may give information regarding immunoglobulins directed towards tumour antigens and so be more meaningful than the levels of all immunoglobulins as measured in the peripheral blood.

Of even more interest is the detection of immunoglobulin-bearing cells (B cells) within the tumour. These can be detected using immunofluorescence techniques. A frozen section of the tumour is stained with an antiserum to antihuman Ig usually made in rabbits or goats and conjugated with fluorescein isothiocyanate. By using conjugated antisera against the different Ig types the number of B cells bearing IgG, IgM and IgA can be quantified. Again it is more likely that when consistent results are available from this work they will reflect more clearly humoral responses directed specifically against the tumour cells.

Complement

If the blocking factor described in the sera of patients with cancer is an antigen–antibody complex then it would be expected to bind complement. From this one might expect to find lower than normal levels of complement in cancer patients as is the case in some other diseases where immune complexes are formed. Many methods exist for measuring complement activity and the levels of the various complement components. The simplest is probably an immunodiffusion technique which measures the concentration of C_3. Studies in cancer patients, however, have failed to show any depletion in complement activity, and in fact higher than normal levels have been reported in some cancer patients. Again it should be stressed that the local tissue levels of complement may be of more importance than systemic levels.

Measurement of 'Specific' Immune Response

The specific immune competence of a patient's lymphocytes toward a particular antigen (e.g. the response of a cancer patient's lymphocytes to his own tumour) can be measured in a number of ways both *in vivo* and *in vitro*.

In vivo TESTS

In 1964 Hughes and Lytton reported that patients with cancer showed delayed hypersensitivity reactions when extracts of their own tumour were injected intradermally. This finding has been corroborated many times since using more modern methods of tumour antigen preparation. A novel method of measuring the functional capacity of leucocytes *in vivo* in cancer patients has been exploited by Black and Leis (1971). They cut a frozen section of a patient's breast tumour and applied it to an abraded portion of the patient's forearm. When the frozen section was removed and stained, it was found that lymphocytes, monocytes and polymorphs had all invaded the frozen section. The degree of invasion has been shown to correlate well with tumour stage and was highest in patients with early *in situ* cancer.

In vitro TESTS

It was mentioned earlier that when lymphocytes react with an antigen they liberate various lymphokines, become transformed into blast forms and begin to multiply. This stimulation can be measured *in vitro* by incubating lymphocytes with extracts of tumour cells or whole tumour cells that have been inactivated by irradiation or by treatment with mitomycin C.

The usual incubation period is from 5–7 days before tritiated thymidine is added. Stimulation levels are normally much lower than those obtained using mitogens. This probably reflects the size of the clone of cells capable of reacting with the stimulating antigen. Positive stimulation has been reported in breast, colon carcinoma and malignant melanoma patients; however, the low levels of stimulation reported as positive in some cases make interpretation of the results obtained difficult (Vanky *et al.*, 1971).

As well as measuring the lymphocyte stimulation occurring, the liberation of lymphokines can also be assayed. One of these, migration inhibition factor (MIF) inhibits the migration of macrophages and peripheral leucocytes. Originally, this test was assayed using guinea-pig macrophages as the indicator cell in a two-stage test. Firstly lymphocytes were incubated with antigen and the supernatant fluid (which will contain lymphokines if the lymphocytes react to the particular antigen being tested) collected after 3 days. Macrophages were obtained from guinea-pigs by injecting oil into the peritoneal cavity and collecting the peritoneal fluid 24 hours later. The macrophages were washed and taken up in capillary tubes which were then sealed and centrifuged. The portion containing packed macrophages was cut and placed in a small well containing medium and the supernatant fluid. The wells were then sealed and incubated overnight. Normally macrophages can be expected to migrate rapidly out of the capillary tube into the medium. A decrease in the area of migration in wells containing supernatant fluid compared to the area in wells containing tissue culture medium alone indicated the presence of the lymphokine in the supernatant fluid (Figure 4.8). More recently a one-step test has been developed using peripheral blood leukocytes as both the lymphokine-producing cells and the migrating cells.

In this test if the leukocytes react with the antigen (tumour extract) the

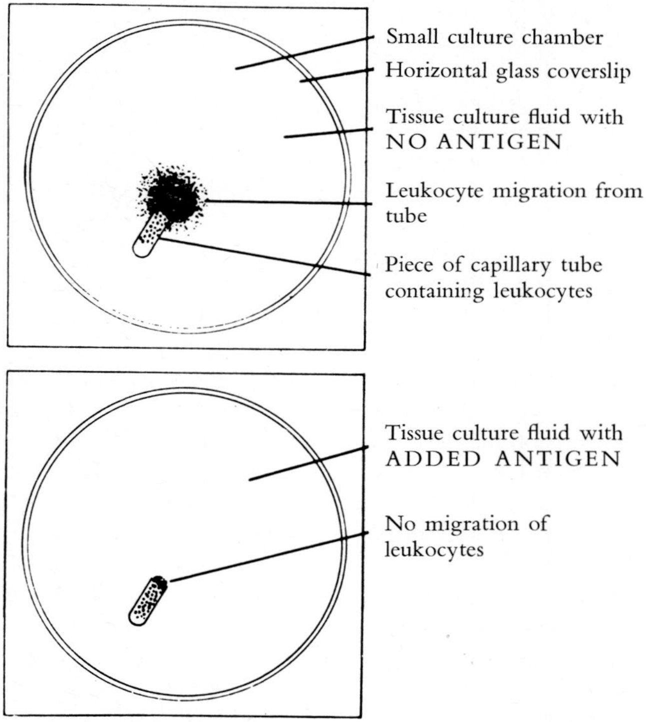

Small culture chamber
Horizontal glass coverslip

Tissue culture fluid with
NO ANTIGEN

Leukocyte migration from tube

Piece of capillary tube containing leukocytes

Tissue culture fluid with
ADDED ANTIGEN

No migration of leukocytes

Figure 4.8 Leukocyte migration inhibition test

migration is less than that in control wells containing only medium. In practice, a migration of less than 80% of the control values has been found to represent significant inhibition and therefore to indicate a specific immune reaction. This test has been found to correlate well with delayed hypersensitivity skin tests with many antigens, e.g. DNCB (Whitehead et al., 1974).

Using this test Cochrane et al. (1972) have found that 60% of breast cancer patients react to at least one of a battery of breast cancer antigens. In comparison only 20% of controls were positive. Similar results have been obtained with malignant melanoma and colon carcinoma. Originally crude extracts of the tumour were used as antigen but recently formalinized tumour cells or frozen sections of the tumour have been described as being satisfactory.

A second lymphokine released by activated lymphocytes causes leukocytes which would normally adhere to surfaces to become non-adherent. This forms the basis for a simple test of specific lymphocyte function (the leucocyte adherence test) (Halliday and Miller, 1972). In essence, lymphocytes are incubated with tumour extracts and a drop of the leukocyte suspension is placed on a haemocytometer and the number of cells counted. The haemocytometer is incubated in a moist atmosphere for 60 minutes at 37 °C, the coverslip gently floated off and the non-adherent cells gently washed away. A new coverslip is then placed on the haemocytometer and the number of cells adhering is counted. This number is compared with a control preparation of leukocytes in medium. Using this technique a very good correlation between a positive result and tumour presence has been obtained.

In some ways the most definitive method commonly being used to detect a specific immune response to tumours is the cytotoxicity test (Figure 4.9). It has been found that immune lymphocytes are able to kill target cells against which they are responsive. Cells derived from tumours are cultured in the wells of microculture plates and lymphocytes are added to the wells and the plates are incubated for 48–72 hours. At the end of this period the plates are carefully washed and the remaining cells stained and counted. A reduction in the number of cells in wells to which lymphocytes have been added compared to the wells containing cells plus growth medium alone indicates cytotoxicity. In practice one can either use cells obtained from biopsies and hope that they will attach to the bottom of the well sufficiently for the test to be performed or one can use cell lines derived from tumours. Except for the case of malignant melanoma very few cell lines have been derived from solid tumours. The majority of cells that are obtained on culturing are fibroblasts. Careful checks should be made on any cells obtained in culture before

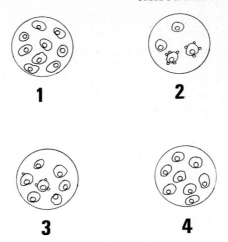

Figure 4.9

1. Tumour cells are grown in the wells of microculture plates

2. Tumour cells + patient's lymphocytes. Many tumour cells have been killed and lymphocytes are adhering to other cells

3. Tumour cells + patient's serum + patient's lymphocytes. There is a reduction in the amount of killing due to the blocking activity of a factor in the patient's serum

4. Tumour cells + normal lymphocytes. This control is necessary to test the sensitivity of the tumour cells to the presence of lymphocytes. There is often a small reduction in tumour cell numbers

they are accepted as tumour cells and used as target cells in cytotoxicity tests. The original studies (Hellström *et al.*, 1971) used short-term cultures of tumours as target cells. Recent studies have shown that normal lymphocytes are often capable of killing tumour cells at the lymphocyte to tumour cell ratios usually used (up to 5000:1 has been described but 500:1 or 1000:1 are more commonly used). Because of these findings the significance of earlier results claiming specificity in the test in a number of tumour systems is now the subject of much debate.

As well as these techniques for assaying the cellular immune response, the humoral response (production of antibodies) can also be assayed. The most successful technique for detecting antibody to tumour antigen in tumour patients is immunofluorescence. However, the only tumour which has yielded significant results is malignant melanoma. Most commonly smears of tumour cells or tumour cells grown in tissue culture are used as antigen and are incubated with serum from tumour patients and then after washing are incubated with antihuman immunoglobulin conjugated with fluorescein isothiocyanate. Two antigens have been described in malignant melanoma cells. Melanoma cells are claimed to have a common cytoplasmic antigen which is cross-reactive and a membrane antigen which is positive in the autochthonous situation only. One problem with the interpretation of results obtained with the cytoplasmic antigen, however, is the high reactivity of some control sera (Whitehead, 1973). These results tend to suggest that what is being measured is probably a fetal antigen which is being re-elaborated rather than a tumour antigen which has arisen *de novo*.

Serum antibody capable of killing tumour cells has also been shown using a complement-dependent cytotoxicity test in which tumour cells are in-cubated with serum from tumour patients plus complement and the amount of killing of tumour cells assayed. Another test similar to that already described in the K cell assay has been used for the detection of antibody to tumours (Pollack *et al.*, 1972).

As well as these potentially beneficial facets of the humoral response, another facet of the overall immune response needs to be considered.

It was found that when tumour cells were preincubated with sera from cancer patients then lymphocyte killing of these cells was decreased. This phenomenon was termed 'blocking' and was initially believed to be due to the presence of antibody to the tumour which coated the tumour cell and protected it from attack by lymphocytes. Recently, however, it has been shown that if the lymphocytes are preincubated with cancer patients' own serum then blocking is also obtained. This observation suggests that the blocking factor is in fact tumour antigen or a tumour antigen–antibody complex which is present in the serum. The appearance of tumour antigen which has probably shed tumour cell membranes or subparticles of these is of quite considerable clinical importance as it is claimed that blocking factor disappears after surgical removal of the tumour and the reappearance of blocking factor in the serum of a cancer patient may signal the presence of metastases. Blocking factor is most commonly assayed using the lymphocyte cytotoxicity test but has also been assayed in the lymphocyte stimulation test, the leukocyte migration test and the leukocyte adherence test.

The ability to monitor lymphocyte reactivity and the presence of antibody and of blocking factor is of importance in our understanding of the disease process and assumes added relevance when any form of immunotherapy is contemplated.

Immune Competence in Relation to Surgical Disease

CANCER

At present our only concepts of the host–tumour relationship are very vague clinical ones which have been found from past experience to be related to prognosis. In the future, we will probably try to look at this relationship from various aspects:

(a) by assessment of the tumour (looking at such factors as histology, sites of spread and cell kinetics);

(b) by assessment of the host, using the techniques for a measurement of immune competence as described in this chapter; and

(c) at the host–tumour interplay as shown by the interaction of the patient's response to tumour cells (for instance looking at indices of the specific immune response discussed earlier, such as skin reactions to injections of tumour extracts, lymphocyte stimulation by tumour extracts and of interaction *in vitro* as assessed by cytotoxicity studies).

At present the aspects of the host–tumour relationship which are best developed are general immune competence and *in vitro* cytotoxicity. The relevance of specific immunity as shown by cytotoxicity will be discussed in later chapters, but the importance of general immune competence in relation to cancer is discussed here.

It is not easy to review the current situation of research into general immune competence in cancer, because there is rarely concordance of results within the immense amount of work that is being carried out in this field. In many cases, it is possible to identify reasons for this lack of concordance, for example, immune competence varies with such factors as the site or extent of the cancer and may be influenced by different treatment modalities. Hence, the results of immune competence testing can only be considered as meaningful if the following criteria are met:

(i) The patients should be studied in homogeneous groups with regard to tumour site and stage.

(ii) Testing should have been completed before any form of therapy is undertaken (unless the effects of specific forms of therapy are being studied).

(iii) Where cancer groups are being compared to control groups, the control groups should be carefully selected in relation to age, sex, general health and disease status.

In fact there are very few studies which conform to these basic requirements, so many of the discrepancies in the literature can be attributed to the heterogeneity of the patients studied.

What, then, is the state of immune competence in cancer patients? Particularly in the case of tests of cellular immunity, depression is usually found in late stages of the disease. The situation with early cancer is less clear-cut, and many studies have shown no depression before the onset of dissemination. More recent studies of large homogeneous series of patients with cancer of different sites have shown that the amount of depression varies with different types of tumours, as well as being stage-related in some cases. The results of DNCB and Mantoux testing for different stages of cancer of three different sites, breast, stomach, and colon are shown in Table 4.3 (Bolton *et al.*, 1975). Control groups were chosen to conform to

Table 4.3 Mantoux and DNCB response grades in patients with cancer of the breast, stomach and colon

Patient group	Number	Mantoux test grade				DNCB response grade			
		0	1	2	3	0	1	2	3
Breast control	34	33%	9%	36%	21%	9%	0%	21%	70%
Breast cancer	174	44%	19%	27%	10%	19%	12%	34·5%	34·5%
GIT control	47	36%	19%	34%	11%	19%	21%	28%	32%
Colon cancer	40	72·5%	10%	15%	2·5%	60%	10%	27·5%	2·5%
Stomach cancer	45	58%	11%	20%	11%	59%	26%	10%	5%

the above criteria by choosing patients who were suspected on clinical grounds of having cancer of the breast or gastrointestinal tract respectively, but who were subsequently found to have benign disease. In each case Grade 0 is a negative response and Grade 3 a maximal response.

From these results one can draw the following conclusions. Cancer patients as a whole show depression of cellular immunity when compared with an appropriate control group (benign breast lumps for breast cancer and conditions requiring surgery such as peptic ulcer or diverticulitis, in the case of gastrointestinal cancer). The change is very obvious in the case of colon cancer, less marked with stomach cancer and least with breast cancer. In fact with this latter group, the difference is not significant on the basis of simple negative or positive reactions, but becomes so when grade of response is taken into account.

Of interest is the comparison of 'breast' controls with 'gastrointestinal' controls, since the response to the latter is significantly poorer than the former. In fact the overall response with the gastrointestinal *control* group is much the same as that of the breast *cancer* group. This underlines the need to use appropriate control groups, and also suggests that general 'ill-health' will have some effect on cellular immunity.

In all cases DNCB responses show a greater depression than do the Mantoux reactions, suggesting that DNCB is a better means of assessing cellular immunity, but the differences are not great.

The breakdown according to tumour stage (based on Dukes' classification for colorectal cancer) is given in Table 4.4. From these figures, the

Table 4.4 Mantoux and DNCB response grades of comparable tumour stages in relation to site

Stage and site	Number	Mantoux test grade				DNCB test grade			
		0	1	2	3	0	1	2	3
Stages A and B									
Breast	80	39%	24%	27%	10%	14%	9%	40%	37%
Colon	18	72%	6%	22%	0%	56%	11%	33%	0%
Stomach	9	45%	0%	22%	33%	37·5%	25%	12·5%	25%
Stage C									
Breast	70	44%	16%	31%	9%	14%	10%	39%	37%
Colon	11	82%	9%	0%	9%	46%	18%	27%	9%
Stomach	10	50%	30%	10%	10%	78%	22%	0%	0%
Stage D									
Breast	24	65%	13%	9%	13%	50%	29%	4%	17%
Colon	11	64%	18%	18%	0%	82%	0%	18%	0%
Stomach	26	65%	8%	23%	4%	59%	27%	15%	0%

Stage A = Early local disease   Stage C = Lymph node metastases
Stage B = Advanced local disease   Stage D = Distant metastases

following facts emerge. Stage for stage, the changes are the same as seen in the total group, that is, colon cancer shows the greatest depression, breast cancer the least and gastric cancer lies between these two. However, interesting and important variations are seen within the individual cancer groups. In the case of colon cancer, all stages show significant depression as compared to controls, and while there is a trend toward increasing depression with more advanced tumours, the depression is so marked in early tumours (Dukes A and B) that these are not significantly less depressed than the more advanced groups.

Cancer of the stomach behaves differently. While the Mantoux tests show a clear trend toward diminished response with more advanced tumour, the DNCB results differ, patients with disseminated disease having a lower negative rate than patients with lymph node metastases. While numbers in this group are small, the much larger group of breast cancer patients shows clearly a pattern different from the early colon patients. The larger number of cases allows the series to be subdivided further, as shown in Table 4.5. The Stage C cases (with lymph node metastases) fall into two main groups on clinical grounds—small tumours with lymph node metastases (Manchester Stage 2 or $T_{1-2}N_1M_0$) usually treated by surgery, and larger primary tumours (Manchester Stage 3 or $T_{3-4}N_{1-3}M_0$) usually treated by radiotherapy.

Table 4.5 Mantoux and DNCB response grades in relation to breast cancer stage

Stage	Number	Mantoux test grade				DNCB test grade			
		0	I	2	3	0	I	2	3
A	55	36%	25·5%	25·5%	13%	16·5%	7·5%	38%	38%
B	25	44%	20%	32%	4%	8%	12%	44%	36%
C_1	31	42%	19%	29%	10%	26%	10%	42%	22%
C_2	39	46%	13%	33%	8%	5%	10%	36%	49%
D	24	65%	13%	9%	13%	50%	29%	4%	17%
Total	174	44%	19%	27%	10%	19%	12%	34·5%	34·5%
Control breasts	34	33%	9%	36%	21%	9%	0%	21%	70%

For descriptions of Stages C_1 and C_2 see text

While patients with disseminated disease show the greatest depression, those patients with advanced local disease (Stage B and C_2 equivalent to Stage 3 Manchester) have normal responses, and in fact these cases of local advanced disease have a significantly better immune response than the early (Manchester Stage 1 and 2) cases. It is not easy to explain this paradoxical finding, but one suggestion would be that a good immune response has allowed control of dissemination while not able to prevent continued local growth of the primary tumour. The greater depression of immune competence in the early breast cancer cases might be explained by the fact that some of these will already have disseminated cancer, although not clinically obvious because it is still microscopic. Whatever the explanation, these findings are so clear-cut that they cannot be dismissed as due to chance, and it seems that these differences between small and large breast cancers and between breast and colon cancer, must reflect some facet of the biological processes in the host–tumour interrelationship, which are at present not understood. It is of interest that the Mantoux responses do not parallel those of the DNCB test, for the B and C_2 patients show a progressive decrease in Mantoux response.

The related test of PHA responsiveness of lymphocytes (as measured by the dose–response micromethod) is shown in Figure 4.8.

In this study which included both treated and untreated patients at various stages of the disease process, the patient groups have been determined by expected prognosis, taking into account such features as pathology, extent of disease and response to treatment. It can be seen that PHA response shows a direct correlation with expected prognosis and so bears a closer similarity to the Mantoux response than to the DNCB response.

While this depression of immune competence in common surgical solid tumours is of only moderate degree, reports are unanimous that a much greater depression is seen in lymphoreticular malignancies such as Hodgkin's disease and lymphatic leukaemia, though considerable restoration of immunity may occur in response to treatment.

Aspects of immunity other than cellular immune responses have been less well investigated. The circulating antibody response to an antigen such as tetanus toxoid has been shown to be normal in most cases, although some depression is seen in patients with advanced malignancy—depression which is greater than that seen in patients with non-malignant disease with a corresponding degree of general debility (Lytton et al., 1964). Considerable interest has recently been shown in the measurement of serum immunoglobulins, though most reports have been of heterogeneous groups of patients with many types of tumours at all stages of the disease and without always allowing for different types of treatment. Having measured levels of immunoglobulins in groups of cancer patients, it must be realized that serum levels reflect the interaction of immunoglobulin production and destruction, and again may not reflect the concentration throughout the body. In addition, any antibody specific to a cancer antigen—with either cytotoxic or blocking activity—might be expected to comprise a small proportion of the total immunoglobulins, so that considerable changes in specific antibody might occur without being reflected in total immunoglobulin levels, particularly on random sampling. At the same time nonspecific depression of immunoglobulin synthesis might well have a secondary effect on production of specific antitumour antibodies, and such an overall depression of immunoglobulins could be expected to be reflected in serum immunoglobulin levels. One of the largest studies of a homogeneous group has been that of Hughes (1971) who included 127 patients with colorectal cancer in his large study. He found no difference in the mean IgG and IgM levels between cancer and normal controls. He found an increase in IgA in the cancer group, with a sex difference, females showing higher levels than males. Our own results in carcinoma of the colon have been similar although we have also found the serum IgM level to be raised in cancer patients, being highest in those patients with widespread metastases. An interesting finding has been that serum IgM levels are raised postoperatively in both the cancer patients and the controls suggesting a non-specific effect of surgery on serum IgM levels which may be prolonged for up to 1 year.

The monocyte–macrophage system has been extensively investigated by means of the clearance of isotope labelled colloidal particles from the bloodstream by hepatic sinusoidal macrophages. Baum *et al.* (1973) investigated macrophage activity in patients with breast cancer. They found that mean phagocytic activity in patients with localized disease was significantly higher than in those with dissemination. There also appeared to be a linear correlation between tumour size and phagocytic activity when the disease was localized, but this relationship was lost when the disease became disseminated.

WHAT IS THE CAUSE OF THE IMMUNODEPRESSION?

Perhaps the most important aspect of this whole problem is the cause of the immunodepression—since only when the cause is known is it likely that some method of removing the depression will be discovered.

Several possibilities must be considered when seeking the basic causes of the immunodepression seen in cancer patients. The first is that the depression precedes the development of the tumour—and indeed might be responsible for it as suggested by Burnet (1969) in his hypothesis of immune surveillance. If this were so, the immune suppression might be genetically determined or could be transient due to a temporary cause such as a viral infection. It is unlikely that established incompetence of the immune system is the cause of cancer, since depression is minimal or absent in the earliest stages and becomes more marked as the disease advances. On the other hand, evidence is strong that some cases do arise in this way, since there are a number of immune deficiency states which are undoubtedly associated with an increased incidence of cancer. The development of skin cancer in transplant patients on prolonged immunosuppression is an obvious (and surgically important) example (Marshall, 1974).

The next possibility is that the immunodepression is due to the tumour—either the tumour itself or to the secondary effects of the tumour on the general state of the patient. In tumours which result in malnutrition, such as cancer of the oesophagus or stomach, the secondary effects of the tumour must play some part since it is well known that protein calorie malnutrition results in immunodepression. It is equally clear that this is not the sole cause for depression, since stage for stage, gastric cancer produces less depression than colon cancer, while being responsible in general for a much greater degree of malnutrition. One is left with the clear implication that the tumour itself (that is, apart from any secondary effects due to malnutrition) is in some way responsible for at least part of the depression and that the proclivity for producing such a depression varies with different types of tumours, being greater with colonic tumours than breast carcinoma or gastric cancer. The actual bulk of tumour does not seem to bear a direct relation to depression even though a more advanced tumour is likely to be associated with a greater degree of depression.

Just how the tumour can produce immunodepression is the source of much controversy. The most widely held belief is that the tumour produces a lymphocyte depressing serum factor—perhaps a tumour antigen or antibody—which either coats the surface of the lymphocyte or can be taken up by the lymphocyte and interfere with its metabolic activity. A factor coating the surface might mask the antigen receptor mechanism of the lymphocyte cell surface, or might make the lymphocyte more susceptible to destruction by some autoimmune mechanism. The possibilities are legion and the evidence in favour of any one is insubstantial at the present time.

In summary, present evidence suggests that the cause of the depression of lymphocyte function is probably multifactorial. It is likely that at least three factors play some part—pre-existing immunodepression, a direct effect of the tumour itself, and the secondary effects of factors such as malnutrition.

CAN THE IMMUNODEPRESSION BE REVERSED?

To the surgeon concerned with patients, this question is as important as the cause of the depression. As with all other aspects of this subject, the situation is unclear at present and the evidence available is insubstantial.

The first question is whether immunodepression recovers spontaneously on 'complete' removal of the tumour. Analysis of the evidence relating to this is hampered by the fact that one cannot assess the completeness of tumour removal except by prolonged follow-up, and such long-term studies have not yet been reported. Our own experience is that some patients do show spontaneous recovery of dermal delayed sensitivity reactions after operation and that these patients tend to have a good prognosis. More commonly, the preoperative situation persists in the postoperative period, irrespective of the likely outcome of the disease. The paper of McIllmurray et al. (1973) has already received comment.

Given a state of persistent immunodepression, there are many possible ways of attempting to reverse it. At present none of them have been shown to be of proven efficacy in the clinical situation. Examples are attempts to remove 'serum factors' by plasmaphoresis or by enzymatic activity (e.g. with streptokinase); to stimulate greater immune activity by substances like C. parvum or BCG vaccine, and to use empirically some drugs that are thought to be able to reverse immunodepression. An example of the latter group at present under investigation is the antihelminthic drug tetramizole. Much work is in progress on the effects of 'transfer factor' and thymic hormones on reversal of depressed lymphocytic function. Yet another approach is to see whether immunity can be improved by reversing protein/calorie deficiency in gastric cancer, using parenteral nutrition. Present results do not suggest that this approach is effective.

IS GENERAL IMMUNE STATUS RELATED TO PROGNOSIS?

This is not easy to determine from current reports in the literature, since the only way in which a definitive answer to this question can be obtained is by following individual patients until the time of recurrence of their tumour. No comprehensive study of this nature has yet been reported. In patients with advanced cancer, particularly of the head and neck, it has been shown that the inability to produce a DNCB response is usually associated with a poor prognosis but the converse is not necessarily true, since many patients maintain a strong positive reaction right to the time of death. This is particularly true of the patients with breast cancer and melanoma. A final answer to this question should be available in 5 or 6 years time, as current studies progress.

WHAT IS THE EFFECT OF CANCER TREATMENT ON IMMUNE STATUS?

All three common modalities of treating cancer—surgery, radiotherapy and chemotherapy—have been shown to have some depressant effect on immunity.

Surgery

The effect of surgery has been studied most widely in relation to depression of lymphocyte stimulation by phytohaemagglutinin and most studies have shown that even minor operations cause depression of lymphocyte response up to 7 days postoperatively (Berenbaum et al., 1973) with a greater degree of depression from more major operations. In general, it appears that depression has returned to normal within a week or two of operation. Resection of a tumour may also result in a reversal of preoperative immunodepression. McIllmurray et al. (1973) showed this in the case of colon cancer, using the PHA technique as the index of immunity. The situation with skin tests is less clear-cut, and in particular it would seem that surgery has little effect on the DNCB reaction, providing the patient has been sensitized prior to operation. It is quite likely, although not definitely documented, that sensitization is diminished where this is carried out in the immediate postoperative period, and for this reason it is important that all testing be completed prior to surgery.

Little is known of the effect of surgery on other aspects of the immune response. Serum immunoglobulin levels may be affected by surgery, and we have recently shown that serum IgA and IgM levels are raised for long periods—up to 1 year—after colonic resection. The significance of this is not apparent at present.

Radiotherapy

Radiation is known to have profound effects on immunity in the experimental situation, and there is growing evidence that clinical radiotherapy may have significant effects. Stjernswärd *et al.* (1972) reported a persistent lymphopenia after postoperative radiotherapy in patients with breast cancer, with the decrease particularly affecting the T lymphocytes. This depression persisted for up to a year. Possible mechanisms include direct irradiation of lymphocytes flowing through the large vessels during the period of irradiation, thymic irradiation or the development of a serum factor resulting in the destruction of T cells. A similar effect on PHA transformation of lymphocytes is seen after radiotherapy for lung cancer (Braeman and Deeley, 1972) though here most patients showed recovery to pretreatment levels by 6 months.

Chemotherapy

The effect of antineoplastic drugs on immune competence in human cancer patients is poorly understood, and it is difficult to assess the amount of immunosuppression due to treatment in patients with an existing defect of cellular immunity due to their disease. Improvement in a patient's condition may mask depression due to the therapy, and deterioration may exaggerate it.

A large group of patients having combination chemotherapy have been studied in our department (K. D. Jones).* In general it is found that the immunosuppression resulting from a standard intermittent quadruple chemotherapy regime is of only slight to moderate degree, and our experience with breast and gastrointestinal cancers is summarized below.

Lymphocyte numbers: The majority of advanced cancer patients are lymphopenic. Chemotherapy causes further reduction of lymphocyte numbers irrespective of clinical response.

B and T cell proportions: All the patients we have studied have had severely reduced T cell and increased null-cell percentages before treatment. Chemotherapy has had little significant effect on either B or T cells. After 2 months there tends to be a steady fall-off of T cells with concomitant rise in B cells. Inversion of B–T ratio occurs between the 4th and 6th months of treatment. However, some patients have been encountered who maintained virtually normal values for over a year while on chemotherapy. Recovery begins within 3 months of cessation of treatment.

Serum immunoglobulins: No significant changes have been found in any

* Personal communication.

of the immunoglobulin subclasses over periods up to 18 months.

PHA transformation: Our patients with advanced disease usually have severe impairment of lymphocyte PHA responses. Some improvement may accompany improved clinical status, and *vice versa*, provided the concentration of cells in culture is adjusted to a constant value, and is not dependent upon the circulating lymphocyte numbers, in which case depression of the PHA response is more likely to be seen after chemotherapy. However, even in those patients maintaining 'remission' over long periods, we have found progressive depression of PHA responses after approximately 6 months of treatment.

Delayed hypersensitivity skin tests: Few chemotherapy patients have altered their sensitivity to either DNCB or Mantoux and there have been as many increased responses as decreased ones in our series.

WHAT IS THE POTENTIAL PRACTICAL SIGNIFICANCE OF ASSESSMENT OF IMMUNE COMPETENCE?

Knowledge of immune competence of cancer patients could have a number of possible practical advantages in the management of patients with cancer.

(i) It is possible that immune competence testing could be helpful in the differential diagnosis of benign from malignant conditions. An example is differentiating carcinoma of the colon from diverticulitis where a strong positive DNCB and Mantoux reaction would make the diagnosis of colon cancer unlikely. Similarly, knowledge of immune status might suggest that the tumour is at a more advanced stage than is clinically apparent, for instance depressed immunity in breast cancer or melanoma would suggest dissemination (although the converse is not true, since with these malignancies a strongly positive skin test may be maintained in the presence of advanced disease).

Whether immune competence will prove to have clinical usefulness in this way is the subject of many studies at present, and only long-term follow-up of individual patients will provide the answers. At present it seems that they will only give general guidance in certain situations, and it seems unlikely that they will ever have absolute diagnostic or prognostic accuracy.

(ii) Of more practical importance in relation to prognosis is the possibility of delineating a poor prognosis group which may be used as an indication for adjuvant therapy at an early stage of patient treatment, before overt and extensive dissemination has occurred. At present this seems a more realistic proposition than the previous one. Its true place will be dependent not only on the accuracy with which one can predict a poor prognosis group, but rest on the development of efficacious modalities of adjuvant therapy. Trials of both chemotherapy and immunotherapy are at present under way in this situation.

(iii) Studying the effect of different therapeutic modalities on immune competence will allow the choice of a regime which will have an optimal anti-tumour effect with minimal immunosuppressive activity. It is known that different chemotherapeutic agents affect immune competence not only to different degrees but in quite different ways. Similarly, more detailed studies of various types and regimes of radiotherapy may show one to have an advantage over another in relation to immunosuppressive effect. In the case of surgery, should the present long-term studies of the relationship between immune competence and tumour prognosis show immunity to be of importance, then the relative merits of conservative and radical surgery for cancer will also need to be studied in this light.

(iv) Measurement of immune competence should be an obligatory part of all trials of non-specific immunotherapy, such as those using BCG or *C. parvum*. At present such trials are speculative and it is important that data available in animal systems should be confirmed by careful monitoring of immune response in any clinical trials. Similar considerations apply to specific immunotherapy since any favourable response to this form of treatment must obviously depend on the ability of the patient to produce an immune response. Here it is important to monitor specific immunity—e.g. by cytotoxicity or by the leucocyte migration test—as well as general immune competence.

(v) Even more speculative is the possibility of reducing the incidence of cancer by immunoprophylaxis—that is, giving an intermittent boost to general immune competence in an effort to maximize immune surveillance against incipient neoplasms. It has been suggested that the incidence of leukaemia is less in children who have been immunized with BCG. On the other hand, a large prospective survey of patients over some 20 years showed no differences in the incidence of cancer between patients who were Mantoux-negative and Mantoux-positive.

Immune Competence in Relation to Other Surgical Diseases

Much work has been done on the relation of immune competence to transplantation and especially in looking for means of controlling the dosage of immunosuppressive agents by their effect on immune competence—since the minimum dosage necessary to prevent graft rejection would be the desirable dosage. Unfortunately such tests have not proved very satisfactory in practice, and this question is dealt with in the chapters on transplantation.

An interesting possibility is that variations in immune competence may play some part in the aetiology of disease processes. A classical example is leprosy, where the pattern of disease, lepromatous or tuberculoid, seems to be directly related to the allergic status of the patient. At present little is known about the nature of the immune deficiency which allows the severe lepromatous form to develop and both genetic and acquired bases for the deficiency have been put forward. Similarly, much of the tissue damage seen in caseating tuberculosis or tertiary syphilis is probably due more to allergy than to the effects of the micro-organisms.

At the present time one can only speculate on this question, but an interesting example is Crohn's disease. This condition has many features suggesting that an immune element is important in the disease although all attempts to elucidate its aetiology have so far failed. It is possible that a tendency—either inherited or acquired—to react to an antigen preferentially by a particular immune mechanism, or combination of immune mechanisms, might produce the local pathological reactions to an otherwise innocuous antigen. Greater understanding of immune processes may well increase the number of conditions associated with aberrant immune responses, providing explanations for otherwise obscure surgical conditions.

Finally, it has long been believed by many workers that the small lymphocyte has a trophic as well as an immunological function (Loutit, 1962) and so may be important in the general nutrition of tissues. If this is true, the maintenance of immune function may well have much wider implications for resistance to disease than has been considered heretofore.

Perhaps the most striking example of this concept comes from the work of Roberts-Thomson et al. (1974), who compared cellular immune competence (employing a variety of tests) in healthy patients under the age of 20 and in patients over the age of 60. They confirmed previous work showing that all aspects of cellular immune competence studied (recall delayed hypersensitivity skin responses, PHA stimulation and late IgG response to flagellin) were significantly depressed in the older groups—a factor which is frequently ignored in clinical studies of cellular immunity. Of particular interest was the fact that mortality in a group of patients over the age of 80 years was significantly greater over a period of 2 years if they were hyporesponsive to the immune testing compared with those showing a normal response. The excess of deaths was due to bronchopneumonia, cerebrovascular accident and cardiac failure, and no deaths were due to cancer.

These concepts of a much broader significance of lymphocyte function than those usually associated with the strict definition of immune processes is one which awaits investigation in the surgical sphere. If this chapter needs to be rewritten in 10 years' time, cancer may lose its pre-eminence in the discussion in favour of general resistance to all disease.

References

Aisenberg, A. C. (1962). Studies on delayed hypersensitivity in Hodgkin's disease. *J. Clin. Invest.*, **41**, 1964

Anthony, H. M., Templeman, G. H., Madsen, K. E. and Mason, M. K. (1974). The prognostic significance of D.H.S. skin tests on patients with carcinoma of the bronchus. *Cancer*, **34**, 1901

Anthony, H. M., Kirk, J. A., Madsen, K. E., Mason, M. K. and Templeman, G. H. (1975). E and EAC rosetting lymphocytes in patients with carcinoma of the bronchus. I. Some parameters of the test and its prognostic significance. *Clin. Exp. Immunol.*, **20**, 29

Baum, M., Sumner, D., Edwards, M. H. and Smythe, P. (1973). Macrophage phagocytic activity in patients with breast cancer. *Br. J. Surg.*, **60**, 899

Berenbaum, M. C., Fluck, P. A. and Hurst, N. P. (1973). Depression of lymphocyte responses after surgical trauma. *Br. J. Exp. Pathol.*, **54**, 597

Black, M. M. and Leis, H. P. (1971). Cellular responses to autologous breast cancer tissue. Correlation with stage and lymphoreticuloendothelial reactivity. *Cancer*, **28**, 263

Bolton, P. M., Mander, A. M., Davidson, J. M., James, S. L., Newcombe, R. G. and Hughes, L. E. (1975). Cellular immunity in cancer: comparison of delayed hypersensitivity skin tests in three common cancers. *Br. Med. J.*, **iii**, 18

Braeman, J. and Deeley, T. J. (1972). Immunological studies in irradiation of lung cancer. *Ann. Clin. Res.*, **4**, 355

Brown, G. and Greaves, M. F. (1974) Cell surface markers for human T and B lymphocytes. *Eur. J. Immunol.*, **4**, 302

Burnet, F. M. (1969). *Self and Non-self.* (Cambridge: University Press)

Cochran, A. J., Spilg, W. G. S., Mackie, R. M. and Thomas, C. E. (1972). Post-operative depression of tumour-directed cell-mediated immunity in patients with malignant disease. *Br. Med. J.*, **iv**, 67

Greaves, M. F., Owen, J. J. T. and Rath, M. C. (1973). T and B lymphocytes: their origins, properties and roles in immune responses. (Amsterdam: Associated Scientific Publishers)

Halliday, W. J. and Miller, S. (1972). Leukocyte adherence inhibition: a simple test for cell-mediated tumour immunity and serum blocking factors. *Int. J. Cancer*, **9**, 477

Hellström, I., Hellström, K. E., Sjögren, H. O. and Warner, G. A. (1971). Demonstration of cell-mediated immunity to human neoplasms of various histological types. *Int. J. Cancer*, **7**, 1

Hughes, L. E. and Lytton, B. (1964). Antigenic properties of human tumours: delayed cutaneous hypersensitivity reactions. *Br. Med. J.*, **i**, 209

Hughes, N. R. (1971). Serum concentrations of gamma G, gamma A and gamma M immunoglobulins in patients with carcinoma, melanoma and sarcoma. *J. Natl. Cancer Inst.*, **46**, 1015

Loutit, J. F. (1962). Immunological and trophic functions of lymphocytes. *Lancet*, **ii**, 1106

Lytton, B., Hughes, L. E. and Fulthrope, A. J. (1964). Circulating antibody response in malignant disease. *Lancet*, **i**, 69

Marshall, V. (1974) Premalignant and malignant skin tumours in immunosuppressed patients. *Transplantation*, **17**, 272

McIllmurray, M. B., Gray, M. and Langman, M. J. S. (1973). Phytohaemagglutinin-induced lymphocyte transformation in patients before and after resection of large intestinal cancer. *Gut*, **14,** 541

Niklasson, P. M. and Williams, R. C. (1974). Studies of peripheral blood T and B lymphocytes in acute infections. *Infect. Immun.*, **9,** 1

Nind, A. P. P., Nairn, R. C., Rolland, J. M., Guli, E. P. G. and Hughes, E. S. R. (1973). Lymphocyte anergy in patients with carcinoma. *Br. J. Cancer*, **28,** 108

Perlmann, P., Perlmann, H. and Wigzell, H. (1972). Lymphocyte mediated cytotoxicity *in vitro*: induction and inhibition by humoral antibody and nature of effector cells. *Transplant. Rev.*, **13,** 91

Pollack, S., Heppner, G., Brawn, R. J. and Nelson, K. (1972). Specific killing of tumour cells *in vitro* in the presence of normal lymphoid cells and sera from hosts immune to the tumour antigens. *Int. J. Cancer*, **9,** 316

Roberts-Thomson, I. C., Whittingham, S., Youngchaiyud, U. and Mackay, I. R. (1974). Aging, immune response and mortality. *Lancet*, **ii,** 368

Rowley, M. J. and Mackay, I. R. (1969). Measurement of antibody capacity in man. I. The normal response to flagellin from *S. adelaide. Clin. Exp. Immunol.*, **5,** 407

Skinner, J. M., Campbell, A. C., Waller, C., Wood, J. and MacLennan, I. C. N. (1974). Immunosuppressive consequences of the treatment of ulcerative colitis with azio-thioprine. *Gut*, **15,** 828

Steel, C. M., Evans, J. and Smith, M. A. (1974). Physiological variation in circulating B cell:T cell ratio in man. *Nature (London)*, **247,** 387

Stjernswärd, J., Jondal, M., Vanky, F., Wigzell, H. and Sealy, R. (1972). Lymphopenia and change in distribution of human B and T lymphocytes in peripheral blood induced by irradiation for mammary carcinoma. *Lancet*, **i,** 1352

Ting, A. and Terasaki, P. I. (1974). Depressed lymphocyte-mediated killing of sensitized targets in cancer patients. *Cancer Res.*, **34,** 2694

Vanky, F., Stjernswärd, J., Klein, G. and Nilsonne, U. (1971). Serum-mediated inhibition of lymphocyte stimulation by autochthonous human tumours. *J. Natl. Cancer Inst.*, **47,** 95

Whitehead, R. H. (1973). Fluorescent antibody studies in malignant melanoma. *Br J. Cancer*, **28,** 325

Whitehead, R. H., Bolton, P. M., James, S. L. and Roberts, G. M. (1974). An *in vitro* method for assaying sensitivity to 2,4-dinitrochlorobenzene (DNCB) in man. *Eur. J. Cancer*, **10,** 721

Whitehead, R. H., Bolton, P. M., Newcombe, R. G., James, S. L. and Hughes, L. E. (1975). Lymphocyte response to PHA in breast cancer: correlation of predicted prognosis to response to different PHA concentrations. *Clin. Oncol.*, **1,** 191

WHO/IARC Workshop (1974). Identification, enumeration and isolation of B and T lymphocytes from human peripheral blood. *Scand. J. Immunol.*, **3,** 521

Further Reading

Asherson, G. L. (1972). The development of lymphocyte function tests. *Br. J. Hosp. Med.*, **8,** 665

Bloom, B. R. and Glade, P. R. (eds.) (1971). *In vitro* methods in cell-mediated immunity. (New York and London: Academic Press)

Harris, J. E., Bagai, R. C. and Stewart, T. H. M. (1973). Serial monitoring of immune reactivity in cancer patients receiving chemotherapy as a means of predicting anti-tumour responses. In sixth *Leucocyte Culture Congress 1972 Proceedings*, p. 443. (New York: Academic Press)

Kersey, J. H., Spector, B. D. and Good, R. A. (1973). Immunodeficiency and cancer. *Adv. Cancer Res.*, **18**, 211

Levy, M. H. and Wheelock, E. F. (1974). The role of macrophages in defense against neoplastic disease. *Adv. Cancer Res.*, **20**, 131

Lobuglio, A. L. (1973). The monocyte—new concepts of function. *N. Engl. J. Med.*, **288**, 212

Magarey, C. J. (1972). The control of cancer spread by the reticuloendothelial system. *Ann. R. Coll. Surg.*, **50**, 238

Sinkovics, J. G. (1973). Monitoring *in vitro* of cell-mediated immune reactions to tumours. *Method Cancer Res.*, **8**, 107

CHAPTER 5

Immunodiagnosis and Prognosis

D. J. R. Laurence and A. M. Neville

Introduction

The doings of surgery are visible and manifest, while the ways of immunology are obscure. If the surgeon is to be helped as a result of immunological testing, it is essential that the scope and limitations of any test procedures should be well defined. In this chapter we have analysed the established methods and current trends in assisting with the diagnosis and prognosis of human tumours. We have left aside those tests that are of value in other diseases although progress is also being made in this direction.

Before discussing the methods available and their applications, the broad outlines will be considered, giving the requirements for diagnosis and prognosis on the one hand, and the immunological methods that are available on the other. The details of individual assays are described to illustrate the development that has occurred in this area. Most of the tests considered measure peptide and protein markers, and the assays for small molecules, such as steroids and prostaglandins, have not been included.

Requirements for Diagnosis and Prognosis

THE DETECTION OF CANCER

A general test for cancer would distinguish any individual with a tumour from an individual with no disease or with a non-malignant pathology. The tumour should be detectable preclinically as well as in patients presenting with symptoms. If such a test were available, there would also be an urgent need for other criteria to locate the tumour and define it further. Fortunately, some partial solutions to this latter problem already exist and are discussed in this chapter.

The inference of tumour type or location

The cancer test may detect a wide range of tumour types but have practical application to only a few (e.g. the CEA test, page 167). It may be influenced either by the tumour type and therefore help to define the tissues of origin of the tumour or by the site to which the tumour has spread. Both tests are potentially useful but interpretation may be complicated by some common tumours (e.g. lung and breast) secreting substances that are not typical of the tissue of origin (ectopic secretion).

Discrimination between different tumours of the same organ

If a tumour is known to be present at a given site, the test could distinguish between different types, for example, a seminoma and teratoma of the testis (the AFP test) or medullary and follicular thyroid cancer (the calcitonin test, page 160).

Differential diagnosis of benign and malignant growth or malignancy and inflammation

It is required to distinguish between a benign or malignant lump in the breast, or between pancreatic cancer and pancreatitis.

Population screens

There is no immunological method that is at present suitable for screening the general population. A more limited screen of populations at risk may be practicable, e.g. the elderly, patients with minimal symptoms, individuals with a family history of one of the rare familial cancers or individuals who have been exposed to carcinogens.

PROGNOSIS

Immunological tests may show whether the tumour is capable of making the typical products of the tissue of origin or is committed to synthesize other products. This can supplement classical histological examinations which reveal the state of differentiation of the tumour.

Follow-up

Another aspect of prognosis is to establish the extent of tumour spread and whether residual tumour remains after surgery or other treatments. Excision gives an immediate and measurable decrease in tumour mass, and this may correlate with quantitative immunological testing. If a relationship is found the test can be used to measure tumour mass at other times.

The more difficult problem is to detect very small tumours that are on the borderline where treatment is needed or where the body's normal defences might effect a cure.

CHOICE OF TREATMENT

A useful function may be served even if the tests indicate that surgery would serve no useful purpose or that other forms of treatment are unlikely to be useful with present knowledge and techniques. A test that has failed in other respects may still be useful in avoiding an unnecessary operation, or help to decide against a form of treatment that is unlikely to be helpful.

APPLICATIONS IN COMBINATION WITH OTHER METHODS

As immunological testing is a junior partner within the range of diagnostic and prognostic procedures, the methods are unlikely to be used without support from other techniques. They are best combined with other objective methods of assessment both in testing their value and in aiding the patient.

Theoretical objectives

The methods may have long-term benefit in throwing light on the development of cancer, its initiation and subclinical history.

Studies using animal models have revealed that the high antigenicity of tumours may be the result of induction by a single large dose of a carcinogen. When the carcinogen is given in a number of small doses the tumours are less antigenic and more like their human counterparts. In studies using liver carcinogens the AFP test (page 169) has revealed increased AFP production at the time of application of the carcinogen, followed by a decline during the induction phase until the gross development of hepatoma, when the levels again begin to rise.

It is possible to use the immunoglobulin level as a measure of tumour mass in patients with multiple myeloma (Chapter 2). By backward extrapolation and assuming a constant doubling time for the growth of the tumour, it has been suggested that the tumour originates 20–35 years before it becomes clinically manifest.

Immunological Testing

Immunological testing of patients has two broad divisions, (a) tests made on the patients own immune system and (b) tests made with immune reagents obtained by active immunization of other animal species, or in some cases from other patients.

In either case the second component of the immune reaction, namely the antigen, will be of human origin or at least equivalent to a human product.

TESTS WITH THE PATIENT'S OWN IMMUNE SYSTEM

This is an attractive possibility for two main reasons. Firstly the immune system may be expected to contain information that relates to the patient's disease. Secondly, the immune system may be important in assisting cure of the patient when the bulk of the tumour has been removed by surgery or other means. By measuring the immune response it may be possible to predict those patients able to derive most benefit from a given form of therapy. Although it seems very likely that immune mechanisms do act against autochthonous tumours with beneficial results in some cases, it is difficult to translate the effect into practical laboratory tests. One problem is that if immune surveillance operates to eliminate incipient tumours the tumour-free individual may have an immune system already primed to tumour products.

TESTS WITH IMMUNE REAGENTS

These are well-established procedures which are presently undergoing the proliferation of all successful technologies. The success of the reagents depends upon the remarkable specificity and high affinity of an antibody towards the eliciting immunogen. There is a corresponding specificity and sensitivity in the resulting assay procedure. Even when the test system uses cellular immunity initial recognition of the antigen depends upon combination with an immunoglobulin receptor on the cell surface.

In order to exploit the full sensitivity of an assay, radioisotopes are used as indicators during the read-out of the test system. With certain tests it is an advantage to use them with a deliberately reduced sensitivity in order to improve their discrimination at a clinical level.

However, the specificity of antibodies, although great, is not absolute, for it depends on the arrangement of interactive groupings in the binding site of the reagent molecule. Even very non-specific effects can give incorrect results if the test system is not properly controlled.

NATURE OF THE ANTIGENIC COMPONENT

The substances used to test the patient's immune response are assumed to be antigens and, if the reaction is specific this adds weight to the supposition. With the tests using reagents developed in other species the use of the term antigen is in many cases redundant as there are now methods by which most organic substances can be made immunogenic. However, the term is still retained as it has value in the descriptions of methods.

Requirements for Tests

Certain general problems arise in attempting to relate the problems of diagnosis and prognosis with the methods available for immunological testing.

GENERAL TEST FOR CANCER

If such a test can be obtained there must be a special feature of malignant tissue that distinguishes malignancy from all other conditions. There could be a specific 'oncogene' in cells whose activation is required in order to create malignancy. Any typical product of this gene could be a marker substance for all cancer. If malignant tumours are due to one or to a limited group of oncogenic viruses the viral antigens could provide such a test. Although such possibilities have been suggested there is no proof that they occur. In a more general way a specific tumour product could be a consequence of the development of malignancy by whatever cause; possibly as a result of a multifactorial process. If the mechanism expressed itself at the cell surface or as a substance shed into the body fluids a cancer test might result. The substance tested could be a new product only present in malignancy or an incomplete synthesis of a normal product. Examples of these two possibilities might be the cancer basic protein (page 144) and the incompletion hypothesis of Hakomori (1975) which showed that tumour cells can fail to complete their surface glycolipid carbohydrate sequences, so leading to development of new antigenic sites. A change in chemical composition of the external surface of the tumour cell is not essential, for a new structure could result merely from rearrangement with exposure of new antigenic sites.

INAPPROPRIATE PRODUCTION OF NORMAL SUBSTANCES

The tests for specific tumour-types and those of broad specificity depend in many cases on the observations of normal body constituents. Detection of a tumour requires either the presence of an abnormal modification of the normal substance or an inappropriate level of it, but with hormone markers definition of such a level requires consideration of the concentration of those substances that normally control the level (e.g. glucose for insulin, calcium for parathyroid hormone, etc.). Even a normal measurement of the hormone would be inappropriate if the control substances were themselves abnormal. Failure of normal control could be due to the absence of normal receptors or storage facilities in the tumour cells.

Although the term inappropriate is usually applied to hormone markers it may be extended to other cases, for example fetal products found in male or non-pregnant female adults because of synthesis by a tumour of substances normally found only in pregnant females.

EFFECTS OF TUMOUR MASS

Apart from the deficiencies of the cells that result from inappropriate levels
or a change in commission, there are comparable changes which are related
to the mass of the tumour. Medullary carcinoma of the thyroid may contain
5 000 times as much calcitonin as a similar weight of normal thyroid tissue
(page 160). At least part of this difference is due to the relatively small mass
of the tissue of origin (the C-cells) in the normal thyroid. With multiple
myeloma another factor is of importance. Although the mass may be
similar to that of normal myeloid tissue, the tumour is derived from only a
single or very few cells. The mass of plasmocytoma is therefore large compared with the group of cells from which it originated. Leakage from a large
mass of tumour or cell death could contribute significantly to the level of
marker substance obtained.

RE-ROUTING OF TUMOUR PRODUCTS

Tumours derived from epithelial cells that normally abut the external surfaces of the body may no longer be able to perform a secretory function
across the normal surface. Consequently there may be a change in direction
of secretion (from 'exocrine' to 'endocrine') that may result in products ap-
pearing in the blood which are normally secreted externally. The concentration of CEA is higher if the tumour tissue penetrates into the body space or
forms metastases. It has been found that the normal gut epithelium secretes a
substance like CEA into the lumen and such a secretion can be detected in
tissue culture. A similar re-routing may occur due to inflammatory conditions and it is recognized that patients with ulcerative colitis have elevated
levels of CEA as well as antibodies to normal gut mucins.

PROBLEMS OF TUMOUR LOCALIZATION

Selective cannulation of the draining vessels of a tumour is a well established
method for the localization of phaeochromocytomas when catecholamines
are measured at various levels in the vena cava. Similarly adrenocortical
tumours causing Conn's syndrome can be located by monitoring steroid
levels in the adrenal veins. The method has also been used to search for parathyroid adenomata when exploration of the neck is difficult because of
previous surgery.

When considering tumour location the possibility of ectopic synthesis of
hormones and other markers must be borne in mind. Cushing's syndrome
can be caused by a small carcinoid tumour in the thorax that actively
secretes ACTH; removal of it leads to a rapid fall in ACTH level. Recognition of such a growth may avoid unnecessary adrenalectomy.

PROBLEMS OF SCREENING

The requirements of a test for screening the general population are (a) it can detect more common tumours and (b) it should be relatively inexpensive. The tests that have been proposed (MEM or SCM tests, see pages 145 & 144) are lengthy, expensive and difficult to perform. The CEA test has been suggested as a potential screening procedure for tumours of the breast, lung and digestive system as they are associated with positive values. However, the use of this test for screening is made difficult by false-positive and negative reactions. A false-positive indicates the presence of a tumour in a normal individual or a patient with a non-malignant condition: elevated levels of CEA are sometimes found in patients with inflammatory bowel disease and in heavy smokers. Such patients cannot be excluded from the examination as they are expected to have an above average incidence of cancer. Thus the test applied as a screen would detect a large number of cases with non-malignant conditions as well as the few individuals with undetected tumours. In the populations at risk the number of positive cases is much higher than the percentage of individuals in these groups who will go on to have a tumour. Another problem is the existence of false-negative results where the test fails to detect an existing tumour. By increasing discrimination levels to eliminate false-positives the incidence of false-negatives is also increased and the number of cases with localized tumours that would be easily treated by surgery would be very small.

PROGNOSTIC INDICATORS

If a patient is known to have a tumour then the prognosis before treatment depends on determining its malignant potential, and the extent of its spread. Evidence from some animal models suggests that a high rate of shedding of the tumour cell membrane is associated with an increased ability of the tumour to metastasize. There is no definite evidence in man that this is the case. Prognosis with lung tumours that secrete large amounts of ACTH is especially poor and may be related to the immunosuppressive effects of this hormone. It has been shown that the blood of cancer patients may contain circulating tumour antigen or antigen–antibody complexes that can have an inhibitory effect on the cytotoxicity of lymphocytes when tested *in vitro*. CEA is considered to be a component of the external surface of the colon carcinoma cell but there is no evidence that a high CEA level with a colonic tumour of a given Dukes' stage carries a worse prognosis, although accurate staging of the disease is needed to clarify this point. High CEA levels are usually a bad sign indicating extension of the tumour.

CHANGES OF DIFFERENTIATED FUNCTION AND CONTROL

Where a growth has been recognized and is considered to be benign a sudden change in metabolic activity, demonstrated by immunological testing, could be a signal for reassessment of the tumour's malignant potential. An example would be a sudden onset of ectopic secretion of a hormone by a carcinoid tumour.

Some carcinomas lose the ability to produce factors that typify them as they progress. Production of acid phosphatase by prostatic cancer is an example; anaplastic growths contain and produce less of it than well differentiated tumours. Decreasing levels of tumour markers of this type could be a bad prognostic sign. When tumours are hormone-dependent some hormone treatments may also inhibit production of the typical tissue products. A response of this type could be a sign that the tumour cells retain the receptors thus permitting effective therapy. However, in these circumstances the marker levels can no longer be used as an index of tumour mass.

INVASION, SPREAD AND RECURRENCE

In its wider sense the term prognosis includes both the malignant potential of the individual tumour cell and the clinical stage of the disease. For example, levels of CEA are influenced by penetration of serosal surfaces, involvement of lymph nodes and widespread metastases. The detection of very elevated levels of a marker substance might indicate that the patient is more likely to be unsuitable for treatment by surgery alone and in addition requires systemic therapy.

If, following surgery, the level of a tumour index substance fails to fall, the outlook is poor: a marked improvement followed by a subsequent rebound suggests recurrent growth. At this stage the possibility of re-examination by 'second look' surgery could be considered. Much will depend on the sensitivity of the test in its ability to detect local recurrence, and on the probability of this in the group of patients under treatment. If the test is heavily weighted in favour of detection of metastatic growth there will be a tendency to select those patients who will benefit least by a 'second look' operation.

ESTIMATION OF RESIDUAL TUMOUR LOAD

The prediction of future tumour recurrence at the time of apparently complete remission is extremely difficult. It seems that there is no possibility of distinguishing a single tumour cell which has the potential to develop metastases. However, it may be considered whether it is possible to distinguish minimal tumour that might be controlled by the normal defences of the body from a slightly larger load that would require a form of therapy. For example, if 10^4 cells were controlled but 10^5 could establish a tumour, the test would need to be extremely sensitive and specific. Tumour weights in both cases are of the order of a milligram or less and the daily production of a marker substance is unlikely to exceed a few micrograms. The test would have to detect this small amount despite dilution, excretion and the competition of the 7×10^7 mg of the total body tissues and their products.

With choriocarcinoma (p. 158) it has been possible to detect 30 mg or less of tumour within the body by using the HCG assay. Most specialized endocrine tissues have weights in the range 10–10^4 mg and their products can frequently be detected by immunoassays using isotopic labelling. The detection of a tumour weighing 0·1 mg and producing little of its marker substance would be difficult using present methods, even if the marker were sufficiently distinct from the other tissue products to make its detection possible in principle.

COMBINATION OF TESTS

The combination of tests may ultimately provide a better system for diagnosis and prognosis than any single method. Tests based on immunological methods might be used together with chemical measurements, thermography, gamma scans and various other investigations of modern medicine. Attention must be paid to the reliability of the individual methods. The salient question in combining several tests is whether a second or further test detects the 'false-negatives' of the other tests or rejects the 'false-positives'. If results of different tests agree this is helpful, but it must be decided whether as good a result could be obtained by repetition of a single type of test on another occasion.

With certain tumours, e.g. islet cell tumours of the pancreas (pages 161 and 163) and teratomas (pages 159 and 169) the production of a number of marker substances is well documented. With teratomas it has been shown that production of AFP and HCG can vary independently during treatment. This raises the possibility of curing a patient of the marker substance, but not of the disease. In such a case it would be necessary to determine whether therapy is selecting one population of cells and leaving a second to continue to grow.

Use of the Patient's Own Immune System

These methods are carried out with cellular and humoral components of the patient's body fluids. With the cellular systems it is possible to study reactivity of the leucocytes, the effect of this on non-target cells or tissues and finally the specific effects of the patient's cellular immunity that leads to death or to damage of tumour cells. This is not a clear-cut classification as leukocytes may be recruited into activity by a small proportion of activated cells.

LYMPHOCYTE REACTIVITY

Lymphocytes are treated with cancer cells or extracts of tumours and their response is measured.

The lymphocyte stimulation test

Where possible, cells, either dead or alive, are taken from the patient's own tumour and exposed to the effector cells from his own blood. The target cells are treated with an inhibitor of DNA synthesis and the response of the effector cells is judged by an increase in incorporation of thymidine into their DNA. Numerous controls are included to ensure the specificity of the response.

The Cercek SCM test

The challenging material in this test is cancer basic protein (CBP), a substance recognized during the development of the MEM test (see page 145). Treatment of lymphocytes with CBP causes changes in the internal viscosity of the cells which can be demonstrated by measurements of fluorescence polarization. Fluorescein is used as an indicator substance and is introduced into the cells by causing them to hydrolyse fluorescein diacetate. As the fluorescein is continually produced it is necessary to extrapolate the measurements of the various fluorescence components. The leakage of fluorescein from the cells must also be measured.

The authors of this test (Cercek, Cercek and Franklin, 1974) found that lymphocytes from cancer-bearing patients reacted with CBP but not with phytohaemagglutinin. In contrast lymphocytes from patients without cancer and normal people reacted with phytohaemagglutinin but not with CBP.

The original results showed a clear distinction between malignant and non-malignant conditions. Later developments showed a specific response after treating lymphocytes with a tumour of the same type carried by the patient. It was also found that the typical cancer response of the lymphocytes returned to normal after successful removal of the tumour. However, further investigation did not show a clear distinction between patients with malignant and benign breast conditions.

Further investigation of this test is required, to explain the different results obtained by different laboratories. If the results can be confirmed the test would be useful for both cancer detection and determination of the tissue type of the tumour.

EFFECTS OF CELLULAR RESPONSE ON NON-TARGET CELLS OR TISSUES

(i) The leucocyte migration inhibition test (LMI) (see Chapter 4).

(ii) The cutaneous delayed hypersensitivity test (CDH) (see Chapter 4). Both the LMI and CDH tests are of value in studies of the isolation and purification of antigens on tumour cells. Particular attention should be paid to the tumour type specificity of the reaction and the lack of response to normal tissue extracts. It is likely that the application of these tests to the purification and characterization of antigens from tumour cells will provide reagents that can be used to improve the other tests.

(iii) The macrophage electrophoretic mobility (MEM) test. This test originated from observations on the effects of challenging lymphocytes with encephalitogenic factors (EF) which is extracted from nervous tissue. Lymphocytes from patients with neural lesions reacted with EF to produce a macrophage slowing factor (MSF), which reduced the rate of migration of guinea-pig macrophages in an electric field (Shenton and Field, 1975).

When lymphocytes from cancer patients were used in the test they also reacted to EF, but those from normal donors were not reactive. The acid extraction method used to obtain EF was applied to tumour tissue and the resulting substance was called cancer basic protein (CBP). This was found to be more effective in slowing the migration of lymphocytes from cancer patients.

The test requires considerable skill and training, and the results that clearly differentiate tumour bearers from normals have not been obtained by all laboratories. Like the SCM test the MEM test may require further definition before it meets with uniform success, although as originally described it had no false-positives.

CELL-MEDIATED IMMUNITY

In order to test the cytotoxicity of lymphocytes towards tumour cells, a suspension of suitable living tumour cells are plated into wells together with culture medium and allowed to adhere to the well (see Chapter 4). Test lymphocytes are added, the mixture incubated after which the lymphocytes are then removed. The number of tumour cells remaining is an index of lymphocyte cytotoxicity. Alternatively the tumour 'target' cells are pre-labelled with an isotope and the release of this into the suspension is an indicator of damage to the target cells. However, there are a number of problems in interpreting such tests:

(i) In animals there is often no relationship between the ability of the host to reject a tumour and the results of cytotoxicity tests.

(ii) Almost always lymphocytes of normal human subjects are cytotoxic to tumour cells. This cytotoxicity differs between individuals and it appears to vary for different types of tumour target cell.

(iii) The test is usually carried out with a great excess of effector cells as compared with target cells. Such culture conditions may have effects that do not depend on a specific immune reaction.

Cytotoxicity testing of individual patients has given disappointing results for diagnosis and prognosis. A possible exception is with bladder carcinoma cell lines used as target cells to test lymphocytes of patients with this tumour, but even here interpretation of the results depends on the previous history of the patient. When this is taken into account the results seem to have some prognostic value.

SELECTIVE INHIBITION AND BLOCKING OF CYTOTOXICITY

The blood plasma of cancer patients contains substances that are able to inhibit the cytotoxicity test. These inhibitory factors are believed to include antigens, antibodies and complexes between them. Consequently there is a specificity in the ability of the plasma to inhibit certain types of cytotoxic reaction. If the effector cells are treated and then washed the inhibition is believed to be due to antigen or antigen–antibody complexes in the plasma. If the target cell is treated the inhibition is referred to as 'blocking' due to antibody or antigen–antibody complexes.

Inhibiting and blocking factors may be used to improve the specificity of cytotoxic testing. They may also be used as chemical reagents for development of humoral immune assays (see Chapter 4) and if specificity could be maintained it would be a considerable advantage to dispense with the temperamental cellular components of the system.

Changes in blocking and inhibitory factors in the patient's plasma during the course of malignant disease may have prognostic significance. There is an increase in plasma inhibitory factors (antigen) as the tumour enlarges and a decrease after successful surgery or chemotherapy. After complete surgical removal of a tumour, free circulating antibody may appear in the plasma. Although the antibody against tumour cells was originally believed to have a mainly blocking effect on cytotoxicity, it is now recognized that together with K cells it can be an important component of the patient's cytotoxic mechanisms. The K cells are able to attack tumour cells in the presence of antibody that recognizes antigenic sites on the tumour cell surface (see Chapter 1).

Humoral Immune Reagents

The immunological methods that employ immune reagents differ from the methods used to investigate the patient's individual immunity. The main variation is that the reagents employed are common to a group of tumours and can be used for testing many different patients. The scope of serological testing is well known and includes precipitin reactions, complement fixation and recently developed radioimmunoassay techniques. The methods for evaluation of tumour marker substances require the modern adaptations of some of the classical procedures.

PRECIPITIN REACTIONS

These are carried out in gels either in tubes or on plates. One or both re-actants, antigen and antibody, are placed on the edge of the gel. In the single diffusion configuration the gel contains a constant concentration of one reactant while the second reactant diffuses across the field of the gel. With double diffusion the gel is originally free of both reactants. These are placed in wells cut in the gel and diffuse to meet each other in the intervening space. The terms single and double diffusion are easily confused with the one- or two-dimensional diffusion that occurs respectively in a tube or on a plate.

Transport of the reagents in an electric field can also be used either as an additional source of information about the antigens or else as a method of causing the reactants to meet each other, replacing the slower diffusion process.

As in the classical precipitin technique there is a certain optimum propor-tion of the antigen and antibody that results in the most rapid and complete precipitation. When the reagents meet in this proportion a precipitation zone forms in the gel that then acts as a 'sink' or barrier to entrap either component as it enters the zone. If the components of the reaction are well balanced the precipitation zone will remain stationary. A stationary zone will also be obtained if a limited amount of one component diffuses into a constant concentration of the other. When the diffusing component is used up in forming the antigen–antibody complex, the zone will then stop moving. However, if an excess of one component diffuses across a low concentration of the other, the precipitation zone may continue to move as the precipitate re-dissolves in the excess of reagent, to re-form further on.

There are a considerable number of possible combinations of single and double, one- and two-dimensional diffusion or transport and the suggested reading should be consulted for a complete account of them. We will only mention one or two of the more commonly used methods.

The Ouchterlony system consists of an agar layer poured into a Petri dish. Five holes or 'wells' are cut in the agar. The materials to be compared are placed in the four peripheral wells and the reagent against which they are tested is in the central well. If the outer wells contain similar substances in solution at similar concentrations a continuous precipitation line may be formed around the central well. This is known as a reaction of complete identity (Figure 5.1a). If the solutions placed in the outer wells have no

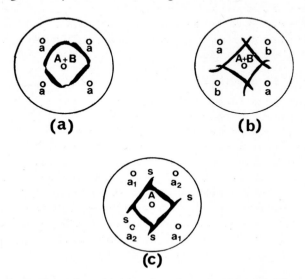

Figure 5.1 Ouchterlony plates. (a) A reaction of complete identity. All samples contain antigen *a* and react with antibody *A*, ignoring antibody *B*. (b) A reaction of non-identity. Antigens *a* and *b* react independently with their respective antibodies *A* and *B*. (c) Reaction of partial identity. Antigens a_1 and a_2 have antigenic determinants reacting with antibody *A* with formation of 'spurs' *S*

reactive groups in common the precipitation zones formed from the individual wells will cross each other without causing a deviation of the individual zones. This is known as a reaction of non–identity (Figure 5.1b). An intermediate case of partial identity is also possible with the formation of a 'spur' or extension of one of the arcs at the point where the two zones meet (Figure 5.1c). False spurs are sometimes found but they are not stable and tend to disappear with time, or if the relative concentration of the substances in the outer wells is changed. This technique is extensively used in studying tumour antigens and in preparatory work to establish other immunoassays.

The immunoelectrophoresis method of Grabar adds a new dimension, for in this test a preliminary electrophoretic separation of the antigens is carried out in agar gel. The gel layer is made on a microscope slide, but various other porous plastic sheet may also be used instead of the gel medium. A well is made at one end of the agar sheet and a trough cut in the agar along the length of the slide. The sample to be tested is placed in the well and an electric voltage is applied across the gel to separate the various components in the sample. At the end of this separation the slide is removed from the electric field and the trough is filled with a suitable concentration of antibody. This diffuses into the agar and reacts with the various antigenic components in the sample. This method is often used to study the serum proteins in order to detect paraprotein markers resulting from multiple myeloma.

When a quantitative estimate of the amount of tumour marker substance is required a single diffusion method is suitable. In the Mancini method a gel layer containing antibody is plated out and wells are cut, into which the test samples are placed. The antigen diffuses out of the well and finally forms a precipitation ring in the gel. The diameter of the precipitation zone can be used as a measure of the amount of antigen that was placed in the well. In the Laurell 'rocket' electrophoresis method the antigens are electrically transported into a gel layer that contains a constant concentration of the antibody. The precipitation zones resulting from this technique appear as sharply peaked comet-like flares (Figure 5.2) in the direction of the electric field. The distance travelled by the antigen before it comes to rest in the precipitate is a measure of the original amount placed in the well. The quantitative precipitin methods are used to study AFP and immunoglobulins produced by tumours.

The gel precipitin methods are inexpensive and the quality of antibody required is not as great as with radioimmunoassay. Some antisera, for example against the heavy chain markers of immunoglobulins, are in short supply and to conserve them a reversed Mancini technique (page 166) may be used. In this method the gel layer is soaked in antigen-containing solution and antibody is placed in the well.

Gel methods can only detect reagents in a concentration greater than $3 \mu g/ml$ whereas RIA methods are at least 1 000 times more sensitive. However, for diagnostic purposes the limited sensitivity may be an advantage, e.g. with the AFP test (page 169) in avoiding a number of false-positive results due to inflammatory conditions. The sensitivity can be increased by radiolabelling one of the reagents and assessing the result by autoradiography or by slicing the gel and counting the pieces.

Rate processes such as diffusion, transport in an electric field and the rate of precipitation all add an extra dimension of specificity to the method. With RIA the kinetic element is not dominant.

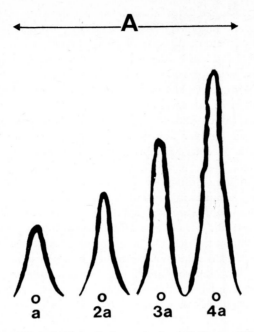

Figure 5.2 Rocket electrophoresis. Antigen *a* in the wells is moved by electrophoresis into a gel containing a uniform concentration of antibody *A*. Increasing amounts of *a* are placed in the wells from left to right

The latex precipitation method is another established technique that is used for estimating HCG and AFP. Like all precipitin methods the results are not expressed on a finely graded scale of response and consequently serial monitoring of levels of marker substances is limited by this feature.

COMPLEMENT FIXATION METHODS

There have been a number of reports describing the application of complement fixation methods to demonstrate elevated levels of AFP and CEA, but clinical follow-up of patients with the technique is limited. Such a test should be cheap to perform and the possible use of radioactively labelled complement components would make it more versatile.

RADIOIMMUNOASSAY (RIA)

This method was developed by Berson and Yalow during studies of antibodies developed in diabetic patients to injections of animal insulin. It was realized that the reaction could be used as a quantitative test for insulin, and the sensitivity and specificity were sufficient to determine levels in normal human plasma or serum without a preliminary extraction. Similar principles were being applied at the same time with the natural binding protein of plasma, e.g. the thyroxin or cortisol binding globulins. As a general description the methods are known as 'competitive binding' assays and the subject is referred to as 'saturation' or 'displacement' analysis.

RIA, though recently developed, is very widely used. It is therefore only necessary to outline the approach and refer the reader to the local expertise for further details. The principle of the method is that a limited number of antibody binding sites exist for which competition occurs between a radioactively labelled antigen sample and unlabelled antigen, that is the substance for which an analysis is required. If there is a greater amount of the antigen in the sample for analysis there will be fewer antibody sites available to bind the radioactively labelled antigen. The sample antigen will therefore displace the labelled antigen or block the antibody sites and prevent the labelled antigen from combining with them. At the end of the assay a separation is made of the labelled antigen which is antibody bound and that which is free or unbound. The assay result is expressed as a ratio of bound/total or bound/free labelled antigen.

Success in radioimmunoassay depends on the quality of the antibody and the labelled antigen. With assay of tumour markers the substance being measured may already be well defined but there is also considerable interest in discovering new and previously unrecognized tumour antigens. The development of an assay for a new tumour substance would need a preliminary purification and characterization, possibly by gel precipitation methods.

Production of antisera suitable for radioimmunoassay is subject to considerable uncertainty as the response of the individual animal being immunized cannot be predicted and many animals may be needed before a single good product is obtained. Small molecules, such as peptide hormones, may be conjugated to a carrier protein in order to enhance their immunogenicity. Adjuvants are commonly used and also booster injections at monthly intervals in order to increase the affinity of the antibody. It has been suggested that higher affinity antibodies are obtained if the immunizing dose of antigen is the minimum required to elicit antibody. For example, anti-CEA antibodies suitable for RIA may be obtained in goats by injection of CEA < 0.05 mg spread over several months of injections.

The first step in testing an antiserum and the labelled antigen is to carry out an antiserum dilution curve (Figure 5.3a). The antiserum is serially diluted with the addition of a small amount of radiolabelled antigen in each tube. At the higher antiserum concentrations the antigen will be bound to

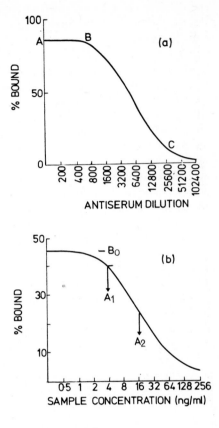

Figure 5.3 Radioimmunoassay control curves.

(a) Antiserum dilution curve. A is the % label that can be bound to the antibody. B is the 'break point' and B–C is the region containing the antiserum dilution giving greatest assay sensitivity.

(b) Standard curve. B_0 is the maximum bound chosen from Figure 5.3a as the working level. A_1 is a 'detectable' level of the substance to be analysed with 10% inhibition of binding. A_2 is in the region of maximum assay sensitivity

the maximum extent, and this provides an estimate of how much of the label is present in antigen that is recognizable by the antibody. A good labelled antigen will be bound more than 70% under these conditions. As the antiserum is diluted further a 'break point' will be encountered at which the binding falls progressively to zero as the dilution is increased. This falling part of the binding curve is the region in which the working dilution of antiserum is located, but the point chosen will depend on the relative importance of various types of experimental error.

An antiserum that can be considerably diluted to its working concentration is economical to use but the dilution is determined both by the affinity of the antibody and the number of antibody molecules in the undiluted antiserum. It is the affinity alone that determines the sensitivity of the assay; this is evaluated at the next step when a standard curve (Figure 5.3b) is determined. To do this solutions of the labelled antigen and the antibody at its working dilution are used and more of the unlabelled antigen is added progressively to the series of tubes. If the antibody is of higher affinity it will need correspondingly less of the unlabelled antigen in order to displace the labelled antigen from antibody binding.

As the original concentration of labelled antigen was chosen arbitrarily without knowing the sensitivity of the assay, it may be necessary to change the amount of label put into each assay tube and repeat the two steps in a second cycle. For example, if the antibody gives a more sensitive assay than was expected an even better result may be obtained if less labelled antigen is used.

The third step in development of an assay is to evaluate a number of pathological samples. It is necessary to obtain a sample of the patient's body fluid, e.g. plasma with a high concentration of the marker substance that is being assayed from a patient with a relevant pathology. It is then possible to test whether there is a parallel dose–response curve between the 'authentic' marker substance that was used in establishing the standard curve and the dilutions of the body fluid. Only if a parallel response is obtained can the assay be used as a quantitative measure and expressed, for example, in nanograms per millilitre (ng/ml). Otherwise the test may be of value either as a ranking procedure or as a quantitative test using the patient's body fluid as a standard in arbitrary units.

It is also desirable during this third stage of evaluation to test body fluids from patients who should be incapable of making the marker substance. The non-specific interference of other factors present in the body fluid can be demonstrated in an RIA procedure for a pituitary hormone by testing the plasma of a patient without pituitary function. The RIA test may also be compared with bioassay if available, or tested by monitoring normal control processes, e.g. the effect of thyroxine on TSH levels. An adjustment of the assay is usually required to ensure that the discrimination level of interest lies on the most sensitive part of the standard curve. Certain marker substances such as HCG and AFP may be found at very varying concentrations in different patients. Some preliminary testing may be required to determine the appropriate dilution in each case.

Radioimmunoassay is a technique in which incubation is continued to the equilibrium point at which the antigen–antibody reaction is nearly complete The rate at which this occurs will be determined by the kinetics of the reaction, but the ultimate outcome will have been determined during the preliminary experiments that define the assay conditions. There are a number of features of the assay that may contribute a kinetic component, but in general the method lacks the specificity that is inherent in the gel precipitation techniques which derive from kinetic effects.

It is frequently required that RIA should decide whether the samples contain the same type of antigen. This is done by noting parallelism between the dose–response curves for the samples. If the curves are not parallel, or if the samples give a plateau at another level at high dose (Figure 5.4), this indicates

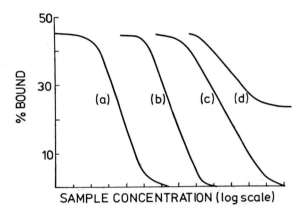

Figure 5.4 Parallelism in RIA. The lower scale represents serial dilution of the samples tested without knowing the absolute concentrations of displacing substances in the samples. (a) Authentic material; (b) sample with parallel response; (c) non-parallel response; (d) as (c) but with incomplete displacement of the label. Samples (c) and (d) are different from (a) but sample (b) is not necessarily the same as (a)

that the samples contain different antigens. However, it is not possible to provide a strict proof of identity by this sort of experiment.

If the RIA system contains a single type of antibody and is arranged to give maximum sensitivity, it is unlikely that any lack of parallelism will be obtained even if the antigens in individual samples are not identical. In practice a proof of non–identity usually depends upon the use of an anti-serum containing a number of types of antibody reactive to different parts of the antigen molecule. A better demonstration is possible if more than one antiserum is available that can detect alternative regions of the peptide or carbohydrate sequence of the antigen.

IMMUNOLOGICAL ABSORPTION METHODS

Techniques of antisera absorption have played an important part in the development of methods for detecting tumour-associated substances. The antiserum raised against a tumour extract may be absorbed by an extract of the normal tissue. In this way the large number of precipitin lines obtained with the original antiserum may be reduced to one or two lines specifically against the tumour extract. In the RIA technique it may be possible to saturate the antibody solution with an antigen, but to retain reactivity towards another antigen of greater tumour specificity.

Although these methods are important during development of a new marker substance, when the purified antigen is available the resulting antiserum may be usable without absorption. A further increase in specificity may then be possible by using chemical modification of the purified antigen which is then used to absorb out antibodies against parts of the molecule that are not tumour-specific. Even antisera from animals that have failed to respond to the tumour-specific substance may be of value as an immunoadsorbant for residual impurities in the antigen.

Surgical and Autopsy Specimens

The preceding discussion has laid emphasis on the testing of the patient's body fluids as this is able to provide a guide to therapy and monitoring of the patient's progress on a continuing basis. These are also applications of immunological methods to define the tumour material itself when this is available from surgical intervention including biopsy or at autopsy.

Evaluation of the tumour provides a two-way interaction between the surgeon and the centre that carries out the testing. By immunological tests it may be possible to characterize the tumour and thereby provide information of value to the surgeon or clinician. Alternatively, surgery may provide the testing laboratory with samples of the tumour. These can be used as the source of marker substances in development of new tests or maintenance of the existing programmes.

As an example of the first approach, application of anti-CEA antibodies to sections will delineate small deposits of CEA-containing cells in the area surrounding a colorectal tumour, thereby helping to define tumour spread and establish staging. Another application is in the study of tumours of the endocrine pancreas and gut with antibodies to the peptide hormones usually associated with these tumours. Together with more general histochemical tests, these are able to detect the 'APUD' cells both in the tumour and as normal components of the gut and pancreas. The gastrointestinal tract has been found to contain a large number of such cells with different hormone secretions. The cells are arranged in a diffuse manner among the tissues responsible for absorption and digestion of food materials. The application of specific tests can demonstrate both malignant cells and also various degrees of hyperplasia of the normal endocrine tissues in the digestive system.

Earlier immunofluorescence techniques used fluorescence labelling of the antibodies specific to the tumour product of interest. Treatment of the tissue section revealed the cells containing the product as fluorescently stained areas. Later it was found to be more economical to attach the fluorescent label to a second antibody able to recognize and combine with the antibody to the product under investigation, the 'sandwich' technique. For example, if anti-CEA antibody obtained in goats is the specific reagent, the indicator substance would be a fluorescently labelled antibody directed towards the goat antibody molecules, e.g. a horse antigoat-IgG antibody. As there are limited numbers of animal species used for developing antibodies, the fluorescence labelling of the second antibodies provides more generally useful reagents that can also be marketed commercially.

The fluorescence methods require a special microscope and there are advantages in the alternative immunoperoxidase staining which can be seen under an ordinary microscope. The fluorescent label is replaced with a peroxidase enzyme that is detected histochemically in the treated section. Ultrastructural studies with the electron microscope are possible with this procedure.

An advantage of many histochemical methods is that the antigen is concentrated within the cell and can be detected there because of its discrete location. This is well demonstrated when staining reveals a few picograms of DNA in each cell nucleus whereas the detection of a similar amount of a substance in a small volume of an extract would require a very sensitive assay system.

The reciprocal arrangement of supply of tumour to the laboratory as a source of test material is equally important. A single large sample of colonic tumour metastatic to the liver can provide several hundred mg of purified CEA. The calcitonin assay was developed by extraction of medullary carcinoma of the thyroid in order to obtain the human hormone as immunizing material and as a source of labelled antigen. Once the amino acid sequence of the substance is established by analytical methods, it is then possible to synthesize it chemically and so become independent of the naturally derived product.

Even when the substance of interest is a product freely available from the normal tissue of origin, the isolation of the tumour product is an important step in determining identity between the normal and tumour-derived substances. A comparison of potencies on a weight basis can overcome the problems of establishing identity by studies of parallelism between the dose–response curves noted above.

Chemical characterization of the marker substances may require even larger quantities of tumour tissues. Further progress in these directions is dependent upon the assistance of the surgeon in providing the source materials if autopsy samples are considered to be unsatisfactory.

Ancillary Methods

The development and evaluation of the assays is aided by a variety of other techniques that have grown up in the course of the last two decades. Mention has already been made of the fluorescence polarization that is the basis of the SCM test. With RIA there are a number of methods that can help in characterizing the substances detected by this assay or establishing that they are indeed of tumour origin. The most important, which are exclusion chromatography and culture of human tumours, are briefly discussed in this section.

EXCLUSION CHROMATOGRAPHY

In this method particles or grains of a gel of carbohydrate or plastic material are required, e.g. dextran or polyacrylamide products of Pharmacia or BioRad. These are usually cross-linked internally to control the swelling of the particles and to make them mechanically robust. Substances of lower molecular weight are able to penetrate the interstices of the gel grains. If a column is made by packing the grains into a surrounding salt solution, the smaller molecules will have access to most of the volume of the column. Larger molecular weight substances are excluded from the grains as they are too large to penetrate the interstices. They can, therefore, only occupy the excluded volume of the column, i.e. the region occupied by the salt solution surrounding the grains. Thus, development of such a column is able to separate substances according to their molecular weights.

Not all the tumour products recognized by RIA have the characteristics of the main product of the tissue of origin. The antibody selects a small region of the total molecule of the tumour product as its recognition site and ignores possible changes elsewhere in the antigen molecule. For example, the RIA may respond to a part of a hormone molecule that is not necessary for biological activity and ignore the region that determines whether the hormone is active or not. The immunoassayable 'hormone' may, therefore, include fragments of the product without biological activity. Another possibility is that RIA may also detect the 'prohormone' that is the precursor of the biologically active molecule. This is usually within the normal gland but can escape when the cells become malignant and lack adequate facilities for 'topping and tailing' the prohormone before secretion.

Exclusion chromatography will detect the prohormone as this will be of higher molecular weight than the normally secreted hormone; similarly, fragments will be detected because of lower molecular weight. Thus, by passing the sample of tumour product through an exclusion chromatography column and assaying the column fractions it is possible to demonstrate abnormal activity of the tumour tissue.

CULTURE OF HUMAN TUMOURS

To make the best use of samples derived from biopsy and surgical removal they may be cultured *in vitro* or *in vivo* in immune-deprived animals. By such techniques, it can be seen whether the marker substance continues to be produced. Cloning of single tumour cells allows studies of variability among the tumour cell population that may be reflected in resistance to therapy as well as in differences in production of the tumour marker substances. The tissue culture medium is an important source of antigens that may give new diagnostic and prognostic indicators for the tumour under study. It has been possible to demonstrate differences between different tumour cells secreting subunits of HCG by cloning them *in vitro*.

Human Chorionic Gonadotrophin (HCG)

One of the greatest successes of application of immunological methods is the diagnosis and follow-up of patients with choriocarcinoma. This tumour is a rare sequel to normal pregnancy but the incidence is greatly increased if there is a history of hydatidiform mole.

The association of gestational and non-gestational choriocarcinomas with HCG secretion was recognized more than 30 years ago. Haemagglutination and latex agglutination immunoassays are available for pregnancy testing but the RIA system provides a more sensitive and quantitative evaluation both for diagnosis and monitoring purposes.

The RIA techniques, available routinely for the past 10 years, do not distinguish between HCG and LH and therefore give false levels due to LH secretion by the normal female during the ovarian cycle. The basal level of LH in the urine is 5–80 IU/24 hr rising to 80–300 IU/24 hr at midcycle. During pregnancy, there is a rapid rise in HCG level to 10^3 IU/24 hr at 6 weeks and 10^5 IU/24 hr at 8 weeks of pregnancy with a peak at about 10–16 weeks.

Levels of HCG in patients with hydatidiform mole are usually in excess of 5×10^5 IU/24 hr. No elevation in the AFP (page 169) level of the plasma is found in cases of mole or choriocarcinoma but a rise occurs in the presence of a living fetus. The HCG level falls slowly after evacuation of a mole but a level above normal may persist for weeks or months after evacuation. Failure of the level to fall progressively towards normal after 4–6 months is a bad diagnostic sign (Bagshawe, Wilson, Dublon, Smith, Baldwin and Kardana, 1973) as is a rising level or values greater than 25 000 IU/24 hr at an earlier time after evacuation. Choriocarcinoma or invasive mole is then suggested and the 6% of women who fall into this class after evacuation can be considered as a group for whom chemotherapy may be beneficial.

In the absence of pregnancy or previous history of mole, a clearly elevated level of HCG must be regarded as suggesting possible choriocarcinoma or other malignancy, e.g. gonadal teratoma, associated with HCG products. The HCG assay is of especial significance in early detection of the tumour when the results of therapy are more likely to be curative. For subsequent monitoring of therapy, a decrease in HCG level is an indication of a reduction in tumour mass. Therapy is continued for some time after the level falls within the normal LH values. Extrapolation of the HCG curve on a log scale can show when the tumour will be likely to be reduced to less than one surviving cell (Figure 5.5). This gives a rational indication of the minimum exposure to drugs that is needed to ablate the tumour.

A further application of the HCG assay is to measure relative levels in the blood and CSF which acts as an indicator of metastases within the central nervous system (Rushworth, Orr and Bagshawe, 1968). In judging the significance of this ratio, account needs to be taken of the lag in response of the CSF levels if the origin of the HCG is from the blood and the blood levels are falling rapidly during therapy.

A recent improvement has been the development of an assay for the β-subunit of HCG. This assay does not respond to LH. It is therefore possible to monitor levels below the background due to the latter hormone. A number of ectopic sources of HCG have been detected in this way with production of the hormone by tumours of the lung and breast (Braunstein, Vaitukaitis, Carbone and Ross, 1973).

There is also an application of HCG assays to assess whether or not syncytiotrophoblastic elements are present in ovarian and testicular tumours. The AFP assay helps to delineate yolk sac elements in these lesions. A possible discordance between these two markers during therapy has already been mentioned.

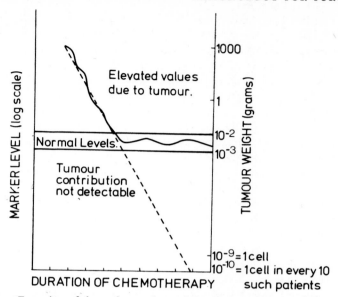

Figure 5.5 Extension of chemotherapy beyond the time when levels return to normal in order to eliminate residual tumour. Continuous line is true course of marker levels and dotted line is extrapolated contribution of tumour substance assuming that the chemotherapy maintains a constant rate of log kill of the tumour cells. After Bagshawe, K. D. (1973). Recent observations related to the chemotherapy and immunology of gestational choriocarcinoma. *Adv. Cancer Res.*, **18**, 231. (By permission of the copyright owners)

Calcitonin

The familial incidence of phaeochromocytoma with frequent bilateral presentation and associated neurofibromas was well documented in 1960. A further association with thyroid cancer was known but considered to result from endocrine effects of one tumour on the development of the other.

The discovery of calcitonin and its association with the parafollicular cells of the thyroid (the C-cells) was made in 1965. It was also observed that the thyroid cancer usually associated with phaeochromocytoma was of the medullary type, and in animals a histological study showed that medullary carcinoma is of C-cell origin. Immunofluorescence staining confirmed the presence of calcitonin in the thyroid C-cells. Both the adrenal medullary cells and the thyroid C-cells are now known to be of neural crest origin.

The scene was then set for considering medullary carcinoma of the thyroid as derived from a tissue within a well-defined hormonal activity. In 1968 it was confirmed that the tumour contains much more calcitonin than the normal thyroid gland and that patients with this tumour have elevated levels of calcitonin in the plasma. The original observations were made using bioassay but by 1970 a RIA procedure had been established. It was then known that the appropriate discrimination level (1 ng/ml) could clearly separate individuals with medullary carcinoma from other types of thyroid cancer and normal individuals.

Further dimensions were added to the test by use of stimulation tests with calcium, glucagon or pentagastrin as provokers of secretion. It was also noted that the C-cells and their accompanying tumours had a high content of the enzyme histaminase and the enzyme levels in patients with the tumour were significantly elevated.

Calcitonin determination is of value in screening the population at risk (Jackson, Tashjian and Block, 1973), such as patients with a family history of bilateral phaeochromocytoma and/or medullary carcinoma. These markers are also of use in detecting residual tumour or metastases in patients following surgical removal of their thyroid carcinomas (Baylin, Beaven, Keiser, Tashjian and Melvin, 1972).

Recent work has shown that patients with metastatic breast cancer also have elevated levels of calcitonin in their plasma (Hillyard, Coombes, Greenberg, Galnet and MacIntyre, 1976). The levels are significantly raised but generally below the values recorded in patients with medullary carcinoma. Few patients with localized breast cancer had elevated levels of calcitonin and tissue culture studies have confirmed the production of calcitonin by both breast and lung tumours.

Gastrin and other Hormones of the Gastrointestinal Tract

An association of non-beta islet cell tumours of the pancreas with multiple peptic ulceration was recognized by Zollinger and Ellison in 1955. They suggested that the ulceration was due to secretion of a hormone by the tumour. At the same time, a condition of multiple endocrine adenomas was recognized, typically affecting the acidophil cells of the pituitary and the parathyroid glands but also with peptic ulceration of the upper gastro-intestinal tract. The condition was familial and the cause of the ulceration was to be found in the pancreas with benign or malignant tumours of the islet cells.

Isolation, purification and characterization of gastrin from antral mucosa was reported in 1964 by Gregory and Tracy. Three years later, these authors found a substance in extracts of tumours giving rise to the Zollinger–Ellison syndrome with biological activity and chemical composition identical with human gastrin.

When RIA for gastrin became available in 1968, it was found that patients with the syndrome had gastrin levels in their plasma that were above the normal range (Zollinger, 1975). Typically, the normal fasting levels of plasma gastrin was 0.2 ng/ml but, with the syndrome, the patients had levels of 0.75 ng/ml or greater. There were also elevated levels in patients with pernicious anaemia but this decreased after an acid load in the stomach. It is necessary to measure gastric acid secretion rate (Stremple and Elliott, 1975). in order to demonstrate an inappropriate gastrin secretion.

Further investigation of the circulating gastrin in patients with elevated levels by exclusion chromatography (page 157) showed that about 50% of the hormone was of higher molecular weight than the product first recognized in Gregory and Tracy's work. The 'big gastrin' contains the earlier described peptide as part of an extended chain.

As a diagnostic procedure, the gastrin assay has detected tumours in four patients with the syndrome that have been found at operation to be small islet cell tumours located in the first or second portion of the duodenum. Antral cell hyperplasia has also been observed in members of families with multiple endocrine adenomatas with increased numbers of the G-cells, known to contain gastrin.

About 5% of patients with functional non-beta islet cell tumours of the pancreas have 'pancreatic cholera', severe diarrhea with no peptic ulceration. The recent isolation of 'vasoactive intestinal peptide' (VIP) from the small intestine of hogs led to an RIA based on this animal peptide (Zollinger, 1975). For normal individuals low values of VIP were found in 22/25 cases while elevated levels were found in 26/28 patients with the diarrhea associated with cancer. The level was elevated in one patient with a lung tumour and the peptide was also isolated from hog lung tissues. As the peptide is present in normal intestinal tissue, it may be that inflammatory conditions of the small bowel could lead to elevations in the VIP.

Other known secretory products of islet cell tumours are gastric inhibitory peptide (GIP), glucagon and secretin (Zollinger, 1975) as well as insulin. Islet cell metastases can also synthesize these peptide hormones. There appears to be a case for screening of families at risk for the associated hormones and follow-up after operation to detect metastases.

Insulin

Patients with islet cell tumours of the pancreas are sometimes found to have depressed fasting glucose levels. The hypoglycaemia may be of sudden onset and can lead to severe symptoms including neurological disturbances (Marks, 1971). However, the disease is very rare and sometimes difficult to recognize.

Although the radioimmunoassay of insulin is the longest established, there is a surprising lack of detection of insulinomas by an elevated level of immunoreactive insulin. The normal levels sometimes encountered are, however, inappropriate when the low glucose level is taken into account.

Other features of the circulating insulin may assist in diagnosis (Gorden, Freychet and Nankin, 1971). In normal islet cell tissue, insulin is first synthesized as a larger biologically inactive molecule, namely proinsulin. Part of the molecule (the C-peptide) is removed prior to secretion of the active hormone. Insulinomas may have less granules in the cells than do normal islet tissues suggesting inadequate storage in the tumour. In tissue culture, the main secretion of insulinomas is proinsulin as opposed to insulin in adjacent normal islet cells. In patients with insulinoma, there is often more than 25% of the circulating immunoreactive insulin and sometimes 60% in the form of the 'big' hormone as revealed by exclusion chromatography (page 157). Normal subjects usually have less than 25% proinsulin in their plasma.

It has been suggested that an elevated proportion of 'big' insulin can be taken as evidence of malignancy and may also be used as a monitor for successful treatment. It is similar but not always identical (Gorden et al., 1971) to proinsulin in molecular size or biological inactivity. A high proportion of the 'big' hormone can also be found in hypokalaemia which may be a consequence of an ACTH-secreting tumour.

Although the majority of the circulating insulin lacks biological activity in some of these patients, the hypoglycaemia accompanied by a normal total insulin level suggests that some part of the insulin secreted could be abnormally active as hormone, a sort of 'super insulin'. There is no evidence that this type circulates as a major component of the total immunoreactive hormone.

Similar observations may be made with retroperitoneal fibrosarcomas, for hypoglycaemia is not always accompanied by elevated circulating insulin levels.

Adrenocorticotrophic Hormone (ACTH)

The occurrence of Cushing's syndrome in patients with bronchial tumours and thymomas was known in 1960 but it was difficult to accept at that time that non-endocrine tumours were able to secrete ACTH. However, within 5 years it had been found, by bioassay, that such tumours contained large amounts of ACTH compared with other body tissues and hormone levels were raised in the blood of patients with the syndrome. The presence of

ACTH in the tumour was confirmed by immunofluorescence which also showed that ACTH in the pituitary was less than normal. Ectopic hormone production by the tumour has since been confirmed in tissue culture and by blood sampling of the arterial supply and venous effluent.

Ectopic secretion of ACTH is associated with many types of tumour, but especially oat cell carcinoma of the bronchus, thymomas, pancreatic islet cell tumours, medullary thyroid and ovarian carcinomas. Sometimes secretion of melanocyte stimulating hormone (MSH), antidiuretic hormone (ADH) and some of the gastrointestinal peptides is also increased. The typical clinical features of Cushing's syndrome do not always appear even when the ACTH level is high, but hypokalaemic alkalosis occurs and raised MSH levels are associated with skin pigmentation.

The first RIA for ACTH was reported in 1964. Levels of ACTH greater than 10 times the upper limit of normal are found in a minority of patients with lung tumours. Asymptomatic disturbances of the diurnal rhythm of hormone secretion and failure of suppression with dexamethasone are found in a large proportion of these patients. Cure of the ectopic syndrome follows complete removal of the tumour, e.g. with bronchial carcinoid or bronchial tumours.

Further analysis of circulating ACTH in patients with the ectopic ACTH syndrome, using antibodies capable of reacting against the amino (N-terminal) and carboxyl (C-terminal) ends of the hormone, revealed excessive numbers of peptide fragments containing the C-terminal end. Peptide fragments have also been described (Orth, Nicholson, Island and Liddle, 1973) in the blood of patients with ACTH-secreting pituitary tumours. There is overlap between the ACTH levels found in the syndrome due to ectopic production and in Cushing's disease due to a pituitary tumour. Levels in the syndrome tend to be higher than those found in the disease, with the very highest levels obtained only in the ectopic syndrome.

A well-defined ACTH-like tumour product is corticotrophin-like intermediate lobe peptide (CLIP). This has the sequence at the C-terminal end of ACTH (from amino acid residue 18 to the end of the chain) that has been found in the pars intermedia of certain animals. Normally, the peptide may be the result of 'tailing' ACTH in order to make MSH. It was isolated from an ectopically producing bronchial carcinoid tumour by Ratcliffe, Scott, Bennett, Lowry, McMartin, Strong and Walbaum (1973). Surgical removal of the tumour resulted in a fall of plasma ACTH from 10 ng/ml to 0.1 ng/ml post-operatively. The level subsequently rose again slightly but the patient was alive and well two years after the operation.

Parathyroid Hormone (PTH)

Little was known about PTH levels in the plasma before application of RIA methods. Studies of patients with chronic renal disease by RIA showed that the levels respond in a very sensitive way to the calcium concentration in the blood. When calcium levels exceeded 9.8 mg/100 ml the PTH was low or not detectable, but levels of 8.3 mg/100 ml or less caused the PTH level to rise sharply with values 10–50 times above normal.

PTH levels are elevated in most patients with primary parathyroid adenomas, but 20% of false-negative tests (Almqvist, Hjern and Wasthed, 1975) with normal blood levels occur. Most of the immunoassayable PTH detected by certain antisera is biologically inactive and elevated levels may persist for several days after surgery with clinical evidence of deficiency. However, the antisera that detect the inactive hormone may be the most useful diagnostically (Silverman and Yalow, 1973).

Selective catheterization has been studied as an aid to location of the tumours by measuring levels of PTH in the veins draining the gland or in metastases. As it carries a risk to the patient, it is usually reserved for those where previous surgical exploration has been undertaken (Davies, Shaw, Ives, Thomas and Watson, 1973).

Ectopic synthesis of PTH may be distinguished from elevation due to an adenoma by relating calcium and PTH levels. However, assays used by various centres differ in specificity and this observation does not appear to be generally confirmed. Severe hypercalcaemia is also found due to tumours (e.g. mammary carcinoma) that do not appear to act by secreting PTH. Other substances such as prostaglandins may be one cause of these effects.

Immunoglobulins (Ig)

Excretion of an abnormal urinary protein by patients with multiple myeloma was reported by Bence-Jones in 1848. During the 1930s, abnormal proteins were also found in the serum of these patients using the recently developed electrophoretic and ultracentrifuge methods. The 'paraproteins' appeared as sharp boundaries superimposed on the normal electrophoretic pattern or as components with unusually large sedimentation constants when studied in the centrifuge.

It is now known that multiple myeloma contains cells like those of plasma and that it is these which are normally the most efficient secretors of immunoglobulins. These are extremely heterogeneous (Hobbs, 1971) because of the ability of each cell to secrete a unique structurally related protein. However, myelomas appear to be derived from one or very few of these cells and during development of the tumour, there is further selection. Each cell tends to keep its unique capability to synthesize one type of Ig during subsequent cell divisions. The source of the Ig (or gammaglobulin) from progeny of a single cell (or clone) has led to a description of the disease as monoclonal gammopathy.

The existence of a tumour-derived Ig is suggested if a deeply staining narrow line appears superimposed on the diffuse background of the normal plasma globulins during zonal electrophoresis on cellulose acetate. The limit of detection using this method is about 20 g tumour as opposed to 1000 g tumour by clinical means. When the tumour has reached these proportions the patient will die after one or two doubling times if the condition is not treated (i.e. in 6 months to a year) (Hobbs, 1971).

A number of confirmatory tests are needed to show that a weak line is an unusually homogeneous product. Antisera to Ig can be obtained that are specific towards commonly occurring 'marker' regions of the peptide chains of Ig: there are four of these in Ig, two larger or 'heavy' chains and two smaller or 'light' chains (see Chapter 2). The light ones have only two alternative markers, κ and λ. The ratio of κ to λ chains in normal individuals is 2:1. The tumour product will contain either κ or λ and so will distort this ratio. There are also a number of markers for the heavy chains.

In immunoelectrophoresis (page 148) the presence of an unusual ratio of the markers and an additional concentration of the Ig at a certain part of the gel will cause deviations in the precipitation zone due to the Ig that can indicate an abnormal component. The reversed Mancini technique is also of value especially if it is applied to the region of a previous zone electrophoretic separation believed to contain the monoclonal product (Nerenberg and Mallin, 1975). A number of antisera specific for different marker regions may be placed in wells in the gel. With a higher concentration of a marker antigen, the corresponding ring of precipitate will have a smaller diameter.

Further confirmation can be obtained from analysis of the urine for Bence-Jones protein. It is now known that this is made up of the light chains of the Ig secreted by the tumour. A low level of the light chains may be detected in the urine of normal individuals that has been concentrated 50-fold or more. The levels are increased in infection or inflammatory conditions. A significant elevation of the Bence-Jones protein level (Perry and Kyle, 1975) with an abnormal $\kappa:\lambda$ ratio helps to confirm the plasma findings and is sensitive to the presence of a few grams of tumour.

The changes in monoclonal Ig levels during therapy are considered to be a good index of tumour mass. If the level remains constant in the absence of treatment over many months, and there is no evidence of invasive tumour, the gammopathy is probably benign. Otherwise, the fluctuations in level during treatment can be taken as a measure of success. A rise in level is a bad sign if the rate of increase is greater than that observed during or after therapy. Changes in the quality of the tumour Ig may indicate selection or mutation of the tumour during therapy.

Carcinoembryonic Antigen (CEA)

This substance was discovered and reported in 1965 by Gold and Freedman. It was found in colorectal carcinoma, both primary and secondary, but was considered to be absent from normal adult colonic epithelium. The first characterization of the substance was by gel precipitation techniques. Subsequently, CEA was isolated and shown to be a glycoprotein containing about 60% carbohydrate and with a molecular weight of 200 000. The finding of CEA in the intestinal tract of human fetuses of approximately 6 months' gestation emphasized the 'embryonic' nature of the antigen.

CEA was not found in other cancers of non-digestive tract origin even when metastatic to the colon or in normal individuals. When a RIA procedure was developed for CEA the substance was found in the plasma of 35/36 patients with colorectal carcinomas and one patient with a pancreatic tumour.

These clear-cut results appeared to offer a screening procedure for colorectal carcinomas but those obtained by later radioimmunoassay methods refuted this possibility.

With current techniques, CEA is detected in the plasma of all classes of individuals irrespective of pathology but is elevated in the presence of a tumour or inflammatory conditions. The levels resulting from tumour are highest and most often above normal for pancreatic, colorectal, lung and breast carcinomas (Table 5.1) but the results are very dependent on the stage of the disease. The highest levels and the most frequent elevations above normal are with metastatic disease. Localized disease leads to elevated levels in a minority of cases and the elevations are usually in the range that

Table 5.1 Frequency of raised plasma CEA levels in some neoplastic diseases

Carcinoma type	Frequency (%) of raised CEA levels
Colon and rectum	73
Pancreas	92
Liver	67
Bronchus	72
Breast	52

might be due to inflammatory conditions. If the discriminating level is raised to exclude the inflammatory conditions, there would only be 10–15% of localized colorectal carcinomas detected.

The main value of CEA plasma estimations is to the follow-up of patients after surgery (Mackay, Patel, Carter, Stevens, Laurence, Cooper and Neville, 1974), who were known to have had elevated CEA levels before surgery or who subsequently developed elevations. There are many examples of the CEA level falling to normal after successful removal of a colorectal tumour. There are also a number of cases where the level did not fall or showed a subsequent rise. From experience in following these individuals, it is now

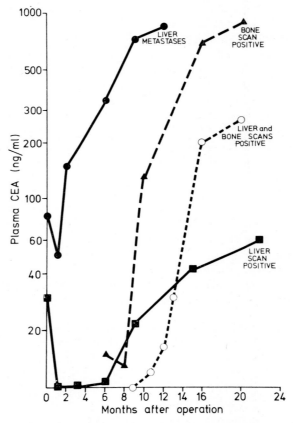

Figure 5.6 Evolution of CEA levels. The rising CEA levels post-operatively give early warning of recurrent disease before other evidence of recurrence is available. From Mackay *et al.* (1974). Role of serial CEA assays in detection of recurrent and metastatic colorectal carcinomas, *Br. Med. J.*, **iv**, 382. (By permission of the copyright owners).

known that the CEA test is able to demonstrate residual tumour or subsequent metastatic spread (Figure 5.6) and may give more than a year's warning before clinical evidence of recurrence is obtained. However, there are also cases where the CEA test gave no previous warning of metastatic growth.

The CEA test has also been used to follow chemotherapy and there are examples with neuroblastoma (Wang, Sinks and Chu, 1974) or breast cancer (Steward, Nixon, Zamcheck and Aisenberg, 1974) where an apparently complete remission was accompanied by a fall in CEA level to normal. More often the test has provided an objective demonstration of the failure of chemotherapy for the solid tumours.

CEA testing of the urine has been found to be helpful in detecting carcinoma but, like the plasma test, inflammation of the bladder can also elevate the urinary CEA levels. Unfortunately, CEA-like material is secreted by ileum used as a substitute bladder after radical cystectomy so the follow-up of these cases is particularly difficult.

Much effort is being made to improve this test by separating subfractions of CEA that are more tumour-specific. From our experience it would be important to carry out a detailed evaluation of any new test, bearing in mind the importance of staging the tumour, before any improvement on existing methods could be claimed.

Alpha-Fetoprotein (AFP)

This protein was first recognized in the blood of human fetuses in 1958. The association with hepatomata was made by Abelev in 1963 by observations on animals bearing liver tumours. Identification was by gel precipitation methods, the antiserum being against mouse fetal blood and absorbed with the blood of the adult animals. In later work, human fetoprotein was observed in patients with hepatoma.

Clinical results obtained up to 1970 were produced by gel precipitation that can detect 3 000 ng/ml AFP. The test was positive for patients with liver cancer but the proportion of such patients that gave a positive reaction varied from 40–85% in different parts of the world. At least some of this variation was due to the age distribution of the patients. In the areas with a higher incidence of positive tests the disease occurred in an earlier age group and for any given locality, the young patients with hepatoma are more frequently positive.

Other types of liver disease and other tumours gave a negative test for AFP in the plasma except in cases with teratoma or in early childhood. Children less than 10 years of age with hepatitis or liver cirrhosis could give a positive AFP gel precipitation test. There were conflicting reports on the presence of AFP in the blood of pregnant women when tested by this method (Abelev, 1971).

When RIA for AFP was established by 1971, there was a 1000-fold increase in sensitivity and the lower limit of detection was 3 ng/ml. It was then possible to show that normal healthy individuals have AFP in the blood but usually less than 20–40 ng/ml. These levels were of course well below the detection limit of the gel precipitation method. During pregnancy the AFP concentration in the mother's plasma rose to within the range 100–1000 ng/ml and this confirmed a living fetus.

Abnormalities of the fetus such as spina bifida caused elevated levels in the amniotic fluid and mother's blood. Congenital deformities resulted in elevations in the newborn but with ataxia-telangiectasia these persisted into early adult life. Non-malignant liver disease, e.g. cirrhosis and hepatitis, gave elevated values (40–1000 ng/ml) and this could be observed in other tumours which had metastasized to the liver. These conditions are associated with regeneration of liver parenchymal tissue but regrowth following partial hepatectomy does not cause a rise in AFP. There are also reports that a minority of primary tumours of the stomach, pancreas and colon without liver metastases may cause elevations within this range.

Even with the most sensitive tests it appears that 5–10% of patients with hepatoma have AFP levels within the normal range. Thus, when the full sensitivity of RIA is available there are a number of false reactions, both negative and positive.

The levels of AFP determined by RIA for patients with hepatoma range from normal ($<$ 40 ng/ml) to 6×10^6 ng/ml (6 mg/ml), but, for any given patient, the value does not usually vary by more than 10-fold during the course of the disease. In these instances there is no correlation between the AFP concentration and prognosis or subsequent response to therapy.

Successful operation can result in a lowered level (McIntyre, Vogel, Princler and Patel, 1972) that may fall to within the normal range. It is considered that for individual patients the change in levels can be related to tumour mass. It is, therefore, possible to use AFP as a guide to the presence of residual tumour, recurrence or tumour growth during therapy (Matsumoto, Suzuki, Ono, Nakase and Honjo, 1974).

AFP has been detected in hepatoma tissue by immunofluorescence methods but not all the tumour cells contain the protein. Tumours which have metastasized to the liver cause AFP to become evident in the host tissue cells and this observation accords with the clinical finding that site of metastasis is an important factor in determining elevations due to non-liver tumours.

As a liver tumour can cause a 5-log increase of AFP level, the test should be valuable for the detection of preclinical hepatoma in those parts of the world where it is common. Surprisingly, screening done in S.E. Africa has failed to detect early preclinical hepatoma in a significant number of individuals. The levels in the native population are sometimes raised but exposure to an urban environment causes a return to normal. This suggests that the elevations may be due to preconditioning factors, e.g. diet. Also, the tumour may grow rapidly, so the chance of detecting an early tumour is reduced. When a tumour is observed clinically, it will be close to the stage at which one or two doublings of mass lead to death of the patient.

The AFP test is of value in detection of malignant teratomas and yolk sac carcinomas. These may be distinguished from seminomas which do not cause elevated levels. In patients with seminoma a positive AFP test might suggest the presence of teratomatous elements that have escaped recognition in the original histopathological material.

References

Abelev, G. I. (1971). Alpha-foetoprotein in ontogenesis and its association with malignant tumours. *Adv. Cancer Res.*, **14**, 95

Almqvist, S., Hjern, B. and Wasthed, B. (1975). The diagnostic value of a radioimmunoassay for parathyroid hormone in human serum. *Acta Endocrinol.*, **78**, 493

Bagshawe, K. D., Wilson, H., Dublon, P., Smith, A., Baldwin, M. and Kardana, A. (1973). Follow-up after hydatidiform mole. Studies using radioimmunoassay for urinary human chorionic gonadotrophin (HCG). *J. Obstet. Gynecol.*, **80**, 461

Baylin, S. R., Beaven, M. A., Keiser, H. R., Tashjian, A. H. and Melvin, K. E. W. (1972). Serum histaminase and calcitonin levels in medullary carcinoma of the thyroid. *Lancet*, **i**, 455

Braunstein, G. D., Vaitukaitis, J. L., Carbone, P. P. and Ross, G. T. (1973). Ectopic production of human chorionic gonadotrophin by neoplasms. *Ann. Intern. Med.*, **78**, 39

Cercek, L., Cercek, B. and Franklin, C. L. V. (1974). Biophysical differentiation between lymphocytes from healthy donors, patients with malignant diseases and other disorders. *Br. J. Cancer*, **29**, 345

Hillyard, C. J., Coombes, R. C., Greenberg, P. B., Galnet, L. S. and McIntyre, I. (1976). Calcitonin in breast and lung cancer. *Clin. Endocrinol.*, **5**, 1

Davies, D. R., Shaw, D. G., Ives, D. R., Thomas, B. M. and Watson, L. (1973). Selective venous catheterization and radioimmunoassay of parathyroid hormone in the diagnosis and localization of parathyroid tumours. *Lancet*, **i**, 1079

Gold, P. and Freedman, S. O. (1965). Specific carcinoembryonic antigens of the human digestive system. *J. Exp. Med.*, **122**, 467

Gorden, P., Freychet, P. and Nankin, H. (1971). A unique form of circulating insulin in human islet cell carcinoma. *J. Clin. Endocrinol.*, **33**, 983

Hakomori, S. (1975). Structures and organisation of cell surface glycolipids. Dependency on cell growth and malignant transformation. *Biochim. Biophys. Acta*, **417**, 55

Hobbs, J. R. (1971). Immunocytoma o' mice an' men. *Br. Med. J.*, **2**, 67

Jackson, C. E., Tashjian, A. H. and Block, M. A. (1973). Detection of medullary thyroid cancer by calcitonin assay in families. *Ann. Intern. Med.*, **78**, 845

Kabat, E. A. (1956). *Blood Group Substances*. (New York: Academic Press)

McIntyre, K. R., Vogel, C. L., Princler, G. L. and Patel, I. R. (1972). Serum αfetoprotein as a biochemical marker for hepatocellular carcinoma. *Cancer Res.*, **32**, 1941

Mackay, A. M., Patel, S., Carter, S., Stevens, U., Laurence, D. J. R., Cooper, E. H. and Neville, A. M. (1974). Role of serial CEA assays in detection of recurrent and metastatic colorectal carcinomas. *Br. Med. J.*, **4**, 382

Marks, V. (1971). Diagnosis of insulinomas. *Gut*, **1**, 835

Matsumoto, Y., Suzuki, T., Ono, H., Nakase, A. and Honjo, I. (1974). Response of alpha-fetoprotein to chemotherapy in patients with hepatomas. *Cancer*, **34**, 1602

Nerenberg, S. T. and Mallin, J. (1975). Characterization of monoclonal gammapathies, a new approach. *J. Lab. Clin. Med.*, **86**, 266

Orth, D. N., Nicholson, W. E., Mitchell, W. M., Island, D. P. and Liddle, G. W. (1973). Biological and immunological characterisation and physical separation of ACTH and ACTH fragments in the ectopic ACTH syndrome. *J. Clin. Invest.*, **52**, 1756

Perry, M. C. and Kyle, R. A. (1975). The clinical significance of Bence-Jones proteinuria. *Mayo Clin. Proc.*, **50**, 234

Ratcliffe, J. G., Scott, A. P., Bennett, P. J., McMartin, C., Strong, J. A. and Walbaum, P. R. (1973). Production of a corticotrophin-like intermediate lobe peptide and of corticotrophin by a bronchial carcinoid tumour. *Clin. Endocrinol.*, **2**, 51

Rushworth, A. G. J., Orr, A. H. and Bagshawe, K. D. (1968). The concentration of HCG in the plasma and spinal fluid of patients with trophoblastic tumours in the central nervous system. *Br. J. Cancer*, **22**, 2

Shenton, B. K. and Field, E. J. (1975). The macrophage electrophoretic mobility test (MEM). Some technical considerations. *J. Immunol. Methods*, **7**, 149

Silverman, R. and Yalow, R. S. (1973). Heterogeneity of parathyroid hormone: clinical and physiologic implications. *J. Clin. Invest.*, **52**, 1958

Steward, A. M., Nixon, D., Zamcheck, N. and Aisenberg, A. (1974). Carcinoembryonic antigen in breast cancer patients. Serum levels and disease progress. *Cancer*, **33**, 124

Stremple, J. F. and Elliott, D. W. (1975). Gastric determinations in symptomatic patients before and after standard ulcer operations. *Arch. Surg.*, **110**, 875

Wang, J. J., Sinks, L. F. and Chu, T. M. (1974). Carcinoembryonic antigen in patients with neuroblastoma. *J. Surg. Oncol.*, **6**, 211

Zollinger, R. M. (1975). Islet cell tumours of the pancreas and the alimentary tract. *Am. J. Surg.*, **129**, 102

Further Reading

Axelsen, N. H. (1975). Quantitative immunoelectrophoresis. *Scand. J. Immunol.*, Suppl.2

Bagshawe, K. D. (1973). Recent observations related to the chemotherapy and immunology of gestational choriocarcinoma. *Adv. Cancer Res.*, **18**, 231

Crowle, A. J. (1961). *Immunodiffusion*. (New York and London: Academic Press)

Ellison, M. L. and Neville, A. M. (1973). Neoplasia and ectopic hormone production. *In* R. W. Raven (ed.), *Modern Trends in Oncology*, Volume 1, Chapter 8. (London: Butterworths)

International Atomic Energy Agency (1974). *Radioimmunoassay and Related Procedures in Medicine*. Volumes I and II (Vienna: IAEA)

Laurence, D. J. R. and Neville, A. M. (1972). Foetal antigens and their role in the diagnosis and clinical management of human neoplasms: A review. *Br. J. Cancer*, **26**, 335

Rosen, S. W., Weintraub, B. D., Vaitukaitis, J. L., Sussman, H. H., Hershman, J. M.

and Muggia, F. M. (1975). Placental proteins and their subunits as tumor markers. NIH Conference. *Ann. Intern. Med.*, **82,** 71

Moore, M., Nisbet, N. W. and Haigh, M. V. (eds.) (1973). Immunology of malignancy. *Br. J. Cancer*, Suppl. 1

Sonsken, P. H. (ed.) (1974). Radioimmunoassay and saturation analysis. *Br. Med. Bull.*, **30,** part 1

Stevenson, G. T. and Laurence, D. J. R. (eds.) (1976). Report of a workshop on the immune response to solid tumours in man. *Int. J. Cancer*, **16,** 887

Williams, C. A. and Chase, M. W. (eds.) (1971). *Methods in Immunology and Immunochemistry.* Vol. III. *Reactions of Antibodies with Soluble Antigens* (New York and London: Academic Press)

CHAPTER 6

Immunogenetics of Tissue Rejection

J. A. Sachs

Advances in the field of transplant immunology have resulted in only limited success in solving the problems related to organ grafting. Part of the difficulty lies in finding suitable animal models. By applying the special considerations of a particular species it is possible to obtain experimental models which take both genetic and biological requirements into account. For instance, our knowledge of the fine structure of the chromosome in the mouse makes it very suitable for studying immunogenetics particularly in relation to *in vitro* testing and skin grafting. Larger animals, generally more amenable to surgery, are more appropriate for certain *in vivo* testing such as organ grafting but we are handicapped by the lack of understanding of their immunogenetics and the availability of pure inbred strains. The constant interaction of knowledge gleaned from the mouse experimental model and human clinical experience has led to some considerable advances in the genetics of transplantation immunology. As more animal models become available, the dangers inherent in extrapolating conclusions derived from one or two species, phylogenetically some distance apart, to general biological phenomena will be avoided. Fortunately, the more extensive our knowledge of the transplantation system in different mammals becomes, the closer the homology amongst them appears to be.

Gorer (1956) first showed that certain antigens that could be distinguished on red cells in different strains of mice were also located on tissue cells and appeared to be responsible for determining the fate of tumour transplants. These strong histocompatibility antigens (a term coined by Snell to describe antigens which relate to transplant reactions) were subsequently found to be controlled by a gene region with multiple alleles known as H2. Rejection of tissue grafts between strains of mice identical for the H2 region but differing for other chromosomal regions indicated the presence of at least 15 other H-loci. This H2 locus was unique in that it appeared to control both tissue antigens which could elicit rejection and red cell antigens which were definable serologically. Thus, the facility for testing red cell antigens could be used to determine the susceptibility of donor to host tissue. A second important feature of the H2 region was its control of more rapid rejection of incompatible tumours than the other non-H2 histocompatibility systems in the mouse. The region controlling the H2 antigens is located on chromosome 17.

In man a highly polymorphic system was identified on leukocytes, first by leukoagglutination test and subsequently by the complement dependent microlymphocytotoxic test. These antigens, also present on tissues, appeared to correlate with the rejection of kidney grafts or experimental skin grafts between closely related family members analogous to the rejection of tumours in different mouse strains. This genetic region controlling lymphocyte cell surface antigens and antigens determining rejection of disparate kidney grafts is the HLA (Human Lymphocyte locus A) system with obvious similarities to the H2 system in the mouse. Such major histocompatibility systems (MHS) have been identified in all mammalian laboratory animals investigated, e.g. H1 in the rat, DLA in dog, etc. each controlling serologically defined antigens and strong transplantation antigens.

After rejection of an organ or tissue there is no difficulty in establishing that certain donor and recipient histocompatibility antigens were incompatible inducing an immune response in the host which led to rejection and failure of the transplanted organ. The identification of the major transplantation antigens has proved more difficult than would have been predicted a decade ago. As our knowledge of the gene region controlling the MHS unfolded in both man and mouse, so the transplantation antigens and the genes controlling them managed to avoid the battery of *in vitro* tests which established a variety of new markers on the cell surface, e.g. serologically defined, MLC and CML determinants. Even those markers initially thought to be controlled by one and the same gene locus controlling transplantation antigens subsequently have proved to be at best merely closely associated with the elusive transplantation antigens. At the biochemical level our knowledge is also limited, and the transplantation antigens in both man and mouse have been isolated only in relatively crude form with contamination by those very determinants which have previously confused our knowledge of the controlling gene structures.

In this chapter I will be concerned with relating the complexities of the ABO and HLA systems in man to tissue rejection with special reference to kidney grafts, focusing particularly on antigen systems defined by *in vitro* testing. Theoretical considerations of the relationship of H2 structures in the mouse model to the biological function of tissue rejection will be applied to support certain concepts formulated in humans. Finally, the technique of tissue typing will be described in detail as an appendix.

The problems bedevilling successful kidney transplantation are essentially immunological. Only through the empirical use of immunosuppressive therapy—azathioprine and steroids—has kidney transplantation become an acceptable alternative treatment for terminal renal failure in spite of the added morbidity and mortality induced by these drugs. Unfortunately the graft survival in transplants is predictable only in monozygous twins or HLA identical sibling donors from live, closely related individuals. Notwithstanding the increased experience of the surgeons, more stringent conditions for accepting potential donors and improved preservation techniques, results obtained with cadaver kidney transplants are even more disappointing. Consequent loss of a kidney, whether early or late after grafting, makes the choice of transplantation over chronic haemodialysis a hazardous one, and the vagaries of the rejection phenomenon make it impossible to predict the outcome of the individual kidney transplants with the exception of the above select group.

ABO and Other Red Cell Blood Group Systems and Kidney Transplantation

The corresponding ABO specificities identified on red cells are detectable on the cells of fixed tissues as well (Kabat, 1956). Kidney grafts from an ABO incompatible donor are almost invariably rejected in a hyperacute fashion (Gleason and Murray, 1967; Khastagir *et al.*, 1969), indicating the overriding importance of these histocompatibility antigens in renal transplantation, although cases of ABO incompatible grafts functioning have been reported (Shiel *et al.*, 1969). (It is interesting to note that ABO incompatibility is not an absolute contraindication in bone marrow grafts illustrating the dangers of attempting to apply rules relevant for one tissue to another.) ABO incompatibility between donor and recipient is now a *sine qua non* before transplantation and easily obtainable through standard ABO blood grouping. This severely limits the donor selection for certain recipients as Group O patients are restricted to kidneys from Group O donors and Group A recipients may not receive Group B donors and *vice versa*.

Even though our knowledge of the ABO structures extends to the molecular level it is not possible to state categorically that the ABO antigens are transplantation antigens. Whether these antigens are one and the same or two different antigen systems will not be resolved as even the most erstwhile surgeon would not consider transplanting across an ABO barrier and since there is no direct equivalent of the ABO system in other animals there is no further experimental data available on this question.

No strong histocompatibility properties have been accorded to any other blood groups except by Ceppellini (1968) who thought that the P blood group may be implicated in skin and kidney transplantation.

HLA Major Histocompatibility System

The first relevant group of antigens determined on white cells were serologically defined by leukoagglutination in 1954. The serum from a multitransfused patient agglutinated the white cells of some individuals and not others (Dausset, 1954). Only after the introduction of the microlymphocytotoxic test (Terasaki and McClelland, 1964), a highly reproducible complement dependent test, was the antigenic system more clearly elucidated. Using more indirect techniques such as absorption studies with different tissues and fluorescent antibody labelling, it was possible to demonstrate the corresponding antigens on cells of fixed tissues as well as lymphocytes (Walford, 1968).

Each laboratory initially developed their serology with sera and cells from local individuals and in order to obtain uniformity in both nomenclature and antigen definition, International Workshops—so-called Histocompatibility Workshops—were held at regular intervals with the purpose of elucidating the HLA system with particular reference to serological specificity. At the Workshop in 1970 (*Histocompatibility Testing*, 1970), eleven HLA antigens were given WHO designation, i.e. HLA 1, 2, 3, 5, 7, 8, 9, 10, 11, 12 and 13, with many more antigens not clearly defined. Based on the observation that no individual had more than two antigens from each series or a total of more than four it was postulated that there were two gene loci controlling these antigens, the first series determining antigens HLA 1, 2, 3, 9, 10 and 11 and the second series, HLA 5, 7, 8, 12 and 13. These two genes are closely linked (cf. below) and we know now they are located on Chr 6 (Lamm et al., 1974). Since we inherit one chromosome from each parent, each individual will have four HLA antigens, two from the first series and two from the second series.

The segregation of HLA antigens in the following family illustrates the genetics of the HLA system. The phenotype of the father is HLA 1, 2, 8 and 12 and the mother HLA 3, 11, 7 and 13—both with two first series and two second series antigens. The phenotype of the offspring are:

HLA 1, 3, 7, 8 / HLA 1, 11, 8, 13 / HLA 2, 3, 7, 12 / HLA 2, 11, 12, 13 / HLA 1, 3, 7, 8.

If the first and second series antigens were on separate chromosomes, the distribution in the children of the antigen associated with HLA 1 from the first series could be either 8 or 12 from the second series.

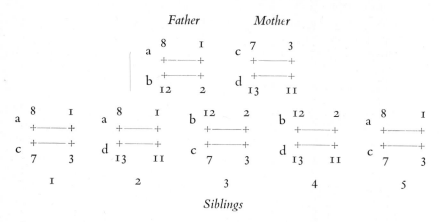

Siblings

Since HLA 1 from the first series and HLA 8 from the second series are always together in the father and three children, in this family the HLA 1 and 8 are clearly linked close together and constitute one paternal haplotype. HLA 2 and 12 constitute the second paternal haplotype and HLA 3 and 7 and HLA 11 and 13 the two maternal haplotypes. In the genotype of the family diagrammatically represented above, 'a' and 'b' refer to the paternal haplotypes and 'c' and 'd' to the maternal haplotypes. This family and data from many other families indicates, therefore, close linkage between first and second series. The distance between the two can be estimated by the frequency of crossing-over which is between 1 and 3%.

The number of different specificities defined in the Tissue Immunology Unit, London Hospital Medical College for the first and second series are given below:

First Series

HLA 1, 2, 3

HLA 9 ⎡W23
       ⎣W24

       ⎡W25
       | W26
HLA 10 | ★★10.3
       ⎣★★10.4[Fe 55]

HLA 11

W19 ⎡W29
    | W30
    | W31
    | W32
    ⎣W19·6

W28

Mo★

Second Series

HLA 5	W5	W15	W27
5A**	W5A**	W15A**	MWA**
7	W5B**	W16	TY
7A**	W10	W17	
8	W10A**	W18	
12	W10B**	W21	
13	W14	W22	

Third Series

Aj (T1); **Hu (T2); **C1 (T3); **Cr (T4)

*W = designation refers to Workshop 1972 antigens not given official designation

**local antigen definitions

What appeared to be a complex system before 1970, simple in 1972, is now obviously more complex again. Antigens such as HLA 9, 10 or W10 previously thought to be single homogeneous entities are now split into at least two or more different specificities.

HLA Cytotoxic Antibody, Cross-match and Kidney Transplantation

Antibodies used to define the HLA specificities are obtained essentially from human serum following immunization by allogenic (foreign) human tissue from different sources. About 10–15% of pregnant or postpartum women develop antibody against paternal HLA antigens in the fetus. A similar proportion of patients exposed to repeated blood transfusions will develop cytotoxic antibodies, often multispecific, in response to stimulation by the HLA antigens on white cells. Some investigators have made oligospecific antisera by matching donors and recipients of skin grafts for three out of the four antigens (Kissmeyer-Nielsen and Thorsby, 1970). Where a rare or undetected antigen is present in a volunteer donor, matching a recipient for the other three donor antigens may result in an antibody identifying a much needed rare or new HLA specificity. Doses of skin, whole blood or white cells seem to be equally efficacious for immunization schedules. Similarly a rejecting kidney may produce cytotoxic antibody, detectable particularly after transplant nephrectomy, directed usually at mismatched antigens in the donor.

Kissmeyer-Nielsen et al. (1966) observed that the cytotoxic antibody directed at donor antigens would cause hyperacute rejection of the transplanted kidney. Patients in chronic renal failure are particularly at the risk of pretransplant cytotoxic antibody production as they are subject to repeated blood transfusions. The cross-match procedure, where donor lymphocytes are tested against patient's sera, is a method derived to eliminate the hazard of transplanting a kidney into a patient whose serum contains antibody directed specifically at the donor antigens. Antibody levels tend to vary in accordance with the time interval that has lapsed since the last stimulation and may disappear altogether. However, a patient whose current serum sample is negative in cross-match will still reject a kidney from a donor whose cells react with serum samples taken previously. Two further measures may be used to protect the patient against hyperacute rejection: (1) donor cells should be tested against a number of serum samples especially those shown previously to have a high antibody titre; (2) patient's sera should be prospectively screened at appropriate intervals against a panel of lymphocytes from individuals especially selected to cover all HLA antigens. Identifying the specificity(s) of the patient's antibody will allow the elimination of potential donors from consideration if they possess the antigen with the same specificity, and at the same time in the presence of multispecific antibody alert the physician to the possibility of a positive cross-match. By doing so, alternative recipients can be considered at the same time, thus avoiding further delay in dispatching the cadaver kidney elsewhere in the event of a positive cross-match.

From the practical point of view it is incumbent on the tissue typists to provide the most sensitive test possible to ascertain the antibody status and specificity of the patient, ideally through a selected panel as well as donor cells. It borders on negligence to persist in using a technique known to be less sensitive than the standard tests suggested by the NIH (see Appendix 1) particularly in the cross-match procedure. Indeed many centres are attempting to increase the sensitivity of their test by prolonged incubation to detect antibody subliminal in the conventional procedure.

In theoretical terms, the production of HLA antibodies in response to rejection of transplanted tissue gives credence to the concept of HLA antigens acting as transplantation antigens, which is further supported by the association of hyperacute rejection with a positive cross-match between donor cells and serum from the patient. Although humoral antibody, either HLA or ABO, appears to be active in hyperacute rejection, chronic rejection is thought to be a cell-mediated immune response. The development of humoral cytotoxic antibody to a rejected kidney could be merely coincidental to cell-mediated rejection but not necessarily associated with it.

HLA Matching and Live Related Transplants

Conclusive clinical evidence for a strong association between these sero-logically defined HLA antigens and transplantation antigens was given by results of Singal *et al.* (1969). Donors and their closely related recipients were retrospectively and prospectively tissue typed and classified into three groups on the basis of HLA haplotype matching: HLA identical siblings, e.g. siblings 1 and 5 in the above family; mismatched siblings which include both HLA semi-identical siblings, e.g. 1 and 2 or 3 and 4 or parent–child combinations; completely mismatched siblings, e.g. 1 and 4. The actuarial graft survival in the two groups were compared:

	Actuarial graft survival		
	1 year	*2 years*	*4 years*
HLA identical sibs:	92%	92%	92%
No:	48	29	
HLA mismatched sibs:	78%	67%	43%
No:	34	18	

These two groups were selected entirely on the basis of the matching for the HLA region as defined serologically and the difference in results reflect directly on the compatibility or otherwise of this chromosomal region. The survival in the HLA identical group is highly significantly different from the other group and indicates the overriding importance of the MHS in kidney graft rejection. However, even recipients of an HLA identical kidney graft require immunosuppression which may abrogate the effect of apparently weaker or minor histocompatibility loci outside the MHS, analogous to the numerous non-H2 minor histocompatibility loci in mice.

However, the HLA identical siblings share not only the same genes con-trolling the serologically defined HLA antigens, but also all the genes in the region in close proximity within the MHS. The evidence from HLA identical sibling transplants established only that the MHS region is of over-riding importance, and it was still an open question as to whether the HLA antigens *per se* were the actual transplantation antigens or merely markers for them.

HLA Matching and Cadaver Kidney Transplants

Unlike HLA identical siblings, unrelated individuals found to be HLA identical for the four HLA antigens are unlikely to be identical for all the other polymorphic antigenic systems controlled by the MHS. If the HLA antigens are the true transplantation antigens, then matching for them in un-related pairs should provide the same success rate achieved by the HLA identical siblings. If, however, associated regions in the MHS control the relevant antigens, then graft survival should be similar to that between completely mismatched siblings!

Logistics of Matching for Renal Transplantation

There is a $1:4$ chance that two siblings within a family will be HLA identical which means they inherit the same paternal and maternal haplo-type. In 1971 when testing for 13 HLA antigens we reported that a minimum pool size of 250 would be required for two unrelated individuals to be identical (Festenstein *et al.*, 1971). Now, with more than 30 different antigens identified, the chances of obtaining a full HLA match would be consider-ably smaller, or a much larger pool size would be required. In the last few years many different populations have been tissue typed and their phenotype and gene frequencies ascertained (*Histocompatibility Testing*, 1972). Some antigens occur much more frequently than others—gene frequencies of different HLA specificities in a Caucasoid population have been established. Also antigens of the first and second series may be associated together more frequently than could be expected on the basis of their individual frequencies. For example, in a Caucasoid population HLA 1 has a gene frequency of 0·120 and HLA 8 of 0·120. If there were random occurrence of first and second series antigens, HLA 1 and 8 should occur with a frequency of 0·014, i.e. 0·12 × 0·12 together. In fact this figure is 0·052 because these two antigens are more often associated. Certain tissue types are therefore quite common, e.g. HLA 1, 2, 8, 12, and the chances of these individuals finding an identical donor is much higher. Likewise certain phenotypes occur rarely and the chances of an identical donor is considerably lower.

The selection of a suitable identical donor is further limited by the require-ment of ABO compatibility for the recipient. The Group AB patient will have access to all donors irrespective of their ABO status, whereas the Group O individuals will be limited to Group O donors and their chances will be reduced to under 50% of the total number possible.

Collaboration in Renal Transplantation

Van Rood (1967) first suggested that only by pooling tissue typing informa-tion on a large number of patients awaiting kidney transplantation would it be feasible to match suitably cadaver donors to the best advantage to the patient. In 1969 there were four collaborative schemes in Europe and several others in the United States and Australia. The two main aims of these centres were to provide their patients with the best possible match grade and to avoid wastage of kidneys, particularly from B or AB donors for whom the number of recipients are severely limited.

Each of the four centres in Europe have from 400–600 patients actively awaiting transplantation, and the combined European size could approach 2000. With improved preservation techniques and harvesting kidneys from 'beating heart donors', kidneys can be exchanged within and between centres without jeopardizing their viability. In a recent report, Eurotransplant Foundation (1974), a negligible difference was found in actuarial graft survival of 394 kidneys used in the donor centre compared to 884 kidneys used outside the donor centre. The three other main centres are Francetransplant, Scandiatransplant and in the U.K. the London Transplant Group (LTG) and now the Organ Matching Service in Bristol. Active collaboration between the centres has resulted in about a third of patients in Europe receiving a well-matched kidney, but the figure of approximately 10% of the total receiving full house identical kidneys is still disappointingly low.

Assessment of Match Grade

Within a family, donor and recipient share either two, one or no haplotypes and therefore four, two or no antigens. If a parent is homozygous for a particular antigen, siblings may have the same antigens from different haplotypes. Similarly, if both parents fortuitously share an antigen, an offspring can be matched for one antigen with no haplotype identity, or three with one haplotype identity.

Siblings

In the family above, sibling 2 and 3 share only one haplotype but three antigens. Similarly sibling 3 has three antigens in common with the father.

Even in the presence of undetected antigens it is often possible to establish haplotype identity between siblings.

When matching cadaver kidneys, some centres are guided by antigens in common between donor and recipient and others by the number of incompatibilities present between the two. If all four antigens could be identified in the donor, the difference between the two methods would be merely one of nomenclature. When, however, only 13 antigens were identified (albeit antigens with a relatively high frequency) many 'blanks' were present. With four antigens defined in the donor none or one incompatibility with the recipient corresponds to a four or three antigen match, whereas in the presence of 'blanks' in the donor and perhaps the recipient as well, no incompatibility may not correspond to a four or even a three antigen match.

We felt that matching for identicals is a more objective criteria for establishing match grade; that in the presence of undetected antigens the match grade put forward was a workable minimum value. In this system there are five possible match grades—four, three, two, one and none—corresponding to the number of antigens in common. The match grades used generally to describe incompatibilities are A, referring to identical phenotype between donor and recipient; B, phenotype compatibility between donor and recipient, and C, D, E and F referring to one, two, three and four incompatibilities between donor and recipient respectively. The A match could conceivably be two incompatibilities if only two antigens were defined and similarly the C match could refer to three antigens in common. Some centres, knowing the gene frequency of the different HLA antigens and 'blanks', calculated the probability of an incompatibility (or full match) by first considering the possibility of homozygosity for the antigen detected in the presence of a 'blank', and the likelihood that the donor and recipient are identical for the same 'blank' antigen.

The expectation that by matching the cadaver kidneys for HLA antigens with those of the recipient might lead to the same success achieved from HLA identical sibling donor transplants has not been realized. Reports on the role of HLA matching vary, with centres in Europe tending to be considerably influenced by matching and centres elsewhere tending to be relatively indifferent. No centres found that matching is harmful although some claimed it made no difference. There is no doubt that collaborative schemes serve a function in helping to utilize cadaver kidneys which may otherwise be wasted. The point in question becomes, does matching *per se* provide a service that favourably influences the outcome of a graft to a degree that makes the exercise worthwhile? It is with this point in mind that the issue will be further discussed.

HLA Matching and Cadaver Kidney Graft Survival

In 1971, 2 years after the LTG was established, we presented preliminary data on the favourable influence of HLA matching on the survival of 128 selected cadaver grafts (Festenstein et al., 1971). The analysis was based on matching for identity and appeared to validate our concept, arbitrarily established, of a well-matched kidney (four and three antigens in common) and an indifferently matched kidney (two, one or no antigens in common). Our subsequent reports have been based on analysis of the total number of cases without exclusions. In addition, the antigen definition has become more precise and an increasing number of antigens have been found, considerably raising the accuracy and the level of matching. In our most recent report (Sachs et al., 1974) the fate of 468 kidneys followed from 1 month to 5 years were assessed. In the same year a joint report with Francetransplant presented data on 918 cases (Dausset et al., 1974). In both series the well-matched kidneys did significantly better at 6 months, 1 year and 2 years than the indifferently matched kidneys, and a rank order of graft survival according to match grade was attained. A more recent analysis from Scandia-transplant Report (1975) with the emphasis on the fate of full house donors, where antigen identity could be established unequivocally, confirmed these results. It is interesting that in their series only 21% are indifferently matched and the rest, in their terms, are well matched. However, they assess the antigen W19 as a single entity whereas in the LTG and Francetransplant compatibility is required for the individual specificities, i.e. W29, W30, W31, W32 and W19.6 (see p. 178). Therefore some of their match grades could be reassessed at one category lower.

Opeltz et al. (1974) re-examined the influence of matching on 1708 cadaver transplants. They used a variety of different assessments to test the value of HLA matching. Where they related the number of antigens in common to graft survival the 81 well-matched kidneys certainly did better than the combined indifferently matched group of kidneys, except for the full house identity group at 12 months, where only a small number of cases were at risk. The rank order of survival is related directly to the match grades 4 + 3 vs. 2, 1, 0 at 3, 6 and 12 months, i.e. 71% vs. 66%; 65% vs. 58% and 56% vs. 50%. Belzer et al. (1974) state categorically that matching for HLA antigens does not matter. In their series, they were not able to show any favourable influence of matching. Nevertheless on closer examination their results are not contradictory to ours! They had no full house identicals, only 23 out of 200 cadaver grafts were matched for three antigens and the rest were matched for two, one or no antigens, all of which match grades we consider to be indifferent.

To assess whether good matching matters requires a sufficient number of cases in each group to draw comparisons. In San Francisco 23 cases were well matched, i.e. 3/4 compared to 177 indifferently matched, little enough cases in the former group. This same group gives the best survival results at 6 months and 1 year, but the curve suddenly takes a rapid drop due probably to the loss of two cases when only five were at risk. It remains to be seen whether this trend will be maintained in a subsequent analysis with more cases considered in this group. It is possible to envisage that in the future with the addition of say five new cases, one of which might have failed, the percentage drop will be from 40 to only 30. If the two failures occurred with 25 cases at risk the percentage drop would then be only eight. Actuarial curves provide an informed basis for comparing two functions: % survival and time interval at risk in relation to graft survival, only if sufficient number of cases are being considered in each group. On the other hand they can be quite misleading if the period of time extends beyond that where a large enough number of cases are being considered. In this circumstance one may see the spurious sudden drop in a graph which diverts the attention away from the overall picture. For this reason Opeltz et al. (1974) confined their statistical analysis to 3, 6 and 12 months time intervals even with a 5-year follow-up period.

Our original finding that matching for HLA identity has a favourable influence on graft survival has now been substantiated by many centres in Europe and the United States involving a large number of transplants (Dausset et al., 1974; Eurotransplant Report, 1974; Opeltz et al., 1974; Sachs et al., 1974 and Scandiatransplant Report, 1975). In the combined data from France and the LTG totalling 918 cases (Dausset et al., 1974), the % survival at 2 years was 58% in the well-matched group compared with 40% in the indifferently matched group, a difference which is both statistically highly significant and of clinical relevance.

Belzer and Salvatierra (1974) report a 2-year survival figure of over 50% without the benefit of good matching. They advocate a regional transplant organization primarily concerned with effective preservation and utilization of local cadaver kidneys within the region by a team of highly trained surgeons backed up by a good tissue typing service. We feel that this is excellent as far as it goes. What is necessary is that other centres acquire the expertise and skill of the team in San Francisco and that the latter team should reap the further benefit of good matching. In this way it should be possible to keep the 2-year survival figure well over 50%. Nevertheless, these calculations would still not be sufficient to predict the outcome of individual kidney grafts, well matched or otherwise, and further attempts have been made to isolate individuals who are either most at risk to reject, or more liable to retain a kidney graft. To this end the effect of various additional parameters on graft survival have been examined.

HLA Matching Retransplants

In our own data (Sachs *et al.*, 1974), although only 24 well-matched and 15 indifferently matched retransplants were assessed, the clinical difference in the survival rate at 3, 6 and 12 months was striking, i.e. 91% *vs.* 33%; 86% *vs.* 26% and 73% *vs.* 13%, the latter being statistically significant $p < 001$. This suggests that patients who have rejected or lost a previous transplant should receive only a well-matched kidney.

Matching for First *vs.* Second Locus Antigens

The value of matching for second locus antigens *vis-à-vis* first locus antigens is still controversial. In our own data (Sachs *et al.*, 1974), and that of Van Rood's group, van Hooff *et al.* (1972), in the total group matched for 3 antigens, those matched at the second did significantly better than those matched at the first. In our combined data with France (Dausset *et al.*, 1974), however, no significant difference between the same two groups was observed, although when measuring in all cases the total number of second locus antigens *vs.* first locus antigens mismatched, the less of the former the better the survival grade. Opeltz *et al.* (1974) found no difference in first or second locus matching employing a number of different assessments.

Although the evidence is not overwhelming, we think it is sufficient to specifically select three out of four match grade with second locus matches as the next priority after full house matches.

Matching Patients with Cytotoxic Antibodies

Although most patients on chronic haemodialysis are exposed to HLA sensitization through pregnancies, and particularly blood transfusions and previous transplants, only a proportion develop cytotoxic antibodies in their serum.

The results from the various different centres all show a poorer prognosis in these patients with preformed antibody particularly for indifferently matched kidneys. One explanation may be due to hyperacute rejection of a certain proportion of kidneys in this group as a result of the presence of subliminal antibody in the patients' serum directed at donor antigens which escaped detection at the time of cross-match. Ting *et al.* (1973) retrospectively tested pretransplant serum samples with donor cells in a technique more sensitive than the conventional test and showed the presence of antibody previously found to be absent. Also Belzer (1974) reported in a series of 20 patients with multispecific antibodies a graft survival of 80%, and related this success to a highly sensitive cross-match technique which reduced the possibility of a subliminal positive cross-match. However, Terasaki *et al.* (1974) pointed out that the difference in graft survival between patients with and without antibody is apparent after 3 months and at 1 year. This indicated to them that the patients were 'responders', i.e. the immune system responded to the allograft over a period of time which explains the continuous graft loss. The presence of cytotoxic antibody in the patient's serum indicates merely that the patient is a 'responder' and not that the antibody is directed against donor antigens which would result in hyperacute rejection.

Responders and Non-responders

The 40% of badly matched kidney grafts which survive 2 years could be explained by unresponsiveness on the part of the recipient to the HLA transplantation antigens. This may be similar to the observation in certain women after repeated pregnancies and in patients after repeated blood transfusions who fail to produce cytotoxic antibody. The difficulty is how to segregate the potential responders from the non-responders before transplantation. Terasaki *et al.* (1974) suggest that patients subjected to repeated transfusions, i.e. those who had been on haemodialysis for longer than 1 year, and did not have antibodies, were considered unresponsive because of their excellent survival rate—80% at 1 year. On the other hand, only 30% of the grafts in 50 patients who had never received a blood transfusion survived 1 year (Terasaki, 1974). This indicated to him that the non-responsiveness in the former group was induced through transfusion. His findings that patients who had rejected a previous graft tended to retain a second graft at least as long as the original suggested further support for the concept of induction of unresponsiveness.

Patients in the LTG and Francetransplant combined series (Dausset *et al.*, 1974), were divided arbitrarily into those who had received 0–20, or more than 20 blood transfusions, not comparable to the analysis from Terasaki's series. Both groups gave essentially the same results. When the 2 groups were further divided into those patients with antibodies and those without, those with > 20 transfusions and antibodies did significantly worse than those with 0–20 transfusions and antibodies.

The possibility that blood transfusion *per se* can lead to enhancement and prolong graft survival in potential non-responder individuals suggests that blood transfusion could conceivably be given therapeutically to induce the state of non-responsiveness. However, were such a patient to be a responder, the risk of graft failure would be even greater. Also the evidence for induction of enhancement is only statistical, and unfortunately no one has been able to correlate an *in vitro* test for immune responsiveness with graft survival.

Third Series Antigens

Recently another group of serologically defined antigens have been identified by the microlymphocytotoxic test controlled by a gene locus closely linked to the second series and nearer to the first than the strong Lad locus (Low *et al.*, 1974).

```
—+————+——+——+——  Chr. 6.
MLC      2nd  3rd  1st
```

Only four different specificities have been detected to date, and many individuals possess no identifiable third series antigens at all. All four seem to be very closely associated with second series antigens. Conventional HLA matching for kidney transplantation has not to date taken third series antigens into account. It is therefore possible that mismatches for these antigens may influence graft survival. So-called full house identical matches in cadaver transplants are not necessarily compatible for third series antigens. Preliminary data (Sachs and Festenstein, 1975) from the LTG shows, however, that graft survival does not appear to depend on or be markedly influenced by compatibility for third series antigens.

MLC Antigens

When lymphocytes from two random individuals are left in culture for several days under defined conditions, the cells transform into blasts and multiply (Bach and Hirschorn, 1964). This capacity for cells to stimulate each other in culture can be measured quantitatively, as proliferating cells have an increased rate of DNA synthesis and therefore thymidine incorporation. If radioactive thymidine is added into the culture, a quantitative measure of the degree of stimulation can be obtained from the amount incorporated into the test cells.

Whereas the cells from random individuals and siblings differing for one or more haplotypes almost invariably stimulated each other in culture, cells from HLA identical siblings rarely did so. About 10% of cell cultures from two unrelated HLA identical individuals failed to stimulate in culture. These points indicate the the MLC determinants are controlled by the MHS (HLA identical siblings do not, as a rule, stimulate) and that the locus controlling them is different from the HLA antigens (HLA identical unrelated individuals usually, and siblings occasionally, stimulate each other). The fact that occasional HLA identical siblings do stimulate each other suggested that crossing-over can occur in parental haplotypes independently of the serologically defined antigens and therefore the MLC locus is not between the first and second series. In informative families where crossing-over has been observed between the first and second series antigens, stimulation has occurred between those siblings differing only at the second series and not between those differing at the first series indicating that the MLC locus is distal to the second series.

These MLC or lymphocyte activating determinants (Lads) are candidates for the transplantation antigens, as both systems are detectable on cell surfaces, associated with the MHS and differ from the HLA serologically defined antigens.

The MLC determinants are unlikely to be the transplantation antigens *per se* as in the face of strong stimulation between donor–recipient cells, grafts survive and *vice versa*. Evidence from experimental skin grafts in outbred populations and families show varied results. Van Rood *et al.* (1973) reported a more prolonged skin graft survival in HLA identical unrelated individuals with a relatively low index of stimulation. In informative recombinant families, Sasportes *et al.* (1973) showed a correlation with prolonged skin graft survival and negativity in MLC, but no correlation with combinations where stimulation was observed, whereas in other recombinant families, Ward and Siegler (1973) found prolonged skin graft survival in the face of negative MLC activity.

Our own results (Sachs *et al.*, 1974), with few cases considered, indicate a non-significant correlation between cadaver kidney graft survival and low or absent stimulation. By employing two-way cultures and a stimulation index arbitrarily set at 8 as the dividing line, Cochrum *et al.* (1975) showed a highly significant association between low stimulation and graft prolongation in a retrospective analysis. The MLC technique is too long at this stage to be of practical value in matching cadaver donors and recipients. It is only possible to accumulate data retrospectively to establish whether Lads may play a more decisive role in the future when the technology may be considerably improved.

Practical Application of MLC Test for Related Donors

The selection of the group of siblings identical for the MHS and the corresponding transplantation antigens is readily established by HLA tissue typing without the need for recourse to MLC typing. However, 1–3% HLA identical siblings will stimulate in culture and it would be of fundamental interest to know the outcome of grafts between two such siblings. If the hypothetical transplantation genes are proximal to the crossing-over, the siblings are in effect only haplo-identical; if, however, transplantation genes are distal to the crossing-over, the siblings remain identical for the transplantation antigens.

The MLC test can be practically applied to selecting the best available donor from haplo-identical sibling or parent–child pairs, i.e. to identify the relative who stimulates the recipient the least. Belzer's group extend the use of the MLC test to selecting preferentially a cadaver kidney over a kidney from a haplo-identical family member who strongly stimulated the recipient in MLC.

The MLC is a prolonged, time-consuming test with results frequently equivocal, reminiscent of the early days of tissue typing and in the same state *vis-à-vis* its relationship to graft rejection. Its true value will only be assessed when the technique is adjusted to give reproducible reliable results within a considerably shorter period of time, a role adequately served at present by HLA serology.

Lymphocyte Dependent Antibody Test (LDA)

The test is based on the release of ^{51}Cr from labelled target cells after incubation with antibody and (effector) lymphocytes in the absence of complement, relative to that released by control mixtures without serum or lymphocytes. False-negative results may occur when the target and effector cells share HLA antigens. In the mechanism proposed for the LDA test, the IgG antibody binds to the target cell, and the presence of normal lymphocytes (effector cells) which have receptor sites for the Fc fragment of the bound IgG antibody induces lysis in the absence of complement. The LDA test is considerably more sensitive than the conventional microcytotoxic test (CMT) and it is not yet clear whether it may also recognize qualitatively different antibody (McClellan, 1972). In attempts to correlate the specificity of the LDA and CMT tests, lymphocytes from the serum donor, whether pregnant women, recipients of blood transfusions or other tissues, or a cell pool of several individuals, have been used. Other manœuvres have been suggested by Descamps et al. (1975) to overcome certain technical problems which they consider to be responsible for explaining some of the conflicting results from different laboratories particularly relating to transplanted patients. Jeannet et al. (1975) found a few cases where in a retrospective analysis, the pretransplant sample was negative in CMT, but the LDA test positive. These patients rejected their kidney acutely. They also studied the eluates of rejected kidneys and found 6 out of 22 eluates which were positive in LDA but negative in CMT. Descamps et al. (1975), on the other hand, found that LDA activity was more prevalent in patients doing well (40 to 4% frequency) whereas the CMT was frequently positive in the serum of patients with poor function (20 to 55%). It is unlikely that variation in technique is solely responsible for the discordant results from the two centres. The LDA test is a useful adjunct to CMT for cross-matching as its increased sensitivity will reveal donor-specific antibody missed by the conventional test. The role of LDA in identifying cytotoxic or enhancing antibody in post-transplant serum samples needs further investigation.

Cell-Mediated Lymphocytes (CML)

An additional function associated with MLC activation is the generation in the responder cell the capacity to lyse selected target cells homologous with the stimulatory cells. This is the basis of the cell-mediated lympholysis test in which specific lysis of PHA transformed lymphocytes by cells activated in MLC occurs (Lightbody *et al.*, 1971). PHA transformed cells freshly labelled with ^{51}Cr, are incubated for varying periods with the effector cells previously sensitized in MLC for 5–6 days. The CML activity is a measure of the % ^{51}Cr release in the test mixture compared to maximum release achieved by artificial methods, e.g. freezing and thawing, of the test cells.

In CML tests between family members with informative crossings-over between first and second series or second and the MLC region, Eijsvoogel *et al.* (1973) found that (1) siblings identical for both HLA and Lad determinants did not generate CML killing against each other, (2) siblings differing for second series HLA antigens but identical for Lad determinants and *vice versa* also did not generate CML whereas (3) siblings differing for HLA and MLC determinants did generate CML. On the basis of these results he proposed that the MHS controlled CML, and that two regions are involved, one identical with the strong MLC locus, the sensitization phase, and the other identical with, or close to, the region controlling the serologically defined antigens. He and other workers subsequently showed that killing could be obtained between unrelated HLA identical individuals as well as those differing for second and first series antigens, suggesting that either the HLA antigens are established as homogeneous in unrelated individuals only by the sera available and not by CML testing, or that the genetic control is located in a region close to the serologically defined antigens. Festenstein has proposed that the region controlling the effector phase in CML is distinct from the strong MLC determinants in the mouse model, and designated this region the effector cell system (ECS). There is no reason to suppose that a similar ECS region may not exist in the MHS in man close to the MLC region.

A number of authors have proposed that CML is the *in vitro* model of the homograft reaction, the two phases corresponding to the sensitizing or afferent, and killing or effector, respectively. Extrapolating back from the mouse model, high and low CML activity did not correlate with skin or heart graft survival in selected combinations (Festenstein, 1975). There is insufficient clinical or experimental data in humans to indicate whether CML activity directly correlates with graft failure, and since the test is even more intricate than the MLC, its practical usefulness is even more limited.

Theoretical and Practical Considerations on Histocompatibility

Each mammalian species so far investigated has a number of histocompatibility regions one of which, the major histocompatibility system, is of overriding importance in graft rejection. Also within the MHS of these species are regions which control antigens determined on the cell surface by serological, MLC and CML techniques. In man our knowledge of the histocompatibility antigens and the antigens defined by *in vitro* tests developed more or less simultaneously in the last decade, and only recently has it become apparent that each is controlled by separate genetic regions within the MHS. Transplantation antigens are not apparently detected by serological or any other *in vitro* testing. How then can we explain the relative success of well-matched cadaver kidneys?

Linkage disequilibrium has already been mentioned as occurring between the three serologically defined groups of HLA antigens. Some specificities of the first and second are closely associated and some of the second and third are likewise associated. Second series antigens HLA 7, 8 and 12 have respectively both first series antigens HLA 3, 1 and 2 and MLC determinants 7a, 8a and 12a associated together. Van Rood found in the retrospective analysis of the Eurotransplant data, Eurotransplant Report (1974), that haplotype matching for HLA 1–8, 2–12 and 3–7 had a striking influence on graft survival with 100% survival (9 grafts) from full house identical donors. Unfortunately this beneficial effect of haplotype matching was not found in our own data (Sachs *et al.*, 1974) nor in the data from Scandiatransplant (1975). Nevertheless, the hypothesis of linkage disequilibrium between the histocompatibility antigens in the MHS and one or other of the *in vitro* markers does indicate a mechanism for the improved graft survival obtained with well-matched cadaver kidneys. The likelihood is that matching for HLA (or MLC) increases the probability by association of the histocompatibility antigens being matched as well.

Ward and Seigler (1973) on the basis of an analysis of data obtained from members of a family with a recombination within the MHS, found no correlation between skin graft survival, HLA compatibility and MLC stimulation. In comparison with results from other families with informative MHS recombinations, they considered that the variations in the MST for skin grafts in relation to MLC and HLA loci could best be explained on the basis of multiple transplantation loci, of which at least two are within the MHS.

Within the H2 region (MHS in mouse) it has already been established that there are three regions controlling different serologically defined antigens, the D, the K and the Ia regions, at least two Lad regions and a number of histocompatibility regions; in addition there are more than 30 non-H2 histocompatibility regions of varying strength. A number of serologically defined antigen systems, as well as a single region controlling strong MLC stimulation (Festenstein, 1973), has also been found outside the MHS. In spite of repeated attempts, no one has yet been able to show that either serologically defined or MLC determinants are capable of inducing graft rejection *per se*, although one report has indicated an association between a non-H2 serologically defined antigen and prolonged skin graft survival (Sachs *et al.*, 1973). The prospect therefore of finding an *in vitro* test to detect the transplantation antigens for matching in clinical transplantation looks unpromising, and our only means of detecting incompatibility for donor–recipient histocompatibility remains the actual tissue rejection.

The prospect of being able to select out recipients most likely to reject their kidney on the basis of their inherent capacity to respond to allografts is also not encouraging. The danger of sensitizing the patient rather than inducing unresponsiveness makes the use of blood transfusion too risky as a means of selecting these individuals prospectively. The therapeutic use of blood transfusion for chronic renal failure has decreased considerably and there are many patients now who have never received blood at all. If Terasaki is correct, this group of patients, now increasing, is a relatively poor risk.

The LDA test is encouraging as a more sensitive test for screening pre-transplant samples for cytotoxic antibody. Positive results obtained from post-transplant patients may be associated with a propensity to retain the graft, whereas positive results with the conventional test may be associated with graft rejection. This concept should be treated with caution as the reverse results were obtained from antibody eluted from rejected kidneys.

We have currently no means of predicting the outcome of individual cadaver kidneys for a given recipient, but the probability of prolonged graft survival can be increased by:

(i) Vigorously screening the patients' serum for preformed cytotoxic antibody against a selected panel, and raising the sensitivity of the cross-match against donor cells.

(ii) Ensuring that all recipients, but particularly the patient who has had a previous transplant or cytotoxic antibodies, receive a well-matched kidney.

The Fine Structure of the MHS with Particular Reference to Disease Susceptibility and Ir Genes

The MHS region was assigned to chromosome No. 6 in a family with a pericentric inversion (Lamm *et al.*, 1974).

The individual gene products of the MHS in man are identified essentially on cell surface membranes by a variety of different techniques. There are more than 10 such markers, including at least three which are serologically defined—first, second and third series; at least two defined by MLR, LD2 and LD1, the Chido and P blood group systems on red cells and a biochemical marker, PGM3. The location of each system in the MHS has been determined by conventional genetic methods, utilizing the frequency and distribution of the antigens in random populations, their segregation within families, and ultimately definite evidence of linkage through crossings-over which, occurring in parental chromosomes during meiosis, are transmitted and detected in the offspring. The frequency of crossings-over between two antigenic systems or markers determines their distance apart, and their relative positions to each other are presented diagrammatically below.

Well established markers of the HLA major histocompatibility system

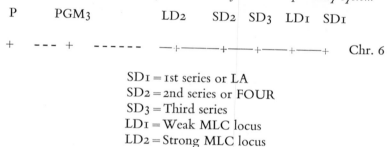

SD1 = 1st series or LA
SD2 = 2nd series or FOUR
SD3 = Third series
LD1 = Weak MLC locus
LD2 = Strong MLC locus

The clinical relevance of the MHS has recently been extended to beyond that of organ transplantation. A number of diverse diseases have become associated with gene products of the MHS. For instance, over 90% of patients with ankylosing spondylitis possess antigen W27 although there are more than 16 other antigens belonging to the second series (Brewerton *et al.*, 1973; Schlosstein *et al.*, 1973). Similarly 70% of patients with multiple sclerosis possess 'LD 7a' which has a normal distribution of about 10% in healthy individuals (Jersild *et al.*, 1973). Several other diseases have either a high association with particular HLA second series specificities or a less significant correlation (*Transplantation Reviews*, No. 22, 1974). Nevertheless it should be remembered that by far the majority of diseases have *not* shown a correlation with the MHS antigens.

The association of two particular conditions with the MHS has given some indication of the possible mechanisms:

(1) Deficiencies in C2 (Friend *et al.*, 1975) and C4 (Rittner *et al.*, 1975) components of complement have suggested linkage between HLA and the genes controlling the quantitative blood levels.

(2) Seven families have been investigated in which individual members respond to ragweed pollen by the production of high titre reagin which induces hay fever allergy (Levine *et al.*, 1972). One of the genes responsible is closely linked to HLA. In the mouse model certain strains can be shown to respond with high or low antibody titres to artifically prepared or natural antigens due to immune response genes situated in the H2 complex (McDevitt and Benacerraf, 1972). Other H2 genes control the susceptibility to viral infections and tumours (Lilly, 1972). Similar immune response genes have been found in the MHS systems of rats (Gunter *et al.*, 1972) and chimpanzees (Dorf *et al.*, 1975). The ability of allergic individuals to respond with high titre reagins to ragweed pollen may be analogous in humans, to high and low titres obtained in some animals in response to synthetic polypeptides. It remains to be seen whether the susceptibility to other diseases associated with the HLA complex is due to immune response genes *per se.*

In our view these susceptibility genes may be located at various regions within the MHS according to the disease involved. Thus, one of the gene loci responsible for susceptibility to ankylosing spondylitis is located very close to that controlling the second series group of antigens and the corresponding allele appears to be in close linkage disequilibrium with W27. Similarly

Other genes located in the major histocompatibility system

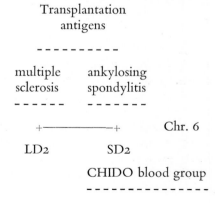

the disease susceptibility determinant in the gene locus close to the LD2 locus relating to multiple sclerosis is in strong linkage disequilibrium with the 'LD 7a' allele. The genes directly responsible for tissue or organ rejection have also not been specifically located and there is no convincing evidence to suggest that they are identical with any of the existing HLA markers. From clinical cadaver kidney programmes, the more favourable outcome of cadaver kidneys matched at the second locus may favour the localization of the transplantation antigens close to the second series.

Appendix 1

Microlymphocytotoxic Test for HLA Antigens

INTRODUCTION

This is a complement-dependent test employing immune sera and lymphocytes as target cells. Only the method of separating lymphocytes from whole blood and the basic procedure of the test, a modification of the NIH procedure, as used in the Tissue Immunology Unit, The London Hospital Medical College, is discussed.

LYMPHOCYTE SEPARATION

We prefer to use blood defibrinated by our own experienced staff, or blood anticoagulated with sodium citrate immediately after withdrawal and recalcified and defibrinated within 24 hours by us in the laboratory. In the latter procedure for each 10 ml of blood, 1 ml of 3·8% sodium citrate is required. To recalcify, 0·6 ml of 10% calcium gluconate solution and one drop of thrombin 50 units/ml needs to be added immediately before defibrinating. We generally defibrinate by gently rotating the blood by hand in an appropriate size Ernmeyer flask with 6–10 glass beads for 10 minutes. The defibrination process eliminates platelets which also carry HLA antigens and could interfere with the reaction. It is also possible to use heparinized blood—contaminating platelet can be either left or removed more tediously by differential centrifugation.

LYMPHOCYTE PREPARATION

Eight ml of defibrinated blood is layered on 1–2 ml of Ficoll–Triosil reagents (Harris and Ukaejiofo, 1970), in 10 ml test tubes. After centrifugation at about 2000 g for 15 minutes at room temperature lymphocytes are harvested from the layer between the serum and the Ficoll–Triosil reagent, washed at least twice in excess of buffered saline and resuspended at a concentration of

$1\cdot5 \times 10^6$/ml in CFT buffer (oxoid). One ml of whole blood provides usually 1×10^6 lymphocytes from a healthy individual.

ANTISERA

One μl of 120 highly selected antiHLA sera defining all the HLA specificities are added separately to individual wells in a microtitre 'Terasaki'
plate (Falcon) under a thin film of liquid paraffin to prevent evaporation.
For convenience 80 such plates are poured at one time, kept frozen at $-40°$ C
and thawed at room temperature prior to use.

COMPLEMENT

For human cells, rabbit serum is our source of complement. It is most important that the efficacy of the complement be previously assessed. We pool
and dispense the serum obtained from the clotted blood of six rabbits into
$0\cdot25$, $0\cdot50$ and $1\cdot0$ ml aliquots which are stored at -40 °C or in liquid
nitrogen. The serum is thawed just before use and any excess is discarded.

METHOD

One μl of cell suspension ($1\cdot5 \times 10^6$/ml) is added to the 1 μl serum drop-
let in each well. After 30 min incubation at room temperature 5 μl of
rabbit serum (complement) diluted $1 + 1$ with CFT solution is added to each
well and the incubation continued for a further 1 hour. Cell death is then
assessed by the use of an inverted phase contrast microscope. We do not
require dye inclusion to define cell death although trypan blue and eosin can
both be used.

The sensitivity of the test is affected by cell preparation, quality and
quantity of the complement and its length of incubation with the cell-
serum reaction mixture. Using excess complement and with the ability to
read the test after a total of $1\frac{1}{2}$, 2 or $2\frac{1}{2}$ hours incubation, we believe we
arrive at the optimal cytotoxicity level for given sera. The standard NIH
technique recommends the use of 5 μl of rabbit serum undiluted. We
have found that diluting the complement with CFT $1 + 1$ is at least as
efficacious.

References

Bach, F. H. and Hirschorn, K. (1964). Lymphocyte interaction: a potential histocom-
    patibility test *in vitro*. *Science*, **143,** 813
Belzer, F. O. (1974). Discussion. *Transplant. Proc.*, **vi,** 37
Belzer, F. O. and Salvatierra, O. (1974). The organisation of an effective cadaver renal
    transplantation programme. *Transplant. Proc.*, **vi,** 93

Belzer, F. O., Perkins, H. A., Fortmann, J. L., Kountz, S. L., Salvatierra, O., Cochrum, K. C. and Payne, R. (1974). Is HL-A typing of clinical significance in cadaver renal transplantation? *Lancet*, **i**, 774

Brewerton, D., Caffrey, M., Hart, F. D., James, D. C. O., Nicholls, A. and Sturrock, R. D. (1973). Ankylosing spondylitis and HL-A27. *Lancet*, **i**, 904

Cepellini, R. (1968). *Genetic Basis of Transplantation in Human Transplantation*. In F. T. Rapaport and J. Dausset (eds.), p. 29. (New York: Grune and Stratton)

Cochrum, K. C., Salvatierra, O., Perkins, H. A. and Belzer, F. O. (1975). MLC testing in renal transplantation. *Transplant. Proc.*, **7**, 659

Dausset, J. (1954). Leuko-agglutinins IV. Leuko-agglutinins and blood transfusion. *Vox Sang.*, **4**, 190

Dausset, J., Hors, J., Busson, M., Festenstein, H., Oliver, R. T. D., Paris, A. M. I. and Sachs, J. A. (1974). Serologically defined HL-A antigens and long-term survival of cadaver kidney transplants. *N. Engl. J. Med.*, **290**, 979

Descamps, B., Dagnon, R., Delray-Sachs, M., Barbinal, C. and Croslier, J. (1975). Lymphocyte-dependent and complement-dependent antibodies in human renal allograft recipients. *Transplant. Proc.*, **7**, 635

Dorf, M. E., Baher, H. and Benacerraf, B. (1975). The major histocompatibility complex of rhesus monkeys (RhL-A): VI. Mapping of RhL-A linked immune response genes. *Transplant. Proc.*, **7**, 21

Eijsvoogel, V. P., du Bois Ria, Melief, C. J. M., Zeylemaker, W. P., Raat-Koning, L. and de Groot-Kooy, L. (1973). Lymphocyte activation and destruction *in vitro* in relation to MLC and HL-A. *Transplant. Proc.*, **5**, 415

Eurotransplant Foundation 1974, Annual Report, p. 20

Festenstein, H., Oliver, R. T. D., Sachs, J. A., Burke, J. M., Adams, E., Divver, P., Hyams, A., Pegrum, G. D., Balfour, I. C., and Moorhead, J. F. (1971). Multicentre collaboration in 162 tissue-typed renal transplants. *Lancet*, **ii**, 225

Festenstein, H. (1973). Immunogenetic and biological aspects of *in vitro* lymphocyte allotransformation (MLR) in the mouse. *Transplant. Rev.*, **15**, 62

Festenstein, H. (1975). Unpublished data.

Friend, P., Handwerger, B., Kim, Y., Reinsmoen, N., Michael, A. and Yunis E. J. (1975). The major histocompatibility region (HL-I) and deficiency of the second component of complement (C2): homozygosity for the MLR-S(CD) gene. *Histocompatibility Testing*, 1975 Ed. (Copenhagen: Munksgaard)

Gleason, R. E. and Murray, J. E. (1967). Report from Kidney Transplant Registry, analysis of variables in the function of human kidney transplants. 1. Blood group compatibility and splenectomy. *Transplantation*, **5**, 343

Gorer, P. A. (1956). Some recent work in tumour immunity. *Adv. Cancer Res.*, **4**, 149

Gunter, E., Rude, E. and Stark, O. (1972). Antibody response in rats to synthetic polypeptide (T.G.)—A-L genetically linked to the major histocompatibility system. *Eur. J. Immunol.*, **2**, 151

Harris, R. and Ukaejiofo, E. O. (1970). Tissue typing using a routine one-step lymphocyte separation procedure. *Br. J. Haematol.*, **18**, 229

Histocompatibility Testing, 1970. Ed. P. I. Terasaki. (Copenhagen: Munksgaard)

Histocompatibility Testing, 1972. Ed. J. Dausset. (Copenhagen: Munksgaard)

van Hoof, J. P., van der Steen, G. J., Schippers, H. M. A. and van Rood, J. J. (1972). Efficacy of HL-A matching in Eurotransplant. *Lancet*, **ii**, 1485

Jeannet, M., Vassalli, P. and Botella, S. (1975). Lymphocyte dependent cytotoxic antibody (LDA) in kidney transplantation. *Transplant. Proc.*, **7,** 631

Jersild, C., Fog, T., Hansen, G. S., Thomsen, M., Svejgaard, A. and Du Pont, B. (1973). Histocompatibility determinants in multiple sclerosis, with special reference to clinical course. *Lancet*, **ii,** 1221

Khastagir, Montondon, A., Nakamoto, S. and Colls, W. J. (1969). Early and late features of human cadaveric renal allografts. *Arch. Intern. Med.*, **123,** 8

Kissmeyer-Nielsen, S., Olsen, S., Petersen, V. P. and Sjelborg, O. (1966). Hyperacute rejection of kidney allografts associated with pre-existing humoral antibodies against donor cells. *Lancet*, **ii, 662**

Kissmeyer-Nielsen, S. and Thorsby, E. (eds.) (1970). Human transplantation antigen. *Transplant. Rev.*, No. 4. (Copenhagen: Munksgaard)

Lamm, L. U., Friedrich, U., Peterson, G. B., Jorgensen, J., Nielsen, J., Therkelsen, A. J. and Kissmeyer-Nielsen, F. (1974). Assignment of the major histocompatibility complex to chromosome No. 6 in a family with pericentric inversion. *Hum. Hered.*, **24,** 273

Levine, B. B., Stember, R. H. and Fotino, M. (1972). Genetic control and linkage to HL-A haplotypes. *Science*, **178,** 1201

Lightbody, J., Bernoco, D., Miggiano, V. C. and Cepellini, R. (1971). Cell-mediated lymphosis in man after sensitisation of effector lymphocytes through mixed lymphocyte cultures. *J. Bacteriol., Virol., Immunol.*, **64,** 243

Lilly, F. (1972). Mouse leukaemia: a model of a multiple gene disease. *J. Natl. Cancer Inst.*, **49,** 927

Low, B., Messeter, L., Mansson, S. and Lindholm, T. (1974). Crossing over between SD-2(four) and SD-3(AJ) loci of the human major histocompatibility region. *Tissue Antigens*, **4,** 405

McClellan, I. C. M. (1972). Antibody in the induction and inhibition of lymphocyte cytotoxicity. *Transplant. Rev.*, **13,** 67

McDevitt, H. O. and Benacerraf, B. (1972). Histocompatibility-linkage immune response genes. *Science*, **175,** 273

Opeltz, G., Mickey, M. R. and Terasaki, P. I. (1974). HL-A and kidney transplants: re-examination. *Transplantation*, **17,** 371

Rittner, C., Hauptmann, G., Grosshans, E. and Mayer, S. (1975). Linkage between HL-A (major histocompatibility complex) and genes controlling synthesis of the fourth component of complement. *Histocompatibility Testing, 1975.* (Copenhagen: Munksgaard)

van Rood, J. J., Koch, C. T., van Hooff, J. P., Van Leeuwen, A., Van der Tweel, J. G., Fredericks, E., Schippers, M. H. A., Hendriks, G., van der Steen, G. J. (1973). Graft survival in unrelated donor–recipient pairs matched for MLC and HL-A. *Transplant. Proc.*, **5,** 409

van Rood, J. J. (1967). A proposal for international co-operation in organ transplantation: Eurotransplant. In E. S. Curtoni, P. L. Mattinz, and R. M. Tosi (eds.) *Histocompatibility Testing 451.* (Copenhagen: Munksgaard)

Sachs, J. A., Huber, B., Pena-Martinez, J. and Festenstein, H. (1973). Genetic studies and effect on skin allograft survival of DBA/2 (DAG), Ly and M-locus antigen. *Transplant. Proc.*, **5,** 1385

Sachs, J. A., Oliver, R. T. C., Paris, A. M. I. and Festenstein, H. (1974). A collaborative scheme for tissue typing and matching in renal transplantation. VII. Relevance of HL-A, donor sex, MLC and other factors on cadaver renal transplants. *Transplant. Proc.*, **7,** 65

Sachs, J. A. and Festenstein, H. (1975). Unpublished data.

Sasportes, M., Lebrum, A., Rapaport, F. T. and Bausset, J. (1973). Skin allograft survival in relation to HL-A compatibility and response to MLC. *Transplant. Proc.*, **5**, 353

Scandiatransplant Report (1975). HL-A matching and kidney-graft survival. *Lancet*, **i**, 240

Schlosstein, L., Terasaki, P. I., Bluestone, R. and Pearson, C. M. (1973). High association of an HL-A antigen, W27, with ankylosing spondylitis. *N. Engl. J. Med.*, **288**, 704

Shiel, A. G., Stewart, J. H., Tiller, D. J. and May, J. (1969). ABO blood group incompatibility in renal transplantation. *Transplantation*, **8**, 219

Singal, D. P., Mickey, M. R. and Terasaki, P. I. (1969). Serotyping for homotransplantation XXIII. Analysis of kidney transplants from parental versus sibling donors. *Transplantation*, **7**, 246

Terasaki, P. I. (1974). Discussion. *Transplant. Proc.*, **6**, 37

Terasaki, P. I. and McClelland, J. D. (1964). Microdroplet assay of human serum cytotoxins. *Nature (London)*, **204**, 998

Terasaki, P. I., Opeltz, G. and Mickey, M. R. (1974). Histocompatibility and clinical kidney transplants. *Transplant. Proc.*, **6**, 33

Ting, A., Hasegawa, P., Serron, S., Reisfeld, R. (1973). Presensitization detected by a sensitive cross-match test. *Transplant. Proc.*, **5**, 813

Transplant. Rev., **4** (1970). Human transplantation antigens. (Copenhagen: Munksgaard)

Transplant. Rev., **22** (1974). HLA and disease. (Copenhagen: Munksgaard)

Walford, R. (1968). *The Isoantigen System of Human Leukocytes*. p. 50. (Copenhagen: Munksgaard)

Ward, S. E. and Siegler, H. S. (1973). Mixed lymphocyte reactions and skin graft survival in an HL-A recombinant family. *Transplant. Proc.*, **5**, 359

CHAPTER 7

Allograft Reaction

J. P. Bramis and R. N. Taub*

Historical Notes

The idea that diseased or worn-out organs might be replaced by new, healthy tissues has always fascinated man. Vague accounts of grafted organs appear even in Greek mythology, exemplified by the chimera, an imaginary monster formed incongruously of a lion's head breathing fire, a goat's body, and a serpent's tail. Ancient treatments such as those attributed to Cosmas and Damian who replaced the leg of a devout person, or the arts of the Chinese doctors, Pien Ch'iao and Hua T'o, who performed cardiac transplants might also be viewed as medical mythology. The 18th-century descriptions by Sir William Hunter of the fate of non-vascularized animal tissues implanted heterotopically in fowls and dogs or orthotopically in humans, also contain some unexplained successes, not necessarily mythological. Attempts to transplant the kidney began in earnest in 1902 when Ullmann reported the first successful experimental organ transfer using Payr's cannulas to achieve vessel anastomoses. The same year, Carrel's publication in Lyon Medicale removed many of the principal technical obstacles to direct vascularization of grafts. Ever since, minor modifications of 'Carrel's vascular patch' have been used for revascularizing organ transplants. Floresco (1905) showed good function of kidneys grafted orthotopically and later to the femoral vessels; the urine outflow drained through a cutaneous fistula. Subsequent kidney experiments performed by workers such as Carrel and Guthrie (1905), Stich (1907), Borst and Enderlen (1909), Unger (1910), and Neuhof (1923) were mainly intended to define optimal

* R. N. Taub is a recipient of USPHS Career Development Award 1-K00034 from the National Cancer Institute.

technical means by which permanent graft survival could be achieved. The early optimism bolstered by these surgical achievements in organ transplantation experiments was soon replaced by the awareness that a destructive process of unknown nature brought about early failure of the graft, even when no technical mishaps could be identified.

In parallel with the development of techniques for vascular anastomoses and transfer of organs, there was rapid development in the field of immunology. As early as 1903, Jenssen suggested that immunological mechanisms might be involved in the rejection of transplanted animal tumour tissue. The discovery of human blood groups by Landsteiner in 1901, and the descriptions of immune changes in tumour-grafted inbred mice by Snell, Little and Strong further conceptualized the possible involvement of the immune mechanism in rejection of transplants. Modern transplantation immunology, however, rests largely on the foundation provided by the work of Medawar and his associates during the 1940s and 50s which described and quantified first and second-set skin homograft rejection and established that transplant rejection is mediated by immunological mechanisms. A comparison of the reactions involved in kidney graft rejection as opposed to skin graft rejection was soon carried out by Dempster and Simonsen in 1953 in dogs. The cellular nature of the reaction was further elucidated by Mitchison in 1954 by adoptively transferring graft immunity from sensitized to intact individuals with injections of living donor lymphoid cells.

It was not long before radiation and antimetabolites, which had shown promise in ameliorating graft rejection in animals, were to be applied to organ grafting in man. Up to 1955, nine kidney transplants had been performed between genetically non-identical donors and recipients, with uniformly poor allograft function. In 1959, whole-body x-irradiation of the recipient afforded the first prolonged survival of a kidney graft which had been performed by Hamburger and his colleagues in Paris. Soon after a similarly treated case was reported by Murray, Merrill and Harrison in Boston. Since then, kidney transplants have been performed in ever-increasing numbers (approximately 23 300 cases as of November 1, 1975).

Allogeneic transplants of the heart have also been performed in increasing numbers, since the first successful operation by Barnard in 1968. Liver transplants have not shown as great a promise as cardiac and renal allografting but experience with these types of grafts is accumulating rapidly. Transplantation of other organs such as pancreas, spleen, lung and small bowel have been attempted for only the past several years, and no significant prolonged benefit has yet been recorded from any of these procedures.

Tissue typing for organ transplantation has advanced rapidly during the past 15 years since Dausset, Payne, van Rood, Walford, Terasaki and others have been compiling the immunogenetics of the histocompatibility loci in man. Its impact on clinical transplantation is increasing steadily.

Basic Definitions and Classification of Grafts

Certain non-surgical terms commonly used in transplantation immunology are defined here.

Immunocompetence—the ability of an antigenically stimulated animal or human individual or cell population to mount an immune response against 'non-self' antigenic substances upon contact. It presupposes an intact, mature immune system.

Humoral immunity—is the response to antigenic stimuli expressed by the ability of lymphocytes and plasma cells to produce circulating serum antibodies against the antigen which provoked the response.

Cellular or cell-mediated immunity—is carried out by immunocompetent cells able to mount a localized immunological attack against the antigen.

Antigen—is any chemical or biological compound able to trigger an immune response. The magnitude of the response correlates with its immunogenicity which in turn varies with the size of the antigenic molecule. The active portion of a macromolecule or cell membrane which is responsible for specificity of the antibodies or cellular response produced is referred to as the antigenic determinant.

Histocompatibility—refers to genetically determined antigenic similarity of a given donor–recipient pair. Complete histocompatibility (i.e. absence of immune response) is not encountered in random-bred populations with the exception of monozygotic siblings.

Chimerism—is defined as the uneventful co-existence of genetically different tissues in the same individual.

Autograft (also 'autologous graft')—is a graft transferred from one part of the body to another within the same individual. Rejection phenomena are absent.

Isograft (also isologous graft, syngeneic graft)—graft exchanged between genetically identical individuals. The immunological behaviour of an isograft is identical to that of an autograft.

Allograft (also homograft, homologous graft, allogeneic graft)—a graft transferred between genetically dissimilar individuals but within the same species. It is the type of graft used most often in clinical transplants which may provoke the full expansion of immunological rejection reactions.

Xenograft (also heterograft, heterologous graft, xenogeneic graft)—a graft transferred between individuals of different species. Rejection reactions are usually even more violent than against allografts.

Transplantation Immunity as an Immunological Reaction

An example of the homograft reaction is observed when a small piece of animal or human skin from one individual is sutured into a prepared graft bed on another individual of the same species, and compared with a similar piece of skin transferred from one site to another on the same individual. The recipient's own skin is vascularized to a pink colour by the third or fourth day and thereafter heals slowly into place. The transplanted skin also is initially vascularized, but soon shows evidence of inflammation with induration and progressively intense erythema, culminating in cyanosis, destruction, and eschar formation (Figure 7.1). These changes show the

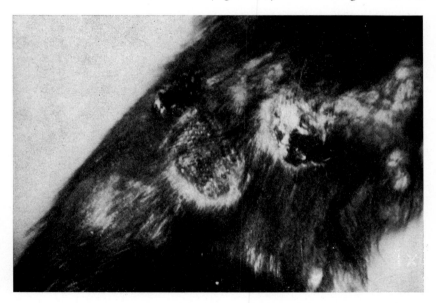

Figure 7.1 Accepted syngeneic (middle) and rejected allogeneic tail-skin grafts on CBA mouse

characteristics of an immunological reaction, namely: (a) *specific*, since tissue grafted repeatedly from the same (but not a different) donor will show accelerated rejection; (b) *reinforced*, since the secondary response is much more violent than the primary; (c) *disseminated*, since hyperactivity to a second graft still ensues no matter where it is placed on the body; (d) *trans-*

acted by lymphoid cells, since during the homograft reaction there is invariably enlargement of the regional lymph nodes and subsequently lymphocytes can be seen to invade the graft. Furthermore, homograft reactivity can be transferred by injecting lymphoid cells from an animal that has already rejected a graft into a potential recipient of a graft from the same donor; and depletion of lymphocytes by immunosuppressive drugs, ionizing radiation or thoracic duct drainage may slow or abrogate the rejection response.

The factors governing the intensity of the primary response to grafted tissue are genetically determined. Acceptance or rejection of the graft is due to genetically determined antigens in the graft itself; these are termed transplantation antigens. The genes responsible for the phenotype of these antigens are called histocompatibility genes and their chromosomal locations (on chromosome 6) are the histocompatibility loci or H-loci. At each of these loci alternative genes or alleles may occur. Histocompatibility alleles are codominant, that is, their products are individually demonstrable in the heterozygote (as with the A and B blood group alleles in man where both antigens A and B are present on heterozygous AB red cells). For this reason, grafts from isogeneic parental strain animals to their F1 hybrids are permanently accepted since the F1 hybrid possesses all the antigens of both its parental strains. (A syngeneic strain refers to a strain where there have been 20 or more consecutive generations of brother–sister matings.) Conversely, grafts from F1 hybrids are promptly rejected by animals of either parental strain since they confront each strain with a set of antigens characteristic of the other strain.

Studies of transplantation antigens are best carried out using skin grafts in small mammals because they are the most exacting of tissues in their requirements for acceptance; they are highly susceptible to even weak levels of immunity and will discriminate finely between histoincompatible animals. Grafts of tissues other than skin, including allogeneic tumour grafts and grafts of solid organs such as renal and endocrine tissues have not been as well studied, and their rejection patterns may be determined by other factors including vascularity and susceptibility to antibodies. Such grafts may occasionally be retained for long periods, despite the fact that a simultaneously placed skin graft taken from the same donor strain may have already been rejected.

The Cellular Basis of Immunological Reactions to Skin Homografts

AFFERENT PATHWAYS

After application of a skin homograft lymphocytes may be sensitized peripherally by making direct contact with the homograft; alternatively, soluble or particulate subcellular units of the homograft may reach draining lymph nodes. One of the experiments showing the former sensitization pathway is that of Strober and Gowans, who passed lymphocytes through a transplanted rat kidney and subsequently showed that such lymphocytes would hasten the rejection of donor strain kidney grafts in recipient strain animals. Also, transplanted kidneys usually contain a resident population of 'passenger leukocytes' which are released into the circulation of the recipient and it may well be that those cells, which are themselves antigenic, evoke the sensitization in the new host.

It has been established that the integrity of the regional lymphatics is an important requirement for the afferent pathway of graft sensitization although lymphatics do not seem to be required for rejection. If a section of skin on the flank of the guinea-pig is deprived of its lymphatic drainage, skin grafted on this undrained area will survive in a prolonged fashion, although it will quickly be rejected if sensitization is evoked by a graft placed elsewhere. The cheek-pouch of the hamster and the brain and testes of mammals generally lack effective lymphatic drainage pathways; both homografts and heterografts have been known to survive for long periods in these sites. In the case of the cheek-pouch bearing transplanted skin, if a state of sensitization is aroused by a second transplantation of skin from the same donor strain to a different, non-'privileged' site, the cheek-pouch skin is quickly rejected indicating that the efferent rejection arm is intact.

CENTRAL PHASE

Sensitized lymphocytes ultimately disseminate sensitivity throughout the body, but they very likely first settle in regional lymph nodes and pro-liferate there. If one excises the regional lymph node draining a homograft earlier than 4 days after grafting, sensitized lymphocytes (i.e. those which will hasten the rejection of grafts in other animals) are present only in this node; after 4 days they are present in other nodes. The population of cells sensitive to skin homografts belongs to the recirculating lymphocyte pool and a specific sensitized population probably results from proliferation at first in the regional node which is then continued in the more distant nodes.

EFFERENT PHASE

Cells of the recirculating pool, many of them newly formed by proliferation either in the lymph nodes or the bone marrow, subsequently reach the skin homograft. At that site, there is initial massive recruitment of normal un-sensitized B and T cells by the sensitized cells. Secondly, there is an attraction of macrophages to the area, probably as a result of the release of macrophage inhibition factor (MIF) by sensitized lymphocytes. Somehow the destruction of the graft is accomplished by all of these cells acting in concert. The complement system may also participate here, perhaps by local direct activation of complement components that are capable of injuring cell membranes.

In order for rejection to take place, lymphocytes must have easy access to the transplanted tissues. The anterior chamber of the eye has long been considered an 'immunologically privileged' site for transplantation, since grafts may be maintained in a viable condition in this chamber without penetration by blood vessels. A number of workers have shown, although not consistently, that both homografts and heterografts will survive for extended periods in this site. Once the graft is vascularized, however, it is only a short time before rejection ensues.

THE ROLE OF SPECIFIC ANTIBODIES IN SKIN ALLOGRAFT REJECTION

It is known that during the process of sensitization to allografts of skin, large amounts of antibody are produced which will specifically react with donor tissue. At the time that cellular proliferation goes on in the regional lymph node there is also intense plasmacytosis indicating that antibodies are being produced. Humoral antibody as such does not greatly influence survival of skin allografts, although antibody has been shown capable of destroying rat skin xenografts placed on mice. It is to be emphasized that skin allografts are rejected by an almost pure mechanism of delayed hypersensitivity or cellular immunity, whereas rejection of other grafts such as kidney or heart probably takes place by both humoral and cellular types of immune mechanisms.

Grafts of Tissues other than Skin

Grafts of dead or preserved tissue (homostatic grafts) are used frequently in surgery to replace diseased segments of bone and blood vessels. For example, ground chips of *bone* taken from animal donors or even from autochthonous bone marrow will not become vascularized after implantation into a surgical wound; nevertheless, the supporting stromal collagen may be retained for long periods, and can serve as a framework for the gradual ingrowth of host tissues. Preserved non-viable *vessels* such as freeze-dried rabbit aorta or tannic-acid treated human umbilical cord, may be sutured directly to living tissue, and over ensuing months the supporting collagenous framework may be colonized by host-supporting tissues and endothelium. Freeze-drying or chemical preservation generally destroys most of the specific antigens so that the recipient is not sensitized to later grafted skin or other tissues from this skin graft donor.

Corneal grafts are considered to be homovital grafts since the cells of the graft may survive intact after transplantation. Corneal grafts are antigenic, and are promptly rejected if transplanted to sites other than the anterior chamber of the eye. Within the anterior chamber, they are relatively protected from the efferent arm of the rejection response because it is difficult for lymphocytes to penetrate through the aqueous humour in the anterior chamber. If the immunological insulation of the cornea is breeched, for example by a blood vessel from the iris which had extended to touch the rim of the graft, this is followed by rapid rejection and opacification.

Similar statements apply to *grafts of cartilage*, in which the individual cartilage cells may remain alive for long periods after transplantation of a crushed cartilage specimen. These cells are also insulated from the action of the sensitized lymphocytes by the thick layer of mucopolysaccharide which surrounds each cell. *Endocrine tissues* were once thought to be poorly antigenic and relatively easy to graft, but it is more likely that most endocrine grafts will be rejected as other tissues. Recently, a recipient of a parathyroid allograft required maintenance chemotherapy with azathioprine and prednisone to prevent rejection and to avoid derangement of calcium metabolism.

Fetal grafts usually do not carry the same surface antigens that are carried by adult tissues, and consequently may sensitize only weakly against subsequent grafts of adult tissues from the same donor. However, such grafts will sensitize to fetal tissues of the same strain animal. Some theories of malignancy include the idea that the surface antigens on tumour cells consist largely of embryonic components which have reasserted themselves on the cell surface. Animals sensitized with fetal tissue may show evidence of sensitization to tumour grafts as well.

Types of Kidney Graft Rejection

The combination of humoral antibody acting on the vasculature of the transplanted kidney, together with cellular infiltration by lymphoid cells, produces the characteristic histological and pathological features of *acute*, *hyperacute*, and *chronic* renal rejection.

In the unmodified recipient of a renal allograft, acute rejection of the transplanted kidney usually takes place between the 8th and 14th day. In the early days of renal transplantation, most patients who received renal transplants underwent a 'rejection crisis' between one and two weeks after transplantation, even though these patients were receiving immunosuppressive drugs. Both cellular and humoral components can be identified in biopsies of such kidneys. Characteristically, there is diffuse infiltration of the entire renal parenchyma by small and large lymphocytes, macrophages, and small numbers of plasma cells. Especially heavy infiltration is found around the smaller afferent arterioles. In some specimens there may be slight swelling and minimal increase in cellularity, and mesangial thickening in the glomerulus. These changes, however, are usually absent or very slight (Figures 7.2 and 7.3).

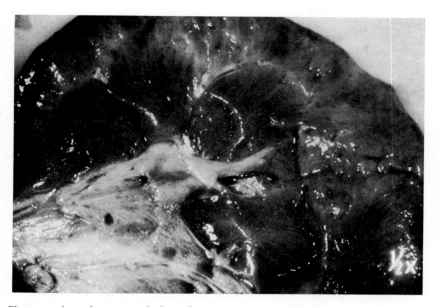

Figure 7.2 Acute human renal allograft rejection, 12 days postoperatively. Note streaks of peritubular haemorrhage and areas of cortical ischaemia and haemorrhage

The timing of early acute rejection is probably a reflection of the kinetics of a primary immune response to the allografted tissue. Approximately one week after sensitization a population of sensitized lymphocytes re-enters the grafted organ, and there is elaboration of humoral antigraft antibody. The pathophysiology of acute rejection may therefore be delayed or altered by the concomitant administration of immunosuppressive agents, such as azathioprine, prednisone, or antilymphocyte globulin. Cellular infiltration may be much less prominent. Immunofluorescent studies would still demonstrate the presence of antibody and complement in the smaller arterioles and the glomeruli, although little histological glomerular change would be evident (Figures 7.4 and 7.5).

The counterpart of the secondary immune response which occurs in patients who may have already been sensitized to specific graft donor antigens is *hyperacute rejection* (Figure 7.6). In extreme cases the kidney may become

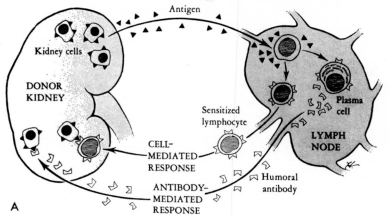

Figure 7.3 Afferent and efferent arms of immune rejection of the allografted kidney. Subunits of donor kidney antigen contact sensitized lymphocytes which ultimately leads to proliferation of T and B cells within the draining lymph node. Populations of sensitized lymphocytes are produced which infiltrate the graft. Also, humoral antibodies are elaborated which injure graft vascular endothelium (see below). From Bellanti, J. A. (1972). *Immunology* (Philadelphia: W. B. Saunders)

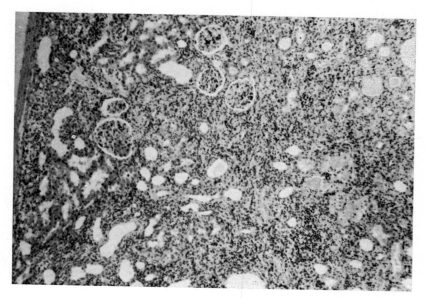

Figure 7.4 Acute rejection of the rat kidney. There is marked infiltration of the entire renal parenchyma by mononuclear cells, with some accentuation of the infiltrate in the area of small peritubular arterioles

cyanotic and cease to function shortly after implantation, indeed, even on the operating table. This type of rejection may proceed by a final common pathway analogous to what is seen in the Schwartzman phenomenon in animals with local paradoxical coagulopathy of the renal vessels. In this case,

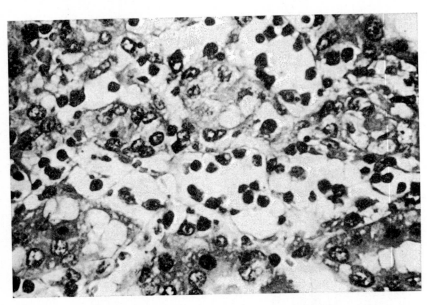

Figure 7.5 High power view of infiltrate in rejecting human renal allograft showing a few polymorphonuclear leukocytes, many small lymphocytes and plasma cells

antibodies in the recipient circulation react directly with donor endothelium and this is followed by deposition of circulating platelets, vessel rupture, and thrombosis and haemorrhage (Figure 7.7). Histologically, the pathological picture seen in hyperacute rejection is acute thrombosis of the medium and smaller arterioles, parenchymal haemorrhage and infiltration with neutrophils, and renal cortical necrosis. The gross appearance of these kidneys is very similar to what is seen in eclampsia. Histologically, there is haemorrhagic necrosis with thrombosis of larger arterioles (Figure 7.8).

If the initial episode of acute rejection is bypassed with the use of immunosuppressive agents, *chronic rejection* may occur over a long period of time, and this is characterized clinically by a progressive deterioration in renal function (Figure 7.9). Pathologically, there is progressive fibrosis and narrowing of vessels, presumably due to the intermittent deposition of fibrin, and progressive occlusion of smaller vessels (Figure 7.10). It is thought that this

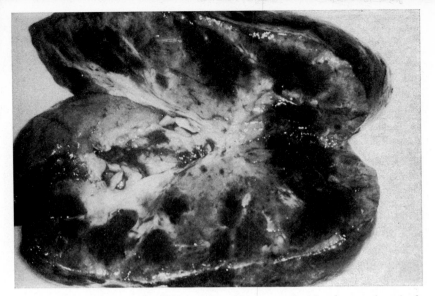

Figure 7.6 Gross photograph of kidney rejected hyperacutely. Note haemorrhage in the medulla region with ischaemic change in the renal cortex

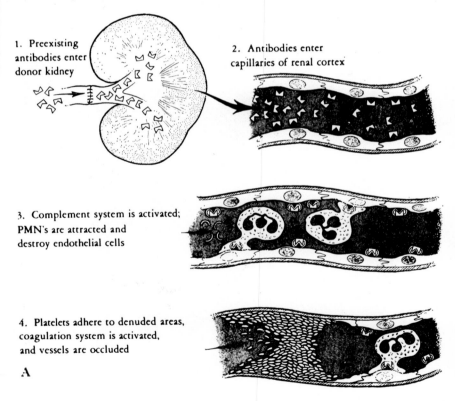

1. Preexisting antibodies enter donor kidney

2. Antibodies enter capillaries of renal cortex

3. Complement system is activated; PMN's are attracted and destroy endothelial cells

4. Platelets adhere to denuded areas, coagulation system is activated, and vessels are occluded

A

Figure 7.7 A schematic illustration of the sequence of events in hyperacute rejection. Taken from Bellanti, J. A. (1972). *Immunology* (Philadelphia: W. B. Saunders)

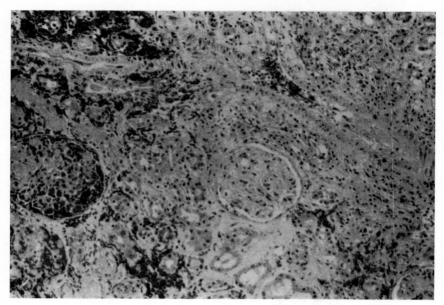

Figure 7.8 The hallmarks of hyperacute rejection are shown in this section of human kidney. There is marked haemorrhage and acute inflammation of the smaller vessels

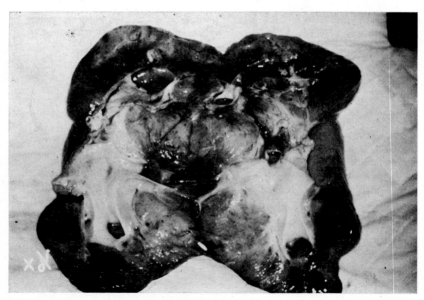

Figure 7.9 Surface of chronically rejected human kidney. The capsule strips with difficulty due to microscopic scarring of the surface leaving the pebble grain shrunk in appearance

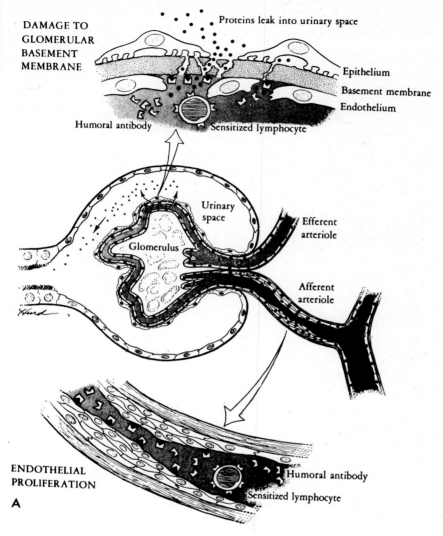

Figure 7.10 Diagrammatic representation of the events in chronic renal allograft rejection. There is both damage to the glomerular basement membrane and endothelial proliferation due to the combined activities of humoral antibody and sensitized lymphocytes. (From Bellanti, J. A. (1972). *Immunology* (Philadelphia: W. B. Saunders)

type of rejection is due to the persistence of low levels of serum antibodies directed against the graft (Figure 7.11).

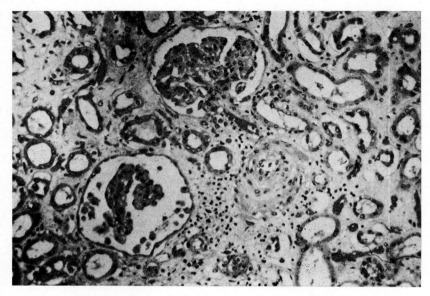

Figure 7.11 The chronically rejected kidney shows a relatively sparse infiltrate. There is endothelial proliferation of the arterioles and some early changes in the glomeruli

Transplantation of Organs other than Kidneys

For reasons that are not well understood, the kidney has been the easiest organ to transplant. To date over 23 300 grafts have been done, and 9 500 recipients are alive with functioning grafts, the longest for over 19 years. Attempts to transplant other organs have been far less successful.

Transplantation of the *liver* has been attempted in a number of cases; initially, none of these patients survived more than a month after transplantation, since the doses of immunosuppressive agents required were too high to allow the patient to fight off infection successfully. More recently, the use of antilymphocyte globulin has permitted survivals up to 6 years in some infants and over 4 years in a few adults after hepatic transplantation. Of over 240 such operations, 29 patients are now alive with functioning grafts. It is interesting in this connection that in certain experimental animals, allografted liver is as easy or easier to maintain than the kidney. In the pig, the liver can be transplanted easily and will survive without any immunosuppression at all. The reason for this is unknown.

Transplantation of the *heart* is beset with difficulties arising from a violent intractable immune reaction. Rejection of the heart is pathogenetically similar to acute rejection of the kidney and is likely due primarily to serum antibodies. Here, even the advent of antilymphocyte globulin has not proven of sufficient value to allow routine transplantation. Nevertheless, there are now at least 50 survivors of cardiac transplantation of over 280 heart transplants, the longest for over 7 years.

Transplantation of the *lungs* as well as combined operations in which the *heart and both lungs* were transplanted have been attended with uniform failure, no patient having survived longer than 10 months. There have been a few instances of attempted transplantation of the *larynx* and of the *pancreas*, but little long-term success has been reported. Of 47 transplants, only 2 are alive with a functioning graft; the longest survival has been $3\frac{1}{2}$ years. In a few cases, attempts to transplant the *adrenals* have been made; in one case, in the early 1950s, a startling success was obtained. However, this has not been repeated or confirmed. There has been one report of a functioning *parathyroid* allograft maintained by immunosuppression in a patient already bearing a grafted kidney.

The transplantation of haematopoietic cells or *bone marrow* transplantation has occupied the attention of clinical haematologists since 1957, both as a tool for restoring diseased marrow of leukaemia or aplastic anaemia patients, and also as a means for inducing chimerism with donor cells allowing tolerance to be induced to a later graft of a solid organ from the same donor. Bone marrow transplantation requires little or no surgical expertise, since a proportion of bone marrow cells infused intravenously as a single-cell suspension will 'home' to haematopoietic organs. Nevertheless the problems associated with marrow grafting have been formidable. First, bone marrow cells have been shown to be exquisitely sensitive to the presence of even small amounts of pre-existing alloantibody (including blood group antibodies). Thus, successful marrow transplantation has proved extremely difficult in patients who had previously received blood transfusions or showed even barely detectable levels of antibody against the infused cells. This has necessitated that near-lethal doses of agents such as total body irradiation and cyclophosphamide are therefore required to generate the immune suppression needed for a marrow 'take'.

A second important complication of marrow transplantation is *graft-versus-host disease*. Bone marrow contains precursors of immunologically competent cells which then mature in the new host. These cells may become sensitized to host antigens and elaborate an immune response directed against the host tissues. If the host is immunoincompetent (as are most patients given immunosuppressive agents prior to marrow transplantation) he will be unable to reject these cells and will consequently suffer graft-versus-host disease.

There may be severe changes in the skin (exfoliative dermatitis), involvement of the liver (cholestatic hepatitis), diarrhea and enteritis, and severe prolonged cellular and humoral immune deficiency culminating in death from over-whelming sepsis.

In order to treat graft-versus-host disease, it is necessary to continue immunosuppression with methotrexate or antilymphocyte globulins for a prolonged period after transplantation. Since both of these agents may depress stem-cell function, the dose must be carefully calculated to allow recovery of haematopoietic cells while simultaneously suppressing lymphocyte activity.

Although over 250 attempts at bone marrow transplantation in man had been recorded up till 1968, there had been no clear evidence of even a single 'take' of the graft. Since that time there have been increased numbers of accepted grafts documented by chromosomal marker studies in patients prepared for marrow transplantation by near-lethal doses of cyclophospha-mide or total body irradiation. So far, the greatest success has been obtained in patients with congenital immunological deficiency disease where there is a defect in rejection of homografted tissues. Immunocompetence was restored to a variable degree after successful marrow grafting. A few successes have also been obtained in adults with aplastic anaemia, and some recipients have survived longer than 3 years with functioning donor haematopoietic cells. A number of graft 'takes' have also been obtained in patients with acute leukaemia, especially after pretreatment with large doses of donor blood cells followed by intensive short-term chemotherapy with cyclophosphamide. However, this procedure will not cure leukaemia; in some cases the trans-planted cells themselves have undergone leukaemic transformation.

Transplantation of the *spleen* has been attempted in very few instances in man, primarily to provide a source of immunocompetent cells in patients with advanced malignancy. No clear-cut benefit was observed, and in one case severe lethal graft-versus-host reaction ensued.

The Nature of Transplantation Antigens

IMMUNOGENETICS

The immunological reaction to transplants is directed against genetically determined foreign substances on the transplanted cells; very likely most of the polypeptide and glycoprotein which forms the cell membrane may be antigenic. As with the blood group substances which vary in their ability to cause strong transfusion reactions, only certain of these substances cause dif-ficulty by stimulating the recipient to reject the graft. Further, just as with bacterial antigens, the type of immune response engendered by different surface antigens may be mainly either humoral (i.e. a stimulus to the B cell system) or cellular (delayed hypersensitivity reaction with little humoral components).

Apart from ABO antigens which may act as strong transplantation antigens, the most important of these substances are antigens of the 'major histocompatibility system' (MHS) which are coded for in the MHS region (see Figure 7.13).

In this region there are three subloci which code for three serologically determined (SD) (formerly HLA, Human Leukocyte Antigen) antigens and at least two lymphocyte-determined (LD) (formerly MLC, Mixed Lymphocyte Culture Antigen) antigens. Serologically determined antigens, as the name implies, are defined by sera obtained from either pregnant women or

MHS PHENOTYPE INHERITANCE

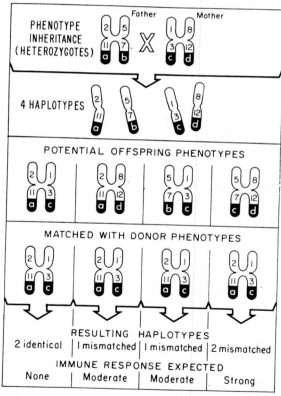

Figure 7.12 Schematic presentation of HLA and MLC chromosomal region with the nomenclature (WHO Nomenclature Committee, 1971) of the different allelic antigens for HLA system. (Modified from Thorsby, E. (1974). *Transplant. Rev.*, **18**, 51

multiply transfused volunteers. By exhaustive testing of panels of antisera by cytotoxicity or agglutination assays against panels of lymphocytes from normal individuals, patterns of specificity and gene frequencies have been developed. The lymphocyte determined antigens do not stimulate antibody formation, but rather stimulate T-cells in the mixed lymphocyte reaction, so that analysis of different specificities defined by these antigens has been a much more difficult task. Hopefully, newer techniques such as automated detection of surface immunofluorescence may aid in directly typing for these specificities as well. The different antigens which can occur at the three SD subloci are shown in Figure 7.13. Thus, each individual would be expected to have a total of six SD antigens, each coded for three MHS subloci on each of two chromosomes. The gene products of each of the three MHS subloci can be shown to move independently on the cell surface by immunofluorescent techniques so that, as in the inheritance of ABO blood group antigens, allelic exclusion does not operate in this system, and inheritance of the SD and LD antigens follows Mendelian laws (Figure 7.12). The best type of transplant is when donor and recipient (both members of the same family) are identical for both SD and LD regions of the MHS.

It is now known that the rejection of tumour grafts and most likely renal, bone marrow, and skin allografts requires the interaction of both LD and SD antigens with both T and B cells. It is thought that T cells are best stimulated by LD antigens and react minimally, if at all, to SD determinants. On the other hand, antibody produced by B cells, as well as *in vitro* B cell-mediated cytotoxicity or cellular cytotoxicity mediated by lymphocyte-dependent antibodies, are all directed against SD determinants. Thus, in the usual sequence of rejection the T cells would be stimulated by LD; stimulated T cells, together with B cells programmed to react against SD determinants, would then interact to induce the latter cells finally to mount the reaction against SD determinants.

The relative influences of SD and LD compatibility matching on the ultimate outcome of renal allotransplantation is presently under investigation. There is some suggestion that in patients matched for LD antigens, a mismatch for SD antigens may only be of importance if the patient has already been sensitized to SD antigens (as by previous renal allografting, pregnancies, or by multiple transfusions of blood during prolonged haemodialysis). The consideration of T and B cell interactions becomes much more important in bone marrow transplantation, where the rejection reaction may proceed in either direction resulting in either destruction of the graft or graft-versus-host disease. It is not inconceivable for example that lymphocytes of the host may be sensitized by the donor graft, and exert a helper effect on graft lymphoid cells in the production of graft-versus-host disease. Host-versus-donor

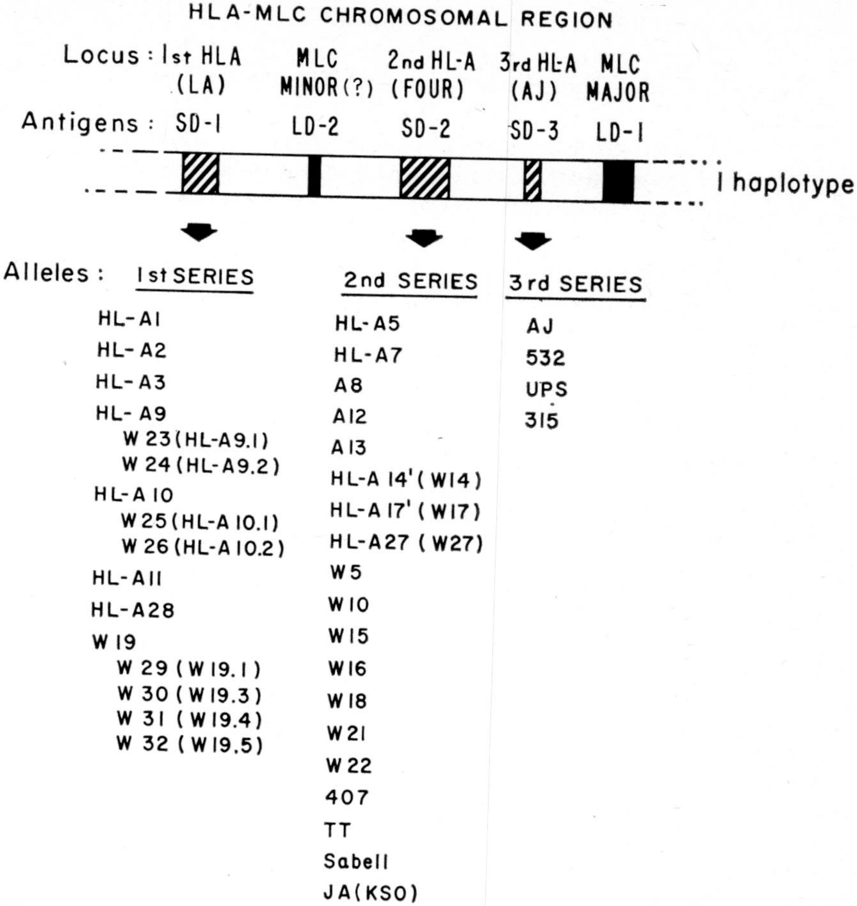

HLA-MLC CHROMOSOMAL REGION

Locus : 1st HLA MLC 2nd HL-A 3rd HL-A MLC
(LA) MINOR(?) (FOUR) (AJ) MAJOR

Antigens : SD-1 LD-2 SD-2 SD-3 LD-1

l haplotype

Alleles : 1st SERIES 2nd SERIES 3rd SERIES

1st SERIES	2nd SERIES	3rd SERIES
HL-A1	HL-A5	AJ
HL-A2	HL-A7	532
HL-A3	A8	UPS
HL-A9	A12	315
W 23 (HL-A9.1)	A13	
W 24 (HL-A9.2)	HL-A 14' (W14)	
HL-A 10	HL-A 17' (W17)	
W 25 (HL-A 10.1)	HL-A 27 (W27)	
W 26 (HL-A 10.2)	W 5	
HL-A11	W 10	
HL-A28	W 15	
W 19	W 16	
W 29 (W 19.1)	W 18	
W 30 (W 19.3)	W 21	
W 31 (W 19.4)	W 22	
W 32 (W 19.5)	407	
	TT	
	Sabell	
	JA (KSO)	

Figure 7.13 MHS phenotype inheritance. Antigens determined by the MHS are inherited in Mendelian fashion, with no allelic exclusion. Thus, any of 32 phenotypes may be realized if both parents differ at all three SD loci, and if LD antigens are taken into account. Assuming the existence of only one LD locus, the chances are 1 in 16 that two siblings will match for both LD and SD

reactivity *in vitro* has been associated with the later development of para-doxical increased severity of graft-versus-host disease after marrow grafting.

Although the presence of MHS compatibility is important to the pro-tection of grafts as shown by the fact that identical members of the *same* family show markedly prolonged survival of exchanged skin grafts, SD identical members from *different* families do not enjoy such prolonged survivals. Thus, there may be many minor determinants of histocompatibility, not coded for by the MHS region, which also play an important. although not pre-eminent, role in graft rejection.

Histocompatibility antigens may be determined by several means including:

(a) *Serologically determined (SD) leukocyte antigens* are assayed for by agglutination or cytotoxicity tests. In these tests lymphocytes are isolated from the peripheral blood and exposed *in vitro* to previously characterized antisera. The ability of an antiserum to agglutinate cells or to promote complement-mediated cytotoxicity is taken as evidence for the presence of the relevant SD determinant on the cell surface.

(b) *Lymphocyte-determined (LD) antigens* are determined by the mixed lymphocyte culture (MLC) assay, in which appropriate numbers of lymphocytes from the prospective donor and recipient are mixed together and incubated for several days in nutrient medium. LD histoincompatibility will incite protein, RNA, and DNA synthesis in the responding set of lymphocytes which can be detected either by morphological change (blast transformation) or by incorporation of radioactive metabolites (e.g. [^{3}H]thymidine). If one set of leukocytes is treated with irradiation or antimetabolites so as to minimize its capacity for DNA synthesis, these cells may still serve to stimulate the reaction; the assay is then termed a 'one way' MLC.

(c) *Test grafting.* The *'third man' skin graft test* was previously used to test the similarity of donor and recipient transplantation antigens by the acceleration of rejection when grafts from the donor and recipient were placed sequentially on a third antigenically indifferent recipient. Accelerated rejection of the second graft indicated prior sensitization by antigens common to the first and second grafts. *Direct placement of a test skin* from a prospective donor onto a prospective recipient has been generally avoided because of the danger of sensitizing to a subsequent renal allograft. However, preliminary testing with skin grafts from several different family members has recently been used as a means for determining which prospective donor excites the weakest transplant reaction and seems to be of value as an aid in organ donor selection.

(d) A variant of the skin graft tests, *the normal lymphocyte transfer reaction* was also used to select the best organ donor from a panel. Lymphocytes from a prospective recipient were injected into the skin of several prospective donors, where they generated a delayed hypersensitivity response in proportion to histoincompatibility. This and similar tests have not proved as reliable, however, as *in vitro* testing and are little used.

(e) Other experimental techniques devised to test histocompatibility prior to transplantation employ chromium labelled donor lymphocytes or lymphoblasts in short-term culture as targets for the action of lymphocytes of the prospective recipient. In some variations of this assay, donor lymphoblasts or cultured kidney cells may first be exposed to recipient serum before lymphocytes are added. The end point of the assay is the ability of lymphocytes with or without added serum to injure the cell membrane of the target cell releasing radioactive chromium into the supernatant. In general, these assays have been unsuitable for prognosticating graft survival, although they may offer techniques for investigating the mechanisms that may be operating during graft rejection.

In renal transplantation, it is assumed that the transplantation antigens present on the surface of peripheral blood leukocytes correspond to those present on the surface of the kidney cells and thus the behaviour of the renal graft might be predicted by determining the compatibility between the leukocyte antigens of the donor and the recipient. This does not always hold, and it is likely that kidney cells may contain additional antigens as well. However, there is some evidence that donor–recipient compatibility for leukocyte antigens may indicate a good prognosis with regard to renal allograft survival.

A mismatch in any of the MSH antigens, so that the donor possesses antigens lacking in the recipient, will unfavourably influence the prognosis of graft survival. It is more difficult to answer whether the degree of incompatibility should be used to select suitable donors, or whether all such mismatched donors are equally unsuitable.

Management of Rejection

The response to homografted tissues may be abrogated by agents which interfere with the sensitization pathway, or with replication of sensitized lymphocytes. Alternatively, they may interfere with the efferent arm of rejection by decreasing the effect of antibodies or sensitized cells on the rejecting graft.

The drugs used most often and in highest dosage for the management of rejection are the corticosteroids, mainly prednisone and predisolone. Their mechanism of action in delaying rejection has not yet been determined. Corticosteroids are lympholytic in certain animals, in whom they may antagonize delayed type hypersensitivity reactions and humoral antibody production. In man their effects on lymphoid cell interactions is less clear. High doses of corticosteroids will cause transient lymphopenia due to redistribution of both B and T lymphocytes from the blood into the bone marrow. Chronic administration of steroids may lower immunoglobulin levels slightly. Nevertheless, administration of corticosteroids can cause a dramatic reversal in all indices of rejection. Lymphoid cell infiltration of the kidney may lyse rapidly after steroid administration, and renal function improves even before there is any detectable drop in the level of antigraft antibodies. Most likely, steroids in this situation inhibit those reactions which are ordinarily triggered in small vessels by the union of antigen, antibody and complement.

The chronic administration of corticosteroids is, at the time of this writing, indispensable for maintaining the function of the homografted kidney. The attendant side-effects of steroid usage including Cushing's Syndrome, peptic ulceration, aseptic necrosis of bone, and heightened susceptibility to infection, have made the reduction or elimination of this type of maintenance therapy an urgent priority of all research in immunosuppression.

Chemical immunosuppressives such as 6-mercaptopurine (6MP) were originally borrowed from the therapeutic armamentarium of the haematologist where they were used in treatment of leukaemia, lymphoma and autoimmune diseases. 6MP and its imidazole derivative, azathioprine, both depress DNA and RNA synthesis in lymphoid cells. In rabbits administration of 6MP may delay the onset of the secondary humoral response to bovine serum albumin or sheep red cells. In man, similar immune effects have been seen in azathioprine-treated patients after immunization with salmonella antigen. The effects of either agent on delayed hypersensitivity and cell-mediated immunity in man have not been systematically studied.

The mechanism of action of azathioprine in maintaining renal allografts is not known. In conventional doses, there are no clear-cut effects demonstrable on lymphocyte populations or immune responses *per se*, and the drug may exert its effects by an anti-inflammatory activity. In a few cases even very small doses of azathioprine, given in conjunction with corticosteroids, have been sufficient to maintain the function of renal allografts. However, if these very small doses were withdrawn, prompt and vigorous rejection ensued.

More recently, cyclophosphamide, an alkylating agent useful in the management of lymphomas and some types of carcinomas, has also been used as an immunosuppressive agent because of its powerful effects on the immune response in experimental animals, and in patients with autoimmune diseases. Its spectrum of activity and toxicity is similar to that of the purine antagonists, with the additional side-effect of possible hair loss. No obvious therapeutic advantage has yet been ascribed to the use of cyclophosphamide rather than azathioprine.

Heterologous antilymphocyte globulin (ALG) is now being used in a number of centres as an adjunct to treatment with corticosteroids and antimetabolites in the management of rejection. Antilymphocyte serum is produced by immunizing horses or rabbits with pooled human lymphoid cells (peripheral blood lymphocytes or thymus-cell suspensions). The resulting antisera are then assayed for activity against human lymphocytes. Irrelevant antibody against human red cells, platelets on glomerular basement membrane may be present and must be absorbed. The globulin fraction of these antibodies (ALG) may then produce significant immunosuppressive effects by direct destruction or inactivation of lymphocytes. In experimental animals antilymphocyte globulin serum has been one of the most potent inhibitors of cell-mediated immunity yet described. Small doses of ALG administered to mice will prolong skin grafts to four or five times their usual survival. Larger doses allow the prolonged survival of xenografted skin.

The impact of antilymphocyte globulin on clinical renal transplantation has been difficult to assess. A controlled study of cadaver renal transplant recipients has indicated that the use of ALG has led to a lower incidence of rejection crisis and better renal function in the treated group. However, overall survival did not appear to be significantly improved. Treatment of acute rejection crisis with an intensive course of ALG has also not been shown to be superior to management with more conventional agents.

Specific Allograft Tolerance, Enhancement and Adaptation

Conventional immunosuppressive agents possess the drawback of suppressing many immune responses in addition to the allograft response, thus compromising host defences against infection and the spread of neoplastic cells. For this reason, many investigations have been concerned with techniques by which specific immune responses may be selectively suppressed.

TOLERANCE

The clonal selection hypothesis of Burnet postulates that those subsets of lymphocytes which ordinarily might give rise to immune reactions against autologous tissue components are eliminated before birth. The experiments of Billingham, Brent and Medawar showed that if animals were infused with large doses of specific antigen (usually in the form of living haematopoietic cells) at a time when the immune system was still 'immature', then acquired immunological tolerance to antigens of the donor would be induced. Subsequent skin grafts from donor strain animals would be accepted, often for the life of the recipient. The presumption was that immature lymphocytes reacting to foreign antigens could not sustain a normal response and would be destroyed or eliminated from the clonal array. Usually haematopoietic or lymphoid cell chimerism was necessary for maintaining the non-reactive state.

Acquired allograft tolerance is very difficult to induce in markedly histoincompatible adult animals. Temporary states of specific non-reactivity may be induced by infusions of allogeneic bone marrow or spleen cells in conjunction with near lethal doses of irradiation or cyclophosphamide or large doses of ALG. Recently, specific depression of transplantation immune response was achieved in rats by implantation of a donor strain spleen directly into the circulation of a prospective recipient of a skin allograft. Here too, tolerance was not permanent unless established across weak histocompatibility barriers.

Tolerance to skin allografts has been achieved in man after induction of haematopoietic chimerism by total body irradiation and allogeneic marrow transplantation. However, the severe risks of marrow aplasia and graft-versus-host disease make this unsuitable for routine use in transplantation. Some recent animal work suggests that intravenously infused donor platelets may substitute to an extent for haematopoietic cells, and when used in conjunction with high doses of cyclophosphamide, may achieve a greater increment of specific immunosuppression than could be obtained by the use of either agent alone.

ENHANCEMENT

A number of recent experiments suggest that the immune response to allografted tissues may on occasion be paradoxically specifically inhibited by the action of certain humoral antibodies or sensitized cells. It is now well recognized that some animals immunized with lyophilized irradiated allogeneic tumour tissue may develop serum antibodies which, rather than exerting a cytotoxic effect on the tumour, served to 'enhance' tumour growth in these animals or even in other passively immunized tumour-bearing recipients. The mechanism of action of these antibodies is unknown although it is likely that their primary effect is exerted on sensitized cells in lymphoid organs rather than on antigenic determinants at the site of the grafted tissue per se. It has been found that some animals made tolerant to skin allografts by neonatal injection of allogeneic bone marrow also show 'enhancement', since their cells retain the capacity for immune reactions against donor antigens, but these reactions are blocked by inhibitory serum antibodies. Similarly, serum taken from rats immunized with allogeneic spleen or renal tissue develop antidonor antibodies in their serum which are capable of paradoxically prolonging the survival of donor strain renal allografts in newly grafted animals syngeneic with the recipient.

Although the development and use of enhancing antisera holds great promise for the future, at present they have not been characterized well enough to be clinically useful. Enhancement of renal allografts in animals is limited to certain strains of rats. Enhancing antibodies may also produce slight or moderate prolongation of skin allograft survival in some strains of rats and mice, but the effect is less than that seen with renal grafts. In man, hyperimmune antigraft antibody directed against SD donor antigens has been used for passive immunization of a prospective recipient of a renal allograft. No definite benefit, however, could be definitely ascribed to this procedure since the patient was treated with prednisone and azathioprine as well.

It is possible that certain sensitized lymphocytes, termed 'suppressor cells', may be mobilized for specific immunosuppression by pretreatment of recipients with donor antigens or specific antidonor antibody. However, suppressor cells have so far been identified only in certain spontaneously occurring human diseases (multiple myeloma, common variable hypogammaglobulinanaemia) and their possible use in clinical transplantation remains speculative.

ADAPTATION

In certain situations, allografts may become established in hosts that are potentially capable of rejecting them by mechanisms different from either tolerance or enhancement. For example, in certain instances when a primary renal allograft has become established, a second allograft placed side by side with the first from the donor was quickly rejected although the first remained intact; in this situation 'adaptation' of the graft is said to have occurred; the well-healed graft had become more resistant to rejection mechanisms. Such phenomena have also been observed, although less often, with grafts of endocrine organs and skin allografts. Graft adaptation may be due to vascularization of the grafted tissue by host endothelium, or to progressive loss of antigenic 'passenger' leukocytes from the grafted tissue.

Teleology and Tissue Transplant Rejection

A biological system as sensitive and specific as that which comprises lymphoid cell populations active in transplantation immunity did not evolve merely to frustrate attempts of the surgeon to graft organs between histoincompatible individuals. It is likely that cellular immune mechanisms in general were meant to deal with localized deposits of relatively insoluble antigenic materials which are relatively resistant to the attack of serum antibodies. The histocompatibility antigens on the surfaces of cells seem to serve as an efficient signal to this segment of immune system which may allow it to distinguish between 'self' and 'not-self' determinants. It has been hypothesized that a system capable of discriminating between homografts and autografts should also be capable of distinguishing antigens on tumour cells from those on normal cells of the host animal, and perhaps the homograft reaction originally served as a means of surveillance of the body against the emergence by mutation of clones of neoplastic cells. The increased incidence of malignancy in patients with congenital immunodeficiency diseases or those given immunosuppressive drugs would tend to support the idea of a role for transplantation immunity in surveillance against neoplasia.

We are indebted to Dr. S. Dikman for some of the microphotographs, and to Ms. V. Dinneny, for excellent preparation of this manuscript which was supported in part by a Grant from the New York State Kidney Disease Association.

Further Reading

Historical

Largiadèr, F. (1970). History of organ transplantation. In F. Largiadèr (ed.), *Organ Transplantation*. 2nd Ed., pp. 2–12. (Stuttgart: Georg Thieme Verlag and New York: I.M.B. Corp.)

Saunders, J. B. (1972). A conceptual history of transplantation. In J. S. Najarian and R. L. Simmons (eds.), *Transplantation*, pp. 3–25. (Philadelphia: Lea and Febiger)

Transplantation Immunology

Billingham, R. E., Brent, L. and Medawar, P. B. (1956). Quantitative studies on tissue transplantation immunity. III. Actively acquired tolerance. *Phil. Trans. R. Soc. (London) Series B*, **239,** 357

Billingham, R. E. and Silvers, W. (1971). *The Immunobiology of Transplantation*. (Englewood Cliffs, N. J.: Prentice-Hall)

Calne, R. Y. (1973). *Immunological Aspects of Transplantation Surgery*. (Lancaster: MTP)

Najarian, J. S. and Simmons, R. L. (1972). *Transplantation*. (Philadelphia: Lea and Febiger)

Rappaport, F. T. and Dausset, J. (1968). *Human Transplantation*. (New York: Grune and Stratton)

Roitt, M. (1974). *Essential Immunology*, 2nd Ed. (Oxford: Blackwell Scientific Publications)

Russell, P. S. and Monaco, A. P. (1965). *The Biology of Tissue Transplantation*. (Boston: Little, Brown and Co.)

Woodruff, M. F. A. (1960). *The Transplantation of Tissue and Organs*, p. 102. (Springfield: Charles C. Thomas)

Transplantation Immunogenetics

Thorsby, E. (1974). The human major histocompatibility system. *Transplant. Rev.*, **18**:51

Histopathology of Renal Transplants

Meadows, R. (1973). Transplantation. In *Renal Histopathology*, pp. 328–356. (New York: Oxford University Press)

Porter, K. A. (1974). Renal transplantation. In R. H. Heptinstall (ed.), *Pathology of the Kidney*, pp. 977–1041. (Boston: Little, Brown and Co.)

CHAPTER 8

Immunosuppression

E. M. Lance

Introduction

The advances over the past several decades in our ability to manipulate immune responses depend largely upon the advent of a wide variety of agents and methods that suppress immunological reactions. Although some of these agents have resulted from careful planning and research, a number of others represent the fallout of the effort to develop chemotherapeutic agents for the therapy of malignancy. Historically, the major impetus for research into the area of immunosuppressive agents was provided by the work of Medawar (1944), who made it clear that the barrier to tissue transplantation was an immunological one. Although the scene is changing, it remains true that the clinical possibilities of organ transplantation still provide the urgency and thrust for continuing research and the largest single outlet for application.

The great success of kidney transplantation as a means of treating chronic renal failure has been achieved only through the advent of potent immunosuppressive agents and this alone assures that immunosuppression is here to stay as a clinical therapy. Nonetheless, current means of achieving this goal are still crude and dangerous justifying application at present to conditions that seriously threaten life. Even within this limited context, there is little cause for smugness, for a critical examination of the results of vital organ transplantation other than kidney leave much to be desired. Either kidneys are 'easy' transplants and require less immunosuppression for success or other vital organs such as heart, lung and liver fail for non-immunological reasons. At the moment the weight of evidence favours the former possibility. Therefore, realization of the full clinical potential for immunosuppression will continue to depend upon progress in the development of immuno-suppressive techniques.

Assuming that the appropriate developments will be forthcoming, the potential for the future is exciting. With the advent of agents or com-bination of agents with high therapeutic indices transplantation of vital organs other than kidney should become commonplace. One would predict further clinical extension of transplantation techniques including the use of skin allotransplants to support the burned patient, and ultimately trans-plantation of non-vital organs for the treatment of endocrine deficiency, congenital limb abnormalities and the ultimate feasibility of xenogeneic transplantation. Although the current drama is centred around the clinical setting of transplantation, a much wider ultimate scope for the application of immunosuppressive agents may be found in the management of patients with a wide group of disorders generally classified under the heading auto-immunity. There is already considerable evidence that the use of intensive immunosuppression may favourably modify the natural history of diseases such as rheumatoid arthritis, systemic lupus erythematosus and more recently, multiple sclerosis. The dangers inherent in the current generation of immunosuppressive agents loom much larger in the mind of a clinician when deciding between therapeutic alternatives for many of the auto-immune diseases. Therefore, the current promising results of experimental trials in this area offer a tantalizing imperative for further research.

In this chapter, we will review in a general way what is known about the agents most commonly employed. We have grouped agents together classifying them according to specificity. Before proceeding to a detailed consideration of these agents, a few general remarks on the potential hazards of immunosuppression seem in order.

Complications of Immunosuppression

The noxious effects of immunosuppressive agents may be considered under two general headings: those that arise as a unique property of the agent itself not necessarily related to its immunosuppressive action, and those which arise as a direct consequence of immunosuppression.

The corticosteroids are often employed in current immunosuppressive regimens either on their own or more usually in conjunction with one of the cytotoxic drugs. Their use is associated with a significant morbidity aris-ing from a multiplicity of actions irrelevant to immunosuppression. Included amongst these are the development of the features of Cushing's syndrome with salt and water retention, hypertension, diabetes and distortion of the physiognomy. Particularly dreaded complications not uncommonly associated with the use of corticosteroids include the induction of severe osteoporosis and associated avascular necrosis of bone leading to disabling collapse of major weight-bearing joints, the facilitation of gastrointestinal ulceration with severe sudden haemorrhages often unaccompanied by the usual prodromata of such conditions, interference with wound healing through retardation of the elaboration and maturation of collagen (a particular problem for the surgeon) and an increased susceptibility to infection as a by-product of general anti-inflammatory effects. Therefore, the use of steroids is truly a double-edged sword representing at once a potent and perhaps indispensable immunosuppressive adjunct and the most significant contributor to noxious sequelae. In children the use of corticosteroids is even more pernicious, for it is a potent inhibitor of skeletal growth.

The cytotoxic drugs produce an entirely different but nonetheless devastating range of complications. These include such relatively trivial but often very distressing manifestations such as alopecia to the dreaded complication of bone marrow depression. These complications arise as the consequence of the mode of action of these agents which generally interfere with the turnover of cell populations. It follows, therefore, that rapidly dividing cell populations are at the greatest risk and the therapeutic range of dosage required for effective immunosuppression is almost coextensive with the range of clinical toxicity.

Turning to the hazards inherent in immunosuppression itself, it has long been recognized that the humoral antibody response is part of the basic defence mechanism against bacterial invasion. It follows that any agent that depresses the ability of the organism to respond in this fashion opens the possibility of increased numbers and severity of infections. Were it not for the possession of potent antibiotic agents, the dangers to patients treated with these agents might preclude their use. With the co-temporal growth and knowledge of the cell-mediated immunities and the advent of immuno-suppressive agents particularly effective in suppressing this category of reactivity, it has become clear that cellular immunity is also of extreme importance in the resistance to many potential pathogens. These include certain bacteria such as the agents of tuberculosis and leprosy, many fungi and viruses as well as a number of parasitic nematodes and helminths. The frequency with which patients with immunological deficiency, either natural or acquired, succumb to bizarre infections with these organisms has been well documented. Therefore, increased susceptibility to infection must be accepted as a direct consequence of non-specific immunosuppression and will manifest itself in proportion to the potency of the agents employed.

Another potential threat even more ominous than infection is the danger of potentiating malignancy. There has been speculation in immunological circles that the natural function of immunity (especially the cell-mediated apparatus) might be the detection and elimination of potentially malignant clones of cells. Although this hypothesis has not been convincingly proven and notwithstanding the conflicting evidence in the literature in which animals treated with continuous immunosuppression failed to exhibit an increased background of malignancies, the now well-documented increased frequency of neoplasia in patients with renal allografts is very disquieting. Particularly disturbing is the implication that there is a direct proportionality between the efficacy of immunosuppression and the frequency of this dread complication. These findings conform to the predictions which might have been drawn from those experiments of nature in which immunodeficiency occurs as a congenital disorder or as a consequence of ageing or auto-immunity. The recent experimental evidence suggests that immunosuppression *per se* may not be a sufficient incitement to the development of malignancy, but that the presence of a concomitant ongoing immune reaction is also required. This will provide small comfort to the clinician who will nonetheless be obliged to apply immunosuppression in precisely such a setting.

These remarks make it clear in which direction skill in immunosuppression must develop. Ways must be found to suppress immunological reactions selectively. The current generation of clinically used agents are a bludgeon to the immune mechanism as they indiscriminately ablate function. We require instruments that dissect out the pertinent reactivities alone and leave the organism with its basic defences intact. To emphasize the importance of this concept, the classification of individual agents and methods has been organized to proceed from the general to the particular, that is one in which the aim of immunosuppression is progressively focused more sharply.

AGENTS OR METHODS THAT DO NOT DISCRIMINATE FOR LYMPHOCYTES

Anti-inflammatory agents

The criteria which we use to measure or assess immunological reactivity at the level of the tissues depend upon the inflammatory response which in itself is completely non-specific. The skin reactions elicited by tuberculin or candida in a sensitized individual cannot be distinguished by the clinical observer. Moreover, tissue damage which results as a consequence of an immunological reaction seems to be mediated through non-specific inflammatory processes. Thus, although immune reactions are themselves highly specific, their manifestations are often non-specific. Inflammation represents the final common pathway for tissue damage initiated by the release of pharmacologically active substances. In the case of immediate hypersensitivities, it is quite clear that when antihistamines or corticosteroids are used to offset acute allergic rhinitis, asthmatic attacks or manifestations of anaphylaxis, these agents act to inhibit inflammation rather than effecting the interaction between antigen and antibody. What remains largely unquantified at the present date is the extent to which the value of agents such as steroids widely used in tissue transplantation as immunosuppressive drugs may, in fact, be making their greatest contribution through their ability to suppress inflammation. A striking example of this possibility is the demonstration that hypnotism can be shown to ablate delayed hypersensitivity skin reactions and to prolong the survival of skin allografts in man. Correlative histological studies make it clear that the underlying immunological events are not effected. Lymphocytic infiltration proceeds on schedule; however, the inflammatory and vasomotor events that make the reaction manifest are forestalled.

Ionizing irradiation and radiomimetic drugs

Irradiation in the form of x-rays was probably the earliest agent demonstrated to suppress immunity. At the beginning of the century it was known that the prior administration of whole body irradiation could suppress the subsequent antibody response to antigen. Some 50 years later it was formally demonstrated that the rejection of skin allografts could also be suppressed by this manœuvre. This order of discovery is not surprising in view of the generalization that irradiation is more effective in opposing humoral than cell-mediated immunities. In common with cytostatic agents, irradiation is less effective when given after immunization and by extension of what is probably the same principle, more effective in opposing sensitization than immunological memory.

Irradiation achieves its immunosuppressive effect in at least two ways. It destroys lymphocytes directly, and it depletes the population of stem cells which are required for replenishment. Within hours after irradiation, histological changes are evident in lymphoid tissue and by 24 hours massive depletion is present. Unfortunately, these effects are not specific for lymphocytes, although they are known to be very sensitive to irradiation. Depending upon the dose of whole body irradiation, other organ systems also suffer damage. The syndromes that appear as the dose of irradiation increases are haematopoietic, gastrointestinal and cerebral. Each of these can be fatal and unfortunately the haematopoietic system has about the same order of sensitivity to irradiation as does the lymphocytic. Therefore, at doses of whole body irradiation that are immunosuppressive, one can expect bone marrow atrophy leading to pancytopenia.

Although in the past whole body irradiation has been used to promote the survival of renal transplants, the relative lack of effect on cellular immunity and the high levels of toxicity proved a discouraging combination and this form of treatment would not be considered seriously for such a purpose today. However, there have been more encouraging developments that use the radioactivity of radionuclides in such a way that the effects are localized to lymphoid tissue. We will deal with these below.

Local radiation has also been used to produce atrophy of lymphoid organs such as the thymus and spleen, often in conjunction with other immuno-suppressive agents. Although the data are few, the evidence does not suggest that these are useful procedures. One use of radiation that has proven bene-ficial in transplantation has been the local irradiation of the renal transplant at the time of transplantation or shortly thereafter and also as a form of therapy for rejection crises. Although there are theoretical reasons why such treatment might be helpful, for example by eliminating donor lympho-cytes which might contribute to host sensitization or to destroy effector cells that have infiltrated target organs, the clinical and experimental evidence does not permit any appraisal of this manœuvre in comparison to alternative forms of treatment.

Cytostatic agents

Agents included in this heading are the antimetabolites and the alkylating agents (purine analogues and folic acid antagonizers). These drugs are often referred to as immunosuppressive agents by second intention. That is, they have entered the clinical armamentarium largely as a by-product of the search for agents effective against malignancy. In fact, most agents used to treat cancer have some immunosuppressive effect. These agents as a class share with irradiation the disadvantage of non-specificity. They have a wide range of undesirable side-effects, and the therapeutic range is virtually co-extensive with the toxic dose range. They are probably too toxic to be used as primary immunosuppressive agents in humans entirely on their own and for the most part are employed in conjunction with corticosteroids. The predominate manifestation of toxicity in common with irradiation, is bone marrow depression.

Cytostatic agents act by interfering with basic metabolic processes neces-sary for cell division, differentiation, or protein synthesis. The purine analogues have enjoyed wide and well-deserved popularity. It is a fair com-ment that the success of clinical renal transplantation is in large measure due to the advent of azathioprine which still constitutes the anchor of most therapeutic regimens. This drug developed from conscious efforts to find a purine analogue which might inhibit cancer growth. 6-MP (6-mercapto-purine was synthesized first, and subsequently the imidazole-substituted azathioprine (Imuran). These agents appeared to block a stage of lymphocyte differentiation, that is formation of the immunoblast, which is believed to be central during the sensitization process. Folic acid antagonists such as methotrexate appear to inhibit a subsequent step: the proliferation of immunoblasts and reconversion into small lymphocytes. The alkylating agents exemplified by cyclophosphamide may act to block differentiation and proliferation of lymphocytes. At any rate these agents have drastic effects upon lymphoid tissue and can produce necrosis within lymphoid organs shortly after administration.

Irrespective of the exact biochemistry involved, all these agents are essentially antiproliferative and, as such, most certainly effect the amplification of the immune response which is necessary to the production of antibody or large numbers of effector cells in cell-mediated responses. It is this feature which makes all such agents more effective when given before or simultaneously with antigen and explains as well the relative inefficiency in presensitized animals. A finding, well documented for the purine analogues, is that the 7S antibody response is much more severely affected than the 19S response. An interesting and highly useful application of biochemistry is relevant to the use of the antifolic agents. Their toxic effects can be largely offset by the subsequent administration of folinic acid and moreover this manœuvre does not reverse the immunosuppressive effect.

Under some circumstances, depending upon such factors as antigen dose and timing, augmentation rather than depression of antibody synthesis has been associated with the administration of cytostatic agents (this applies to irradiation as well). A variety of explanations have been put forth to account for this observation: creation of *Lebensraum*, release of nucleic acids which facilitate the replication of responding cells, or the induction of some sort of compensatory feedback mechanism resulting in an overshoot. Present evidence does not allow a choice between these possibilities. However, this effect must always be borne in mind and could explain some otherwise curious findings in humans.

The fact that these agents can suppress cell-mediated immunity has been demonstrated for both delayed hypersensitivity and tissue transplantation. As a generalization, they are more potent inhibitors of humoral immunity. The prolongation of skin or renal allografts is not terribly impressive when compared for example with the effects achieved by antilymphocyte serum. All cystostatic agents are relatively ineffective in opposing immunological responses in presensitized individuals. There is little to choose between these agents but, however, if one had to make the choice, then cyclophosphamide may have a greater range of effectiveness and slightly higher therapeutic index than the others.

The importance of these agents is twofold. They constitute the main-stays of the current generation of immunosuppressive agents and secondly they can be used to abet the induction of immunological tolerance. In this regard the pioneering work of Schwartz and Dameshek (1952) deserves special mention. They were the first to show that immunologically specific tolerance could be induced in adult animals through the combination of 6-MP and antigen. The ability to use the cytostatic agents as a means for setting the stage for tolerance induction may prove to be the most important application of this class of agents in the future.

AGENTS THAT DISCRIMINATE FOR LYMPHOCYTES

Corticosteroids

We have already indicated that this class of agent exerts anti-inflammatory effects, but it is also clear that the adrenal corticosteroids exert profound and direct effects upon lymphocytes. The interrelationship of the lymphatic and adrenal tissues has been long appreciated, but the detailed mechanisms through which steroids affect lymphocytes still remain in large part mysterious. There is no question that corticosteroids can kill lymphocytes *in vivo*, and lymphopenia in the blood and lymph nodes has often been attributed solely to cell destruction. However, recent work suggests that another mechanism may come into play, namely the driving of lymphocytes from the periphery into bone marrow compartments. Steroids are known to suppress humoral antibody responses in a variety of animal species. Suppression of primary responses is much more effective than that observed in secondary responses and steroids have a maximal effect when given prior to antigen. There is impressive evidence that steroids prolong the survival of tissue allografts. Suppression of the second set response is also well documented. This is in marked contrast to most conventional immunosuppressive agents and also differs from the effect of steroids on the humoral secondary response. In spite of this evidence, there is little direct proof that steroids as commonly used in man are immunosuppressive. Patients treated with corticosteroids at dose levels commonly used to maintain renal allografts have little altera-tion in those aspects of immunological function which have been studied thus far. It may well be that the appropriate tests have not yet been chosen or that the level of sensitivity in our assays is too low. The major use of corticosteroids in the context of immunosuppression is in conjunction with cytostatic agents to support renal allograft survival. The toxicity of steroids is well known and has been reviewed briefly above. The numerous side-effects associated with their use constitutes a major drawback to their application. It has been recently suggested that many of these undesirable side-effects are reduced by administering steroids on alternate days rather than as a steady daily dose. However, the evidence on this point is too scanty to be conclusive.

The future for steroids seems to be as a synergizing agent with other therapies. In this context the remarkable synergy between antilymphocyte serum (ALS) and steroids is of special interest. Steroids are as effective in maintaining a state of immunosuppression induced in mice by ALS as is the continued administration of ALS itself. The explanation for this finding may lie in the fact that while steroids at large doses have a direct lympholytic effect they exert a highly toxic action on young immature thymocytes even at low doses. Therefore, low doses of steroids after ALS serve to prevent regeneration of the recirculating lymphocyte population believed crucial to the rejection of solid allografts.

Surgical ablation of lymph nodes or spleen

Although these procedures have been tried clinically, their major interest lies in what they have revealed about the immune response, since any alterations in responsiveness have been too feeble for clinical exploitation. Lymphadenectomy does impair the rejection of skin grafts within its area of drainage. In view of what is known about the initiation of the immune response to skin allografts, this is not surprising. Although the antigen-sensitive lymphocyte may become initially aware of the presence of graft antigens through direct contact with donor tissues, it is clear that these cells migrate to the regional lymph nodes where they undergo explosive pro-liferation. The descendants of these cells spread throughout the lymphoid tissue of the body and indeed, some probably return to the graft where they participate in the rejection response. It seems likely that a similar course of events takes place during sensitization to other antigens administered via the dermal or subcutaneous routes. A privileged site for the placement of skin allografts can be created by preparing skin pedicles devoid of lymphatic drainage. However, sensitization ultimately occurs. This is also the case for the naturally occurring 'privileged' sites such as the intracranial cavity and the anterior chamber of the eye where no primary lymphatic drainage exists. Although sensitization is much delayed it none the less occurs, presumably because some cells find their way to lymphoid tissue via the bloodstream.

The spleen is the major site for antibody production when antigen is administered via the intravenous or intraperitoneal route. It is possible to design experiments wherein dosage and timing are critical to show that splenectomy can impair the immune response. However, the opposite effect can also be demonstrated and may be attributed to two separate mechanisms peculiar to the spleen. The spleen seems to be a major site for the production of so-called 'blocking' antibodies and under some circumstances ablation of the spleen may accelerate allograft breakdown. More recently, evidence has been adduced to the effect that a subclass of thymus-derived cells which have a propensity to localize in the spleen may exert a regulatory function on the magnitude of both cell-mediated and humoral responses. Thus, it can be demonstrated experimentally that the response to sheep erythrocytes or the graft-versus-host response may actually be augmented following splenectomy. For these reasons the effect of splenectomy is not only sometimes paradoxical, but often unpredictable. In clinical practice it would appear that the opposed functions of the spleen often cancel each other out since there has been no demonstration that splenectomy is of any value as an adjunct to immunosuppression with respect to organ allotransplants, or for that matter that patients who undergo splenectomy for entirely unrelated reasons suffer from inadequate immunological responses.

Asparaginase

The fact that the enzyme asparaginase adversely effects the performance of lymphocytes was first revealed by the demonstration that a factor present in normal guinea-pig serum could inhibit lymphoid leukaemia cells. This agent, subsequently shown to be asparaginase, is now enjoying some vogue in the treatment of lymphatic leukaemias in humans. Lymphocytes appear to have a greater requirement for asparagine than other tissues. Removal of this amino acid from the environment impairs lymphoid performance. The greater sensitivity of lymphocytes to deprivation means that an element of specificity can be achieved in this way. A number of studies have been undertaken to investigate the potential of asparaginase as an immunosuppressive agent. The results are somewhat contradictory and some of the differences probably stem from the difficulty in obtaining pure preparations of standardized activity. There is also the difficulty that asparaginase is usually produced from bacterial sources and the preparations are therefore highly immunogenic. As a consequence of this immunogenicity *in vivo* neutralization is likely to occur. Nonetheless, recent experiments seem to establish that the administration to mice of large doses of asparaginase can inhibit both cell-mediated and humoral antibody formation. The precise mechanism of action has not yet been elucidated nor is it known whether one lymphocyte subpopulation is more susceptible than another. The immunogenicity of asparaginase and the fact that even at high doses the immunosuppression is relatively feeble compared with other immunosuppressive agents, probably indicates that the clinical utility of asparaginase is limited. Nonetheless, the advent of this type of agent is exciting to the clinical immunologist because of the suggestion that peculiarities of metabolism may exist for lymphocytes and, indeed, why not lymphocyte subpopulations which can be manipulated and controlled by specific metabolic inhibitors. Therefore, work in this area will be followed with considerable interest.

AGENTS WHICH DISCRIMINATE FOR MACROPHAGES
Reticuloendothelial blockade

There is overwhelming evidence that macrophages are important and even required for the initiation of humoral antibody formation to some antigens. The exact way in which macrophages participate is still *sub judice*, but it seems clear that they can process antigen or present antigen to lymphocytes in a way that enhances immunogenicity. It is also clear that macrophages participate as effector cells in many types of immune responses, and indeed they are an invariable histological feature at sites of inflammation. The role of macrophages in the initiation of transplantation rejection is less clear. Histological and kinetic studies make it certain that macrophages are present during rejection, but they appear to arrive in large numbers after sensitization has already occurred. However, *in vivo* studies using models of the allograft reaction seem to require the presence of macrophages for sensitization, so that it is best to keep an open mind in this regard. The omnipresence of macrophages during cytopathic immune reactions suggests that interference with their performance should seriously alter the response. In the light of this, it is interesting to note that agents that preoccupy macrophages, for example large amounts of trypan blue dye or colloidal carbon particles, do in fact impair immune responses and delay, for instance, the rejection of skin allografts. This effect, known as reticuloendothelial blockade, is, while clearly demonstrable, rather feeble and escape or rerouting must occur.

Antimacrophage serum

The remarkable success of ALS soon led to attempts to prepare an antiserum directed against macrophages. Although rather glowing reports were made initially it seems that most of the immunosuppression (IS) activity in antimacrophage serum (AMS) could be attributed to the presence of antibodies directed against lymphocytes. Indeed, when rigorous attempts were made by careful absorption to remove ALS activity from AMS, the IS effect also seemed to have been removed. However, monospecific AMS can be quite effective *in vitro* and alters the behaviour of macrophages both with respect to their kinetics and their ability to participate in immune responses. The discrepancy between *in vitro* and *in vivo* activity may be related to the fact that after extensive absorption the titre of AMS activity against macrophages is relatively low or there may be a problem of access to macrophages *in vivo*. That is, the antibodies simply may not be able to reach the macrophages fixed within tissues in high enough titre. The rapid production of new macrophages from bone marrow precursors may also be an obstacle, because any damage caused by AMS could be rapidly repaired. None the less, this serological approach is well worth pursuing. It is clear in mice that cell surface differentiation antigens characterize the different cell types, and there is no theoretical reason why antisera of great specificity and potency could not be developed. The value of such agents would be their selective action and therefore corresponding freedom from noxious sequelae.

AGENTS THAT DISCRIMINATE BETWEEN LYMPHOCYTE SUB-POPULATIONS

Recirculating small lymphocytes

Thus far we have discussed agents or manipulations that affect cells, be they lymphocytes or macrophages, in an indiscriminate way. As a consequence, the IS effects have been rather broad, showing depression of both cell-mediated and humoral immunities. Nevertheless, agents described in the above sections are an improvement over those described in the first, not because they are more potent suppressors of immunity but because they are less toxic to the recipient. We now turn to methods that represent a considerable refinement because they affect predominantly lymphocyte subpopulations. In the past 20 years, it has become clear that lymphocytes, which appear to be a fairly homogeneous population on morphological grounds, are in fact heterogeneous. They can be divided into subpopulations on the basis of several criteria, but one of the most useful distinctions is that some lymphocytes continuously recirculate from the blood to the lymph, while others are predominantly sessile within lymphoid tissue. In the mouse abundant evidence exists to equate the recirculating lymphocyte subpopulation with the thymus-derived, small, long-lived cell chiefly responsible for the mediation of cellular immunities although participating as a helper in some humoral responses. The sessile lymphocytes can be equated with the bone marrow-derived lymphocyte which is the precursor cell in humoral antibody production. Although these distinctions can be made with the greatest clarity in the mouse, the data available in other species suggests that this gross division of lymphocytes into functional subclasses applies as well. In man, the best evidence comes from experiments of nature in which some children are born congenitally deficient in one or the other subclass. There are, for instance, agammaglobulinaemic children missing a functional bone marrow-derived subpopulation who cannot mount humoral antibody responses but are perfectly able to reject skin grafts. Conversely, some children born without a thymus have a specific deficiency in cell-mediated immunity. It will be clear to the reader that to be able to duplicate this set of events in patients at will would have distinct advantages. For instance, in transplant patients the ability to suppress cell-mediated immunity while not disturbing humoral responses might be advantageous, while in patients with malignancy the exactly opposite circumstances appear to be desirable. This type of immunosuppression or, preferably, immunoregulation would be equivalent to the ability of a hi-fi enthusiast to adjust the treble or bass boosts on his equipment to give the precise effect desired.

1. *Thymectomy*. Ablation of the thymus in experimental animals before the peripheral lymphoid system is populated with recirculating T cells has profound IS effects. Such ablations, which are usually performed in the perinatal period, produce animals that are unable to reject allografts and which have deficient delayed hypersensitivity responses. They are also deficient in some humoral antibody responses, namely, those for which the T cell acts as a helper. There animals in an unprotected environment have a very circumscribed life span and are subject to an illness known as runting, which may result from their inability to mount effective protective reactions. Although the exact cause of runting is unknown, this syndrome can be avoided by rearing these animals in a gnotobiotic environment. When thymectomy is performed in adult life, no effect is apparent for many months. This is explained by the fact that the recirculating lymphocyte is a long-lived cell, and there is some evidence in humans that these cells may last for 20 years or more and, indeed, some investigators believe for the lifespan of the animal. Nonetheless, in mice in which although thymic atrophy occurs the thymus appears to be functional into adulthood, there is a gradual depletion of T cells after adult thymectomy, and defects in immunological performance are detectable after a lapse of 6 months. In large mammals, including humans, in which the thymus undergoes rather more complete involution at about the time of puberty, there is little evidence to suggest that immune function is in any way impaired by adult thymectomy. It may be that insufficient time has elapsed at the time of study or that tests of insufficient sensitivity were employed, nevertheless, thymectomy in humans does not appear to be a useful adjunct to immunosuppression. A trial of thymectomy in combination with conventional IS agents in renal transplant recipients did not show any clear-cut gross differences in comparison to controls, although on histological criteria there was a suggestion of less severe damage to the renal allografts of thymectomized patients than to those of controls. The usefulness of thymectomy in humans might have a role in preventing the regeneration of T cells depleted through the use of some of the other agents mentioned later. Such a role has been convincingly demonstrated in experimental animals.

2. *Thoracic duct drainage*. The creation of a fistula via the thoracic duct allows the drainage of recirculating cells preferentially and produces clear-cut depression of cell-mediated responsiveness. Animals so treated show a selective lesion histologically in the lymph nodes and spleen where the so-called thymus-dependent areas are depleted of cells while the non-thymic areas remain normal. Studies in rats, dogs and humans have shown that thoracic duct drainage impairs the rejection of both renal and skin allografts. Indeed, thoracic duct drainage is now currently employed to prepare patients for renal transplantation, although the mainstay of immunosuppression still depends upon conventional agents. Thoracic duct drainage has been an important tool in studying the dynamics of lymphocyte recirculation and also in revealing the pathways lymphocytes take in the execution of their immunological functions. A skin graft placed in the area of drainage of a thoracic duct fistula remains unrejected for as long as the fistula remains open, while a skin graft in the cephalic portion of the animal is rejected normally. This suggests that lymphocytes must re-enter the circulation from the draining lymph node in order to effect rejection. These studies also point out one of the inadequacies of thoracic duct drainage as an IS tool, namely, that there are other pathways, that is, alternative routes by which lymphocytes can avoid exteriorization via a thoracic duct fistula. This in turn may explain the relative inefficiency of thoracic duct drainage in depleting recirculating cells when compared to, for instance, ALS.

Although these features taken in combination with the fact that thoracic duct drainage requires an operative procedure with its attendant risks of complication and that it is sometimes difficult to maintain a continuously draining fistula, combine to make thoracic duct drainage a less desirable way of depleting recirculating lymphocytes than for example ALS. However, it may well be that the synergistic effect of combining thoracic duct drainage with ALS therapy as is currently employed by the Munich group headed by Brendel has certain advantages. They have found that their clinical results seem to be best in patients who have had both thoracic duct drainage and ALS administration as compared to groups of patients who have had only the thoracic duct drainage or ALS singly. Moreover, it appears that thoracic duct drainage prior to the administration of ALS may help in reducing the immunological response to the foreign serum components of ALS or to abet the induction of specific immunological tolerance. There is also the consideration that some patients will be allergic to the foreign proteins represented by ALS and for these patients thoracic duct drainage may be the only practical alternative.

3. *Extracorporeal irradiation of blood (ECIB).* By creating an arteriovenous fistula and effecting a shunt of blood flow through an irradiation chamber, lymphocytes in the circulation can be exposed to damaging doses of irradiation. The advantages of such a procedure are twofold. Toxicity is limited to other blood elements, for example, erythrocytes, and a selective effect on circulating lymphocytes can be achieved. Histological examination of lymphoid tissues after ECIB reveals depletion of lymphocytes in a selective fashion, that is, in those areas normally populated by recirculating cells. Therefore, the effect of ECIB is similar in many ways to thoracic duct drainage. However, the great expense of such apparatus, the necessity for patients to travel to such facilities, the prolonged exposure times required for the delivery of clinically effective doses, and the cumulative damage to erythrocytes, as well as the fact that it hardly seems within the realm of possibility that access could be made available to more than a handful of patients, limits the potential of this method largely to that of a research tool. However, there may well be application in selected problem cases such as the treatment of rejection crisis, an application that has already been tested with some success.

4. *Antilymphocyte serum.* One of the most exciting developments in the field of immunosuppression has been the realization of the remarkable potency of ALS in promoting the survival of tissue allografts. This class of agents had been rather unsystematically investigated since the time of Metchnikoff, but it was not until inhibition of the tuberculin reaction had been shown that the potential for immunosuppression was recognized. Although not the first to report prolongation of skin allograft survival, the work that clearly established ALS as a potent and relatively innocuous inhibitor of graft rejection was performed by Woodruff and Anderson (1963).

The features that distinguish ALS from other IS agents explain why interest in the study and development of this agent continues unabated at the present. ALS may be said to be the first really true IS agent inasmuch as it achieves its effects as a direct result of its effects upon lymphocytes and not as a by-product of some more general antimetabolic action. This specificity undoubtedly contributes to the low toxicity associated with its use. Indeed, ALS can be administered to animals continuously over long periods without significantly altering growth, weight gain, the ability to procreate or to raise normal litters, and without apparent prejudice to health. Moreover, the former occurs at doses that achieve remarkable IS effects. This combination of low toxicity and high potency gives ALS a high therapeutic index.

ALS has been shown to be the most potent inhibitor of cellular immunities.

Delayed hypersensitivity reactions are abolished by quite small doses, and the survival of allografts and xenografts greatly extended. The use of ALS in animal models has made what were hitherto considered difficult transplantations easy, and impossible transplants possible. The graft-versus-host reaction is also susceptible to the action of ALS. In some contexts, modification is best achieved by treatment of the cell donors (rodents), whereas in others, treatment of the cell recipients seems better (primates including humans). ALS can also inhibit the humoral antibody response, especially to those antigens classed as thymus-dependent. There are, however, important differences in the effects achieved in these two arms of the immune response. ALS appears to oppose rejection of all types of transplants effectively, whereas depression of antibody response is restricted to some antigens. Dosage levels of ALS that effectively support the indefinite survival of skin allografts across strong histocompatibility barriers do not prevent the formation of antibodies to antigens contained within the graft, nor alter the antibody response to serum proteins contained in the heterologous ALS itself. ALS is effective in preventing rejection even in presensitized animals and can be shown to abolish memory of prior sensitization under appropriate dosage regimens, whereas ALS is almost without effect in opposing the secondary humoral antibody response. On histological grounds a similar distinction is also evident, for the lesion created by ALS is selective with depletion of those sections of lymphoid tissue associated with cellular immunity (the so-called thymus-dependent areas), while the germinal centres, cortex and medulla, remain intact. This selectivity against cell-mediated immunity distinguishes ALS from other IS agents which, insofar as their usage is associated with discriminative effects, oppose humoral immunity more effectively. In common with other IS agents, ALS can be used to set the stage for the induction of immunological tolerance. By using ALS as the sole IS agent, tolerance to allografts lasting for hundreds of days has been achieved. Although tolerance to xenografts can also be accomplished in a similar way, the results, as might have been predicted, are not as impressive, and it has been found necessary to combine ALS with thymectomy to prevent the rapid loss of tolerance to xenogeneic antigens. The way in which ALS achieves these effects has been the subject of some controversy, but it now seems relatively clear that whatever secondary effects may also occur, the IS action of ALS is achieved by a progressive and selective depletion of the recirculating lymphocyte subpopulation. It is believed that after injection high titres of antilymphocytic antibody are achieved in the blood and extravascular compartment. Lymphocytes present in these peripheral sites are coated with antibody and are either directly killed through an interaction with host complement or opsonized and subsequently ingested by macrophages. Lymphocytes that are obliged to enter the circulation, that is, the recirculating pool, are at greatest risk, while those that remain without the confines of lymphoid tissue (which ALS does not penetrate as heavily) are relatively protected.

Although the site of action of ALS is peripheral, the central stores of recirculating lymphocytes are gradually depleted as members of this compartment are obliged to enter the circulation. This hypothesis now rests on substantial experimental evidence and accounts for the known properties of ALS. It explains why cell-mediated immunity and the humoral response to some antigens that require assistance from recirculating cells are selectively depressed. It also provides an explanation for the fact that the IS effect of ALS outlasts by so long its own metabolic lifetime within the host inasmuch as it is known that the recirculating pool of lymphocytes is regenerated very slowly. Therefore, depletion is only slowly reconstituted. Moreover, the synergy between ALS and thymectomy and small doses of hydrocortisone agents, which prevents or retards regeneration of this cell population, receives a rational base.

ALS may be raised by the injection of the lymphocytes from one species into another. Although potent antisera can be raised by using any source of lymphocytes, certain cell sources have advantages primarily because of the freedom from contaminating cell populations which give rise to undesirable antibodies and which increase the need for absorption. The relevant antibodies in the resulting preparation are the antilymphocytic antibodies of the IgG class. Antibodies that arise as a result of tissue contaminants or in response to antigens shared by lymphocytes and other tissues may be removed without prejudice to the IS potency. While the exact antigenic target of ALS has not yet been identified, it is clear that the relevant antigen or antigens are both tissue- and species-specific, that is, they are differentiation antigens of lymphocytes and are shared by the lymphocytes of all members of the species. Whether or not these antigens identify a lymphocyte subclass has not yet been clearly established, but current evidence suggests that this is not the case.

The use of ALS in clinical practice was pioneered by Starzl et al. (1967) and has now come into rather general use. The greatest clinical experience with ALS relates to its application in the field of clinical organ transplantation and a number of findings attest to its beneficial effects. These include a reduced frequency and severity of rejection crises, a better histopathological and functional status of the transplanted organ, the ability to reverse severe rejection crises and by the inclusion of ALS into the immunosuppressive regimen and ability to lower the overall dose of steroids which are administered. In most clinical protocols ALS is not administered continuously throughout the post-transplant period, but rather is confined to a period of several weeks in the peritransplant phase. More recently attention has been directed towards the use of ALS in the treatment of a variety of so-called autoimmune conditions. Most reports in the literature are limited to rather small series of cases usually covering a wide variety of entities so that it is difficult to be certain that the natural history has, indeed, been altered. However, there have been some outstanding successes reported, particularly with disorders such as sympathetic ophthalmia, the nephritis of lupus erythematosus, dermatomyositis and the management of patients with multiple sclerosis when treated in the acute phase of disease. For the most part these reports are anecdotal and it will remain for properly controlled studies including large numbers of patients with a single entity and followed for a reasonable period of time before the role of ALS in the treatment of these disorders can be established.

Although there is good clinical evidence that ALS is a potent immuno-suppressive agent in humans, when viewed in the context of the spectacular results achieved in experimental models the results seem to be slightly disappointing. There are many reasons why this might be so: the toxicity of earlier preparations which limited their administration in suitable dosage, problems associated with the administration of large doses safely, the immunogenicity of foreign proteins in general and ALS IgG in particular. With respect to this last obstacle there now appears to be a strong ray of hope that the immunogenicity of ALS IgG can be circumvented by the prior induction of immunological tolerance. This approach has been successfully demonstrated in animals a number of times and there are now a number of reports in the clinical literature indicating that by the prior administration of relatively large doses of aggregate-free normal IgG, it is possible to induce a state of specific immunological tolerance so that upon the subsequent administration of ALS IgG no immune reaction occurs. Of course, any contaminating serum proteins other than IgG still present in the ALS preparation upon administration will continue to be immunogenic and therefore this approach requires the clinical availability of ALS IgG in high degrees of purity.

All of the foregoing notwithstanding the most important single obstacle to the rational use of ALS preparations in man has been the lack of a reliable assay for the potency of material generated for use in humans. The most reliable assay in experimental animals is one based upon the ability of ALS to prolong the survival of skin allografts across a known histocompatibility barrier. While some studies have established that similar models in humans can be assessed with similar results, this is not a practicable clinical possibility for general use. The search for a simple *in vitro* test that will predict *in vivo* potency goes on, and many such candidates have fallen by the way-side. Currently, the most promising candidates are the inhibition of rosette formation and various opsonization tests. None of these offers a complete correlation with skin allograft prolongation, but they represent steps in the right direction. At present, ALS is tested by a combination of *in vitro* assays plus an *in vivo* skin allograft assay in surrogate subhuman primates. Since the acceptance of this procedure and with the increasing confidence in drawing upon the results of animal experimentation to guide both the pro-duction, purification and application of ALS, there has been a notable im-provement in the results achieved in clinical trials and there is no reason to assume that the promise inherent in experimental experience will not also be fulfilled in humans.

The enthusiasm many have expressed for ALS is justified in that ALS is certainly a step in the right direction, for it allows discriminate immuno-suppression. However, there is no reason to be complacent, because the dangers in depressing cell-mediated immunity are still formidable. The fore-going remarks on this subject apply with equal force to ALS, that is, one can expect a weakening of host resistance to certain infectious agents such as viruses and fungi and, moreover, there is still an unquantified risk of increasing the background rate of spontaneous neoplasm. There is no way around this problem inasmuch as complications of this kind can be predicted to arise in direct proportion to the potency of the agent used.

Non-recirculating lymphocytes

1. *Bursectomy*. In the same way the thymus serves as a primary lymphoid organ controlling the maturation of the recirculating lymphocyte, so in birds does the bursa of Fabricius act with respect to the cells that mediate the humoral antibody response. These bursa-dependent cells can be deleted as a consequence of neonatal ablation of the bursa with a corresponding defect in the humoral antibody response. There is as yet no known bursal equivalent in mammals, and the corresponding cell population is spoken of as bone marrow-derived to distinguish it from the thymus-derived popula-tion. Several investigators have endeavoured to locate a mammalian bursa equivalent by ablating various portions of gut-associated lymphoid tissue but without convincing results thus far.

It would obviously be an advantage to be able to depress humoral re-sponses selectively, leaving cell-mediated immunity intact in the same way that the converse is true. We have stated that some of the conventional IS agents appear to discriminate slightly in favour of humoral immunity and, more recently, Turk (1972) has produced evidence that cyclophosphamide can, under some circumstances of dosage and administration, produce lymphoid depletion of extreme degree in the cortex, germinal centres, and medullary areas of lymphoid tissue, while leaving intact the thymus-dependent areas. Animals so treated may actually have an augmented delayed hypersensitivity responsiveness which may represent release from the restraint of enhancing antibody formation.

2. *Specific antisera.* In addition to some of the properties already mentioned that can be used to discriminate between lymphocyte subpopulations, there are antigenic differences that can also be used to distinguish these cells. It is probably a general property of differentiation that mature cell lines possess cell surface antigens that are distinctive. These antigens are called differentiation antigens, and antisera specific for these antigens can be raised which have selective actions. In this way, for example, θ is known to be a differentiation antigen of thymus-derived cells, and anti-θ antiserum is selectively cytotoxic for T cells *in vitro*. Because all attempts thus far to exploit this property *in vivo* have failed to reveal any immunosuppressive effect, this agent has not been hitherto mentioned. It is interesting to speculate on the discrepancy between the *in vitro* efficacy of anti-θ antiserum and its total lack of potency when administered *in vivo*. The most likely explanation for this discrepancy is as follows. Although θ is a cell surface antigen specific amongst lymphocytes for the thymus-derived subpopulation, there is broad representation of this antigen in other tissues. For example, θ has been found on epidermal cells and in the brain and on some tumours arising from the adrenals. It is likely that were a thorough search made for the representation of this antigen additional sites would be apparent as well. Therefore, the wide tissue distribution of θ in the body will act as a sponge to absorb any anti-θ antiserum administered *in vivo* removing a large portion of the antibody which might have otherwise been available to react with lymphocytes. However, the *in vitro* treatment of heterogeneous cell populations with anti-θ can be used to depress the subsequent ability of such cells to cause graft-versus-host reactions after transfer to appropriate hosts.

In much the same way, it is possible to raise antisera that are specific *in vitro* for the cell surface antigens of the bone marrow-derived cell. Thus far, for poorly understood reasons, this class of antisera seems not to possess immunosuppressive properties *in vivo*. In experimental animals it has been possible to raise an antiplasma cell serum which after suitable absorption appears to react with differentiation cell surface antigens expressed only on the surface of the plasma cell. Upon administration of such antisera to animals it has been possible to suppress selectively the humoral antibody response to a variety of antigens. Therefore, this type of approach retains considerable appeal because the potential for reagents of this type is so great that continued effort along these lines is well worth pursuing.

AGENTS THAT DISCRIMINATE FOR SPECIFIC REACTIVE LYMPHOCYTE CLONES

Without entering the argument about how the situation arises, it is generally accepted that lymphocytes are not omnipotential with respect to all immunogens. The reactivity of individual cells is confined to one or perhaps several closely related antigenic determinants. This selective reactivity is in turn dependent upon cell surface sensing units which direct the immunological reactivity of the individual cells. According to this notion, antigenic strength may be nothing more than a reflection of the number of potentially reactive cells within the total lymphocyte population. If it were possible to remove selectively just those potentially reactive cells, then immunosuppression with respect to any given antigen or combination of antigens could be effected while leaving the immunological defences of the animal otherwise intact.

Acquired immunological tolerance

The presentation of antigen to animals at a time when their immunological apparatus is immature often results in a state of specific non-reactivity to that antigen when challenged after maturity. Reactivity to other antigens remains unimpaired, so that a specific deletion has been effected from the immunological repertoire. This set of conditions mimics to some extent the state of affairs presumed to act with respect to self-antigens. The theoretical importance of this phenomenon can hardly be over-estimated but does not offer many practical applications, for in clinical settings we deal for the most part with patients who are immunologically mature. Under these circumstances the introduction of antigen ordinarily leads to immunity. There are some notable exceptions to this rule which concern special antigens administered under strictly limited circumstances of route and dosage, but for practical purposes these can be ignored. It was therefore a great step forward when the studies of Schwartz and Dameshek (see the section on cytostatic agents, page 234) established that IS agents used in conjunction with antigen could produce specific tolerance in adult animals. This property already alluded to above is shared by a great many IS agents, with ALS being outstanding with respect to transplantation antigens. The mechanism operating here appears to be one in which IS agents reduce the immunological reactivity to that which obtains in the immature animal, whereupon the antigen is introduced. Reactivity recovering in the continued presence of antigen somehow precludes the development (at least in a functional sense) of the relevant reactive clone. To set the stage, as it were, for tolerance induction, a brief albeit intensive treatment programme is required approaching toxic levels with the conventional IS agents, whereupon antigen is introduced. This more-or-less standard protocol explains both the advantages and disadvantages of this approach since, although the long-term use of IS agents and the attendant hazards are circumvented, the required treatment is fairly drastic. In this sense, the finding that ALS is effective in this context at dosages which, although high, appear to be well tolerated by experimental animals, represents a great advance holding out the hope that such an approach may become clinical reality in humans.

Of course, the ideal solution is to find a way to present antigen so that tolerance is the outcome rather than immunity, a circumstance at present applying to only a very few types of antigen.

Immunological enhancement

Enhancement shares in common with tolerance that the deletion of responsiveness applies to a specific antigen; however, the mediator is not antigen directly but antibody. Antibody interferes with immune responsiveness either by competing with potentially reactive lymphocytes for antigen, or by exerting some central feedback-inhibiting control, or most probably through some combination of these two mechanisms. Enhancement can be achieved either through active immunization of the host with antigen according to certain prescriptions, or through the passive infusion of antibody from one animal to another.

Of great practical significance is the growing realization that the enhancement of antibody may interfere with the expression of cell-mediated immunity and that this may in fact apply to many states of non-reactivity formerly attributed to the mechanism of tolerance. Nowhere does this possibility have greater importance than in the field of clinical cancer research where good evidence exists that such situations may obtain. In the context of tissue transplantation, such a situation might be highly desirable (apart from worry concerning the long-term effects of antibody in damaging tissue and the question of antigen–antibody complexes), but this is clearly disastrous in the context of cancer where cell-mediated responses appear necessary for destruction of solid neoplasms. In this context the desirability of IS agents selective for humoral immunity becomes apparent.

Antigen columns

When a population of lymphocytes known to contain cells capable of responding to a given antigen is passed through a column containing particles coated with that antigen, the effluent consists of cells that have been specifically depleted of reactive cells. The evidence that these cells have actually been retained within the column, rather than having been modified during passage, consists in the fact that reactive cells can be recovered from the column by appropriate washing. This technique remains at the moment an interesting research tool but might, for instance, be exploited in the field of bone marrow transplantation to remove cells with the potential to react to the transplantation antigens of the host and, therefore, avoid the dreaded complication of graft-versus-host disease.

Immunological suicide

1. *Radioactive antigen.* The killing of a specific lymphocyte clone can be effected through reaction with radioactive antigen. This approach takes advantage of the interaction between antigen and cells that have a specific cell surface receptor for that antigen. By labelling the antigen with a beta-emitting isotope in high concentration, it is possible to deliver lethal doses of irradiation to those cells that combine with antigen, while cells that do not make close contact with antigen are relatively spread.

2. *5-Bromodeoxyuridine treatment.* Since one of the consequences of antigen recognition by specifically reactive clones is the process of blast transformation, it is possible by introducing a lethal DNA analogue at the appropriate time *in vitro* to cause irreparable damage to a highly select population of cells.

The approaches discussed in the sections on antigen columns and immunological suicide are at the moment entirely experimental but are included because they point the way to the possible development of techniques that may one day be practicable in humans, and, moreover, approach the ideal of immunosuppression, namely, to delete only the desired specific reactivity without disturbing the general economy of the organism.

MISCELLANEOUS COMMENTS

Because of the great theoretical and potential clinical importance of improving techniques in immunosuppression, the search for new agents and manœuvres will continue to go on. Some rather recent experimental work offers promise for the future. For example, a substance has been identified in peritoneal exudates of experimental animals aroused either through the introduction of non-specific irritants or in response to ascitic tumours which interferes with the recruitment of circulating lymphocytes upon administration to otherwise normal animals. This has the effect of producing a non-specific immunosuppression by interfering with one of the early kinetic events which occurs after immunization through a mechanism quite distinct in its mode of action from that of any other immunosuppressive technique currently available.

Another promising area for future research concerns the differential susceptibility of lymphocyte subpopulations to freeze–thawing damage. It has been found that lymphocyte subpopulations can be selectively destroyed by choosing different cooling and thawing rates and, moreover, that it is possible to stimulate clones of lymphocytes responsive to a particular mitogen or immunogen so as to alter selectively their susceptibility to this kind of damage. Therefore, it is theoretically possible to produce clonal elimination by step-wise stimulation and freeze–thawing and such a technique might be particularly applicable in the processing of bone marrow transplants. Adjuvants are powerful stimulators of the immune response but they appear to differ in their mode of action and their effect upon different lymphocyte subpopulations. It is, for example, possible to select adjuvants which boost the humoral response but depress the cell-mediated response to one and the same antigen. Therefore, paradoxically, it might be useful under some clinical circumstances to employ adjuvants in the immunosuppressive regimen, for example, where the desired effect was to foster active enhancement.

Another stimulating recent report deals with the altogether surprising observation that ALS administered to experimental animals via the oral route is nonetheless immunosuppressive. One might have anticipated that the digestive enzymes would inactivate the relevant molecules prior to absorption, but such does not seem to be the case altogether. An interesting sideline of this observation is that the oral administration of foreign proteins seems to be an effective way to abet the induction of specific immunological tolerance. This observation has considerable practical importance because the continued intravenous or intramuscular administration of ALS does constitute an objection to its long-term application. If it were possible to administer ALS to patients by the oral route without a loss in potency, a very objectionable feature in its application might be removed.

The exploration of regimens that combine several immunosuppressive agents administered together is still in its infancy. The notion that agents differing in their mode of action might be synergistic in their effects while reducing the potential toxicity through a lowering of the dosage requirements for any one of the components is a well-accepted pharmacological principle. No doubt the future will see many more effective combinations of agents than is currently available in the usual clinical protocols. Such has certainly been the case with respect to the multi-drug chemotherapy for malignancy and there is no reason to expect that this principle will not apply to immunosuppression as well.

In this brief review we have attempted to present first of all a rational system of classifying IS agents which indicates the direction it is hoped developments in the future will take. Inasmuch as what is wanted is a much finer and discrete control over immunological reactivity, we personally think that immunoregulation is a more apt term than immunosuppression. In attempting to present a broad view, we have by no means touched all the bases. For instance, we have not discussed items such as the γ_2-globulins, aldactone, the possibilities inherent in antigenic competition, or such poorly understood phenomena as the Liacopoulous effect. Moreover, the abbreviated coverage given any one agent or class has necessitated a very limited and selected presentation of the facts. Although we believe this is permissible where the object has been to deal with general principles rather than details, it is important for the reader to understand that many important details and qualifications pertaining to the subject have been omitted.

References*

Medawar, P. B. (1944). The behaviour and fate of skin autografts and skin homografts in rabbits. *J. Anat.*, **78**, 176

Schwartz, R. S. and Dameshek, W. (1952). Drug induced immunological tolerance. *Nature (London)*, **183**, 1682

Starzl, T. E., Porter, K. A., Iwasaki, Y., Marchioro, T. L. and Kashiwagi, N. (1967). The use of heterologous anti-lymphocyte globulin in human renal transplantation. In G. E. W. Wolstenholme and M. O'Connor (eds.). *Anti-lymphocytic Serum*, p. 4. (London: Churchill)

Taliaferro, W. H., Taliaferro, L. G. and Jaroslow, B. N. (1964). *Radiation and Immune Mechanisms*. (New York: Academic Press)

Turk, J. (1972). Personal communication.

Van Bekkum, D. W. and de Vries, M. J. (1967). *Radiation Chimaeras*. (New York: Academic Press)

Woodruff, M. F. A. and Anderson, N. A. (1963). Effect of lymphocyte depletion by thoracic duct fistula and administration of anti-lymphocyte serum on the survival of skin homografts in rats. *Nature (London)*, **200**, 702

CYTOSTATIC AGENTS

Berenbaum, M. C. (1967). Immunosuppressive agents and the cellular kinetics of the immune response. In E. Mihich (ed.). *Immunity, Cancer, and Chemotherapy: Basic Relationships on the Cellular Level*, p. 217. (New York: Academic Press)

---

* We have indicated in the text specific references in which the work of particular individuals is referred to, but have not undertaken to identify the source for most statements inasmuch as they, to a large extent, reflect our interpretation of the relevant literature. For these reasons, the reader who desires to explore this subject in detail is provided with a general reference list of reviews in the field which contain detailed bibliographies.

Brent, L. and Medawar, P. B. (1966). Quantitative studies on tissue transplantation immunity. VII. The normal lymphocyte transfer reaction. *Proc. R. Soc. Ser. B*, **1–5,** 281

Calabresi, P. and Welch, A. D. (1965). In L. S. Goodman and A. Gilman (eds.). *The Pharmacological Basis of Therapeutics*, 2nd Ed. p. 1345. (New York: Macmillan)

Gabrielsen, A. E. and Good, R. R. (1967). Chemical suppression of adaptive immunity. *Adv. Immunol.*, **6,** 92

Hitchings, G. H. and Elion, G. B. (1963). Chemical suppression of the immune response. *Pharmacol. Rev.*, **15,** 365

Maibach, H. I. and Epstein, W. L. (1965). Immunological responses in healthy volunteers receiving azathioprine (Imuran). *Int. Arch. Allergy Appl. Immunol.*, **27,** 102

Schwartz, R. (1965). Immunosuppressive drugs. *Prog. Allergy*, **9,** 246

Schwartz, R. S. (1968). Immunosuppressive drug therapy. In F. T. Rapaport and J. Dausset (eds.). *Human Transplantation*, p. 440. (New York: Grune & Stratton)

STEROID HORMONES

Medawar, P. B. and Sparrow, E. M. (1956). The effects of adrenocortical hormones, adrenocorticotrophic hormones, and pregnancy on skin transplantation immunity in mice. *J. Endocrinol.*, **14,** 240

Roberts, B. V. (1969). The effects of steroid hormones on macrophage activity. *Int. Rev. Cytol.*, **25,** 131

Schwartzman, G., ed. (1953). *The Effect of ACTH and Cortisone upon Infection and Resistance*. (New York: Columbia University Press)

Travis, R. H. and Sayers, G. Adrenocorticotrophic hormone, adrenocortical steroids and their synthetic analogues. In L. S. Goodman and A. Gilman (eds.). *The Pharmacological Basis of Therapeutics*, 2nd Ed., p. 1608. (New York: Macmillan)

White, A. (1948). Influence of endocrine secretions on the structure and function of lymphoid tissue. *Harvey Lect.*, **43,** 43

Wolstenholme, G. E. W. and Knight, J., eds. (1970). *Hormones and the Immune Response, Ciba Found. Study Group No. 36*. (London: Churchill)

SURGICAL ABLATION OF LYMPHOID TISSUE

Good, R. A. and Gabrielsen, A. E. (1968). The thymus and other lymphoid organs in the development of the immune system. In F. T. Rapaport and J. Dausset (eds.). *Human Transplantation*, p. 526. (New York: Grune & Stratton)

Miller, J. F. A. P. and Osoba, D. (1967). Current concepts of the immunological function of the thymus. *Physiol. Rev.* **47,** 437

Stark, R. B., Dwyer, E. M. and Forest, M. D. (1960). Effect of surgical ablation of regional nodes on survival of skin homografts. *Ann. N.Y. Acad. Sci.*, **87,** 140

Starzl, T. E., Porter, K. A., Groth, C. G., Putnam, C. W., Penn, I., Halgrimson, C. G., Starkie, S. J. and Brettschneider, L. (1970). Thymectomy and renal transplantation. *Clin. Exp. Immunol.*, **6,** 803

Veith, F. J., Luck, R. J. and Murray, J. E. (1965). The effects of splenectomy on immunosuppressive regimens in dog and man. *Surg., Gynecol., Obstet.*, **121,** 299

Woodruff, M. F. A. (1960). *The Transplantation of Tissues and Organs*. p. 102. (Springfield: Charles C. Thomas)

ASPARAGINASE

Broome, J. D. (1968). Studies on the mechanism of tumour inhibition by L-asparaginase. *J. Exp. Med.*, **127,** 1055

Weksler, M. E. and Weksler, B. B. (1971). Studies on the immunosuppressive properties of asparaginase. *Immunology*, **21,** 137

THORACIC DUCT DRAINAGE

Dumont, A. E. (1968). Thoracic duct cannulation. In F. T. Rapaport and J. Dausset (eds.). *Human Transplantation*, p. 482. (New York: Grune & Stratton)

Gowans, J. L. and McGregor, D. D. (1965). The immunological activities of lymphocytes. *Prog. Allergy*, **9,** 1

Tunner, W. S., Carbone, P., Blaylack, K. and Irwin, G. L. (1965). Effect of thoracic duct lymph drainage on the immune response in man. *Surg. Gynecol. Obstet.*, **121,** 334

EXTRACORPOREAL IRRADIATION

Chanana, A. D., Brecher, G., Cronkite, E. P., Joel, D. and Schnauppauf, H. (1966). The influence of extracorporeal irradiation of blood and lymph on skin homograft rejection. *Radiat. Res.*, **27,** 330

Schiffer, L. M., Atkins, H. L., Chanana, A. D., Cronkite, E. P., Johnson, H. A., Robertson, J. S. and Strykmans, P. A. (1966). Extracorporeal irradiation of the blood in humans: effects upon erythrocyte survival. *Blood*, **27,** 831

Wolf, J. S., Lee, H. M., O'Foghluda, F. T. and Hume, D. M. (1966). Effect of circulating blood radiation with an extracorporeal Strontium 90 shunt on transplantation immunity in dogs and man. *Surg. Forum*, **17,** 245

ANTILYMPHOCYTE ANTISERUM

Bach, J. F., Dormont, J., Eyquem, A. and Raynaud, M., eds. (1970). Proceedings of international symposium on anti-lymphocyte sera. *Symp. Ser. Immunobiol. Scand.*, **16**

Lance, E. M. (1970). The selective action of anti-lymphocyte antiserum on recirculating lymphocytes: a review of the evidence and alternatives. *Clin. Exp. Immunol.*, **6,** 789

Medawar, P. B. (1968). Biological effects of heterologous anti-lymphocyte sera. In F. T. Rapaport and J. Dausset (eds.). *Human Transplantation*, p. 501 (New York: Grune & Stratton)

Proceedings of the Conference on Anti-lymphocyte Serum. (1970). *Fed. Proc., Fed. Amer. Soc. Exp. Biol.*, **29,** 97ff

Sell, S. (1969). Anti-lymphocyte antibody: effects in experimental animals and problems in human use. *Ann. Intern. Med.*, **71,** 177

Taub, R. N. (1970). Biological effects of heterologous anti-lymphocyte serum. *Prog. Allergy*, **14,** 208

Wolstenholme, G. E. W. and O'Connor, M. J. A., eds. (1967). *Anti-lymphocytic Serum, Ciba Found. Study Group No. 29.* (London: Churchill)

BURSECTOMY

Good, R. A. and Gabrielsen, A. E. (1968). The thymus and other lymphoid organs in the development of the immune system. In F. T. Rapaport and J. Dausset (eds.). *Human Transplantation*, p. 526. (New York: Grune & Stratton)

Cooper, M. D., Peterson, R. D. A. and Good, R. A. (1965). Delineation of the thymic and bursal lymphoid systems in the chicken. *Nature (London)*, **205**, 143

ENHANCEMENT

Hellstrom, K. E. and Hellstrom, I. (1970). Immunological enhancement as studied by cell culture techniques. *Ann. Rev. Microbiol.*, **24**, 373

Kaliss, N. (1958). Immunological enhancement of tumour homografts in mice: a review. *Cancer Res.*, **18**, 992

Moller, G. and Wigzell, H. (1965). Antibody synthesis at the cellular level. Antibody induced suppression of the 19S and 17S antibody response. *J. Exp. Med.*, **121**, 969

Proceedings of the Third International Congress of the Transplantation Society. (1971). Several papers. *Transplant. Proc.*, **3**, 697

Uhr, J. W. and Moller, G. (1968). Regulatory effect of antibody on the immune response. *Adv. Immunol.*, **8**, 81

TOLERANCE

Dresser, D. W. and Mitchison, N. A. (1968). The mechanism of immunological paralysis. *Adv. Immunol.*, **8**, 129

Lance, E. M. and Medawar, P. B. (1969). Quantitative studies on tissue transplantation immunity. IX. Induction of tolerance with anti-lymphocyte serum. *Proc. R. Soc. Ser. B*, **173**, 447

Landy, M. and Braun, W., eds. (1969). *Immunological Tolerance. A Reassessment of Mechanisms of the Immune Response.* (New York: Academic Press)

Medawar, P. B. (1960). Theories of immunological tolerance. *Cell. Aspects Immunity, Ciba Found. Symp.*, *1959*, p. 134.

Weigle, W. O. (1967). *Natural and Acquired Immunological Unresponsiveness.* (Cleveland, Ohio: World Publ.)

General Reference List of Reviews

COMPLICATIONS OF IMMUNOSUPPRESSIVE THERAPY

Gowing, N. F. C. (1970). Morbid anatomical and histological features of unusual infections. *Proc. R. Soc. Med.*, **63**, 63

Hirsch, M. S. and Murphy, F. A. (1968). Effects of anti-lymphoid sera on viral infections. *Lancet*, **ii**, 37

Hume, D. M. (1968). Kidney transplantation. In F. T. Rapaport and J. Dausset (eds.). *Human Transplantation*, p. 110. (New York: Grune & Stratton)

ANTI-INFLAMMATORY AGENTS

Glenn, E. M., Miller, W. L. and Schlagel, C. A. (1963). Metabolic effects of adrenocortical steroids *in vivo* and *in vitro*: relationship to anti-inflammatory effects. *Recent Prog. Horm. Res.*, **19**, 107

Selle, W. A. (1946). Histamine—its physiological, pharmacological and clinical significance. *Texas Rep. Biol. Med.*, **4**, 138

Sherman, W. B. (1951). The uses and abuses of antihistamine drugs. (2) *Bull. N.Y. Acad. Med.*, **27**, 309

Weissman, G. and Thomas, L. (1964). The effects of corticosteroids upon connective tissue and lysosomes. *Recent Prog. Horm. Res.*, **29**, 215

IRRADIATION

Cronkite, E. P. and Chanana, A. D. (1968). Ionizing radiation. In F. T. Rapaport and J. Dausset (eds.). *Human Transplantation*, p. 423. (New York: Grune & Stratton)

Mathe, G. (1969). Immunodepression by whole body irradiation and chemical cytostatics. *Concours Med.*, **91,** 55

Smith, L. H. and Congdon, C. C. (1968). Biological effects of ionizing radiation. In F. T. Rapaport and J. Dausset (eds.). *Human Transplantation*, p. 510. (New York: Grune & Stratton)

CHAPTER 9

Enhancement and Tolerance

J. W. Fabre

Introduction

The problems of clinical transplantation are to a large extent connected with immunosuppression. The immunosuppressive agents in current use have made possible the excellent advances in clinical transplantation which have occurred over the past decade, but they have well-known and serious short-comings in the areas of safety and potency. There is today real hope that a different approach to immunosuppression, the approach covered by the terms enhancement and tolerance, will make substantial contributions to both the safety and potency of immunosuppression. The purpose of this chapter will be to review the work that has been done in this area with special emphasis on the clinical applicability of the techniques used and the theoretical and practical problems associated with transfer from the experimental to the clinical situation.

Enhancement and tolerance are terms used loosely in the literature, and they are better grouped under the single heading of specific immunosuppression. *Specific immunosuppression* may be defined as immunosuppression directed *only* at the lymphocyte clones responsible for the rejection of the *particular* graft the patient receives, i.e. it is an antigen-specific immunosuppression. It is the most selective form of immunosuppression possible and avoids the immunological and non-immunological complications of the non-specific immunosuppressive agents currently in use.

The reason for the imprecise use of the terms enhancement and tolerance is that they imply a mechanism for the unresponsiveness induced. *Tolerance* is generally defined as unresponsiveness due to *deletion* of the specifically reactive clones. Enhancement implies that the specifically reactive clones are present but are being continuously suppressed, by blocking antibodies, suppressor T cells, etc. As will be discussed at length later, mechanisms in specific unresponsiveness are an area of much controversy. In this situation, the use of the terms is obviously unsatisfactory, but they are too deep-rooted in the language of immunology to be discarded. It is probably best to use the terms enhancement and tolerance in the general sense, without implying mechanism, and it is this approach which I shall follow.

To specifically immunosuppress a host with respect to any particular antigen one may use the antigen itself, antibodies directed against the antigen, or various combinations of the two. In the transplant situation this would involve treatment of a graft recipient with preparations containing donor histocompatibility antigens (*active enhancement*) or with antisera directed against these antigens (*passive enhancement*). Another possibility which has recently emerged is the use of so-called 'anti-receptor' antibodies. On exposure to a new antigen, a host will form antibodies, the antigen-combining site of which will be directed at the new antigen. Since the host in his previous existence will not have been exposed to these antibodies which he has newly produced, the formal possibility exists that he will now form antibodies directed against the antigen-combining site of the anti-bodies to the new antigen. Such antibodies seem to have been demonstrated and, when transferred to fresh hosts, can apparently specifically suppress the antibody response to the initial antigen (Strayer *et al.*, 1974). However, these anti-receptor antibodies are poorly defined and their role in transplant systems is not established, so they will not be considered further.

When considering specific immunosuppression it is useful to keep in mind two phases. The *inductive* phase refers to the time around which the host is being treated and grafted. The *maintenance* phase represents the stage after which the various interactions between host and graft have stabilized. It is impossible to give any clear demarcation between these two phases, but it is nevertheless helpful to think of specific immunosuppression in this way.

The area of main clinical interest is the induction of specific immuno-suppression. It is proposed to begin with a brief historical survey, to then discuss in detail the induction of specific immunosuppression first by anti-body and then by antigen, and to follow with a brief outline of the main-tenance phase of specific unresponsiveness.

Historical Perspectives

The first experiments demonstrating specific immunosuppression were per-formed at the turn of the century by Flexner and Jobling (1906). Their experiments were an attempt to vaccinate against cancer, and when they found that 'vaccination' with heat-killed tumour resulted in the exact opposite of what they had anticipated (i.e. instead of suppressed tumour growth on challenge with live tumour, they observed much more vigorous than normal tumour growth, as a result of active enhancement) they did not appreciate the meaning or the significance of their results.

The key observation was made by Owen (1945). He discovered that cattle twins, as a result of shared vascular connections between placentae, exchange haemopoietic stem cells *in utero*, and that these foreign stem cells continue to proliferate side-by-side with the host's own stem cells to produce red blood cells, etc. throughout the animal's life: a remarkable example in nature of tolerance induction to foreign tissues. It was this observation which led to Burnet's clonal theory of immunity and to his ideas that self-tolerance was the result of deletion of self-reactive clones due to contact with self-components during fetal life (Burnet and Fenner, 1949). Burnet's clonal selection theory provided the essential theoretical framework for the interpretation of studies on specific immunosuppression.

The first demonstration of experimentally induced long-term acceptance of a foreign graft was made in 1953, as a more or less direct result of Owen's observation in cattle and of Burnet's theory (Billingham *et al.*, 1953). Mouse fetuses, *in utero*, were injected with tissues from a foreign strain incompatible at the major histocompatibility locus and as adults were found to accept freely skin grafts from the foreign strain.

The induction of long-term graft acceptance in adult animals incompatible at the major histocompatibility locus was first demonstrated in 1961 (Shapiro *et al.*, 1961). Injection of adult mice with large doses of donor strain spleen cells over several weeks resulted in permanent acceptance of skin grafts in the majority of treated mice. An important observation was made by Kaliss in tumour systems (Kaliss, 1956) who showed that treatment with antisera to donor strain tissues could enhance the growth of tumours as effectively as treatment with the tissues themselves, i.e. that passive enhancement was an effective method for prolonging graft survival.

A large number of studies on the specific suppression of graft rejection was performed in the 1950s and 1960s. Passive enhancement, the more clinically applicable approach, was tested on skin grafts in rodents where its effect in prolonging graft survival was shown to be very weak. Active enhancement was tested mainly with skin grafts in rodents and occasionally with kidney grafts in dogs, with variable but often encouraging results. However, mainly because of the risk of sensitization, active enhancement was not generally regarded as a clinically applicable approach. The turning point came in the mid-1960s with the development of microsurgical techniques for organ transplantation in the inbred rat. These techniques meant that passive enhancement studies, difficult to perform in outbred animals, could easily be done with kidney grafts, and that direct comparisons of skin and kidney grafts would be possible in a variety of situations. By 1970 (Stuart *et al.*, 1968; French and Batchelor, 1969) it was clear that the induction of specific immunosuppression was much easier with kidney than with skin grafts, and, more importantly, that passive enhancement of kidney grafts gave excellent immunosuppression. These findings very much brightened the prospects of applying specific immunosuppression to clinical transplantation.

Induction of Specific Immunosuppression by Antibody (Passive Enhancement)

INTRODUCTION

Of the two approaches to specific immunosuppression, passive enhancement is the safer, and, therefore, the one more likely to find clinical application in the near future. The early clinical steps with passive enhancement have indeed already been taken (Batchelor *et al.*, 1970) but an evaluation of its clinical merit awaits further study. From the discussion which follows, I hope to demonstrate that there is every possibility that passive enhancement will find a place in clinical immunosuppressive regimens in the near future. It will not be possible, for reasons which will become obvious, to use passive enhancement as the sole method of immunosuppression, but it should be possible to restrict the non-specific agents to low dosage and/or short-term use, and thereby avoid the dangers attendant on non-specific immunosuppression.

PRINCIPLE OF THE TECHNIQUE

The principle is in essence simple and is illustrated in Table 9.1. It involves

Table 9.1 **Principle of passive enhancement**

Donor	Recipient	Enhancing serum
DA $(DA \times Lewis)F_1$	Lewis } Lewis }	Lewis anti–DA
HLA 1, 8, 2, 12	HLA 1, 8, 9, 13	? anti HLA 2 and anti HLA 12

treatment of the recipient with antibodies directed against incompatible graft antigens. In inbred animals this presents few theoretical or practical difficulties. Thus, for instance, one would immunize Lewis rats with tissues from the foreign DA strain, harvest the serum at the end of the immunization schedule, and freeze it. A Lewis rat receiving a DA or $(DA \times Lewis)F_1$ graft would be treated at the time of transplantation and for a few days thereafter with this Lewis anti-DA serum. Since in this situation the animals used as donors and recipients for producing the antiserum are genetically identical to the donors and recipients in the transplant experiment, one can be sure that all graft antigens, both major and minor, will be covered by the antiserum. It is clearly impossible to duplicate this situation in outbred populations, such as the human, except in the most devious of circumstances. Any regimen of passive enhancement applicable to cadaver kidney transplantation and relying on complete cover of incompatibilities must rest on accurate tissue typing of donor and recipient and the use of sera raised in unrelated individuals against the incompatibilities detected. This raises serious potential difficulties, mainly because of the recently discovered complexity of the major histocompatibility system (for review see Shreffler and David, 1975).

Until recently, the only known antigens of the major histocompatibility system in the mouse were the so-called SD antigens which almost certainly correspond to the currently defined HLA antigens of the human. In this situation, there is no difficulty in choosing enhancing sera: as shown in Table 9.1, one would HLA type the donor and recipient and choose sera (from multiparous women, polytransfused patients or immunized volunteers) directed against the incompatible HLA antigens. However, in recent years the major histocompatibility system of the mouse has been shown to be an extremely complex genetic region consisting of a large number of closely linked genes coding for many cell surface antigens, in addition to the SD antigens. This degree of complexity is beginning to emerge with the major histocompatibility system of man. It is clear that in this situation antisera directed against the incompatible HLA antigens of the donor will leave uncovered many of the as yet undefined antigens of the major histocompatibility system. Whether all or only some of these additional antigens are important for the rejection of grafts is unknown. Nevertheless, from the point of view of clinical passive enhancement the important question is this: must one wait until the major histocompatibility system of man has been better defined and then, relying on the theory current at the time, use antisera against those antigens which are considered important for graft rejection? The answer, fortunately, is probably no.

It has recently been shown in a rat kidney graft model (Fabre and Morris, 1974b) that one need cover only *some* of the antigens of the major histocompatibility system for effective passive enhancement. Moreover, it seems that no particular group of antigens is important in this respect for it has been possible in the rat to induce passive enhancement with antisera directed, on the one hand, against non-SD antigens only (Staines et al., 1974) and, on the other hand, against SD antigens only (J. R. Batchelor, personal communication). These findings suggest that as long as an antiserum can be shown to interact with some of the incompatibilities of the major histocompatibility system, it will be effective for passive enhancement. If this proves to be a valid generalization, a serious potential difficulty to the clinical application of passive enhancement will be removed and the clinical approach will be considerably simplified. Thus the use of antisera against the incompatible HLA antigens of the donor (Table 9.1) might well turn out to be a legitimate approach, but other assays might prove more useful in choosing sera for enhancement.

The foregoing discussion has centred on the major histocompatibility system. It is well known that numerous other genetic loci (minor histocompatibility loci) are involved in the rejection of skin grafts, and that at least some of these are also involved in kidney graft rejection. Though these minor loci evoke relatively weak rejection reactions, they should not be forgotten. In the human, none of the minor histocompatibility systems has been identified, and the prospect of identifying them in the future seems remote. Quite apart from the practical difficulties associated with dealing specifically with numerous histocompatibility systems, the fact that they have not been identified means that it will not be possible to direct passive enhancement against them. Thus, unless directing passive enhancement against the major incompatibilities in some way also induces unresponsiveness to associated minor incompatibilities, for which there is only very circumstantial evidence, these simple genetic considerations show that supplementary non-specific immunosuppression will be necessary to deal with the minor incompatibilities. However, since they evoke only weak rejection reactions, the non-specific agents should be able to deal with them quite easily on a low dose and/or short-term treatment schedule.

POSSIBLE MECHANISMS

Little is known of the way in which the injected antibody interacts with the graft and with the host's immune system to induce unresponsiveness. The old arguments have revolved around central or peripheral mechanisms, i.e. on whether the antibody acts at the level of the specifically reactive lymphocyte or the graft, respectively. The peripheral mechanisms essentially involve the masking of antigen by antibody. They have been divided into 'afferent' or 'efferent' mechanisms, depending on whether the antigen masking prevents the development of the immune response or prevents an established immune response from destroying the graft, respectively. While antigen masking probably occurs to some extent, especially with respect to afferent inhibition when large doses of antibody are used, it is unlikely to be the essential mechanism. Very small doses of antibody, which seem unlikely to be effective in antigen masking, can induce passive enhancement of kidney grafts in rats (Fabre and Morris, 1973). Moreover, the injected antibody has been shown to attach itself only transiently to the kidney graft. By 24 hours much of it has been lost from the graft (Fine *et al.*, 1973).

If the antibody does indeed act at the level of the reactive lymphocyte, the manner of its interaction and the effect on different lymphocyte sub-populations are unknown. The T cells involved in graft rejection must be suppressed in one way or another. Since passive enhancement also suppresses the antibody response to the graft, either completely or after a transient production of antibodies, helper T cells and/or B cells must also be inactivated. The role, if any, of so-called suppressor T cells in the induction of passive enhancement is unknown.

On the basis of very interesting *in vitro* studies, Diener and Feldmann (1970) have proposed a model whereby antibody might act at the cellular level to cause inactivation. They suggest that the antibody (which is of course bivalent) acts to connect antigen particles and thereby form a lattice with repeating antigen determinants. Such a lattice could cause linkage of the surface receptors of the lymphocyte over a wide area of membrane, and their experiments suggest that such linkage results in non-reactivity. Linkage of receptors, however, seems to be an absolute requirement only for B cell inactivation. Though helper T cells might be inactivated under similar circumstances, it is clear that they can be inactivated in situations where no receptor linkage occurs (Feldmann and Nossal, 1972).

It has been shown that different subclasses of IgG vary in their effectiveness for inducing passive enhancement. For instance, in tumour systems some subclasses have been shown to be completely ineffective (e.g. Kinsky *et al.*, 1972), while with liver grafts in baboons (Smit and Myburgh, 1974) one class of IgG seems to be much less effective than another. These studies suggest that the Fc portion of the antibody might play a role in the induction of passive enhancement. However, pepsin-degraded IgG (yielding $F(ab')_2$ fragments) has been shown to induce passive enhancement (e.g. Myburgh and Smit, 1972), and this tends to rule out a role for the Fc segment. It is possible that different subclasses of IgG vary in their effectiveness because the specific IgG (that directed against donor antigens) is not evenly distributed among the subclasses.

Recently, Enomoto and Lucas (1973) have reported that passive enhancement of kidney grafts was *completely* ineffective in splenectomized rats, and they suggest that the spleen plays an essential, though as yet undefined, role in the induction of passive enhancement. However, in a different strain combination, splenectomy was found not to influence passive enhancement at all (Fabre and Batchelor, 1975a). The reason for the discrepancy in results is unknown. However, though it is clear that the spleen is not an absolute requirement for passive enhancement, it will be interesting if its role in the experiments of Enomoto and Lucas can be elucidated.

VARIABILITY OF EFFECTIVENESS OF PASSIVE ENHANCEMENT WITH DIFFERENT TISSUE GRAFTS

The marked difference in the effectiveness of passive enhancement with skin and kidney grafts is important from both the historical point of view, as previously discussed, and the practical one as well. In recent years the same batches of antiserum have been tested for their ability to enhance passively skin, kidney and heart grafts in the same strain combination (Tilney and Bell, 1974: Fabre and Morris, 1975). Whereas the rejection of kidney and heart grafts was completely suppressed, skin graft survival was prolonged by only 1 or 2 days. The reason for this remarkable difference is unknown though a number of possibilities exist (Fabre and Morris, 1975).

Passive enhancement has been studied mainly with kidney grafts in rats, but studies have also been done with heart grafts in rats (Tilney and Bell, 1974) and liver grafts in baboons (Myburgh and Smit, 1972). Though it is too early to make generalizations, the indications are that passive enhancement will be more effective with organ grafts as a group than with skin grafts.

POTENCY OF PASSIVE ENHANCEMENT AS AN IMMUNOSUPPRESSIVE AGENT

Potency is an important factor for any immunosuppressive agent of potential clinical use. There are two important indices of potency: effectiveness across a wide variety of different major histocompatibility barriers, and effectiveness in presensitized recipients. The results show that, by itself, passive enhancement is only a moderately potent immunosuppressive agent.

The effectiveness of passive enhancement across different histocompatibility barriers

Passive enhancement of kidney grafts has been tested across seven or eight different major histocompatibility barriers in the rat. In all cases it has been beneficial in that it has caused at least some prolongation of graft survival.

Table 9.2 The effectiveness of passive enhancement of kidney grafts across different major histocompatibility barriers in the rat*

Strain combination	Mean ± I.S.D. of blood urea (mg/100 ml) at week:				Survival (days)
	1	2	3	20	
AS2 to DA	42±7	62±11	60±17	45±5	All >300 (4 rats)
(AS × August)F₁ to AS	64±12	146±163	81±35	68±14	All >300 (5 rats)
August to AS	104±64	167±92	201 ±165	—	41, 41, 43, 36, 73
(DA × Lewis)F₁ to Lewis	84±17	201±90	730±75	—	18, 21, 22, 23, 27

* In all strain combinations, untreated recipients have severe acute rejection from which they die, almost invariably in the second week.
Adapted from Fabre and Morris, 1973, 1974a, and Fabre and Batchelor 1975a

However, as illustrated in Table 9.2, there is a broad spectrum of effectiveness. In some strains (e.g. AS2 to DA) it is completely effective. In others (e.g. August to AS), grafts from the F_1 hybrid donor are completely protected, but the rejection of homozygous grafts, though substantially delayed, is not completely prevented. The least effective combination has been the DA to Lewis, where even the F_1 hybrid graft is only transiently protected. Passive enhancement of liver grafts in baboons doubled or trebled the mean survival time of grafts, but they were eventually rejected (Myburgh and Smit, 1972). It is clear that in the clinical situation, where one must assume the worst case, it is not possible to even contemplate the use of passive enhancement without supplementary non-specific immunosuppression.

The effectiveness of passive enhancement in specifically presensitized recipients

Most patients coming to transplantation (at least in the cases of heart and kidney grafts) have had blood transfusions. Some have been pregnant or have received previous transplants. There is, therefore, a real possibility that some, perhaps a significant proportion, are specifically presensitized to the incompatible antigens on the graft they receive. The techniques for detecting specific sensitization to the donor, and therefore of avoiding sensitized donor–recipient combinations, are far from adequate. Thus the efficacy of passive enhancement in the face of specific sensitization would define a clinically important variable.

Attempts to enhance passively kidney grafts in rats previously sensitized against the donor strain have shown that passive enhancement is much less effective or completely ineffective in sensitized recipients, depending on the strain combination tested (Fabre and Morris, 1975). In this respect, passive enhancement is probably no different from other immunosuppressive agents. Nevertheless, these experiments define sensitization as a probable limit to the use of passive enhancement and stress the importance of sensitization as a limiting factor in immunosuppressive therapy.

THE EFFECTIVENESS OF PASSIVE ENHANCEMENT IN CONJUNCTION WITH NON-SPECIFIC IMMUNOSUPPRESSIVE AGENTS

A remarkable synergism has been shown to exist between passive enhancement and antilymphocyte serum (ALS) for the prevention of kidney graft rejection in rats. A brief course of a relatively weak ALS together with passive enhancement, in a strain combination where neither agent alone had any marked effect in preventing rejection, gave complete suppression of rejection in most treated recipients (Batchelor et al., 1972). In more recent experiments, a brief course of a potent ALS in combination with passive enhancement completely protected homozygous kidney grafts across the strongest histocompatibility barrier in which passive enhancement has been tested in the rat (Fabre and Morris, 1974a). These data are very encouraging, especially as they suggest that it might well be possible to use only very restricted courses of non-specific therapy in conjunction with passive enhancement.

ALS and passive enhancement together have given excellent synergism, but not indefinite survival, with skin grafts in mice (McKenzie *et al.*, 1971). It has also been tested with liver grafts in baboons, though here the results were not impressive (Myburgh and Smit, 1973). Whether this represents a species difference in effectiveness, or is due to the use of liver grafts or to the differences in approach used for passive enhancement, is unknown. In any case, in view of the relative ineffectiveness of ALS in the clinical situation, at least as it is currently used, it would be interesting to see if the more accepted non-specific agents were as effective as ALS in combination with passive enhancement. Prednisolone has been shown to augment the effectiveness of passive enhancement with skin grafts in mice (Chutnà, 1971), but it has yet to be tested with kidney grafts.

In specifically presensitized recipients, even the strong combination of ALS plus passive enhancement is relatively ineffective. Passive enhancement together with a short course of a potent ALS could only briefly delay the onset of kidney graft rejection in sensitized rats, most animals dying before the end of the fourth week (Fabre and Morris, 1975). It seems, therefore, that to achieve high success rates by the addition of passive enhancement to clinical immunosuppressive regimens, the avoidance of sensitized donor–recipient combinations will be essential. This could be achieved by preventing the development of sensitization in prospective graft recipients, or by developing better tests for detecting sensitization to donor antigens. The former approach will be discussed in the next section.

THE PREVENTION OF BLOOD TRANSFUSION–INDUCED
SENSITIZATION TO HISTOCOMPATIBILITY ANTIGENS

Blood transfusions represent the most common source of exposure to foreign histocompatibility antigens in patients awaiting kidney and heart transplantation. Most transplant centres attempt to reduce the risk of sensitization by minimal transfusion policies or by giving leukocyte-poor blood. Another possible approach, potentially more efficient, is to use antibodies directed against the histocompatibility antigens of the blood. This approach has been shown in rats to prevent both the lymphocytotoxic antibody response to the blood and its ability to sensitize to kidney grafts

(Fabre and Batchelor, 1975b). The use of antibody to suppress the immune response has been very successfully applied clinically to the prevention of maternal Rh immunization by Rh incompatible pregnancies. Though the problems associated with the use of antibody in the context of blood transfusions and transplantation are more complex, it should be possible to use it after a few simple but essential precautions have been taken. The approach rests on the fact that most HLA antigens are not present in red cells, which are the important cells from the point of view of the transfusion, but that they are present on leukocytes and platelets which are the components of blood which induce sensitization. High titre, broadly cross-reactive HLA sera from multiparous women could be used as the source of antibody, after appropriate tests for serum hepatitis. A cross-match would have to be performed to exclude the presence of antibodies in the serum against the red cells of the blood, since antibody-coated red cells are rapidly destroyed. After absorption of blood and antiserum, removal of buffy coat and supernatant would minimize risks of transfusion reactions due to release of vasoactive substances, etc. from granulocytes and platelets.

Recently, the long-standing controversy over the possible beneficial effects of blood transfusions in clinical renal transplantation has been revived with some interesting data from Opelz and Terasaki (1974). Their data shows that non-transfused patients do substantially worse than those who have been transfused, and they suggest that the blood transfusions are beneficial possibly by inducing a degree of specific immunosuppression. While it is possible that blood transfusions might be beneficial to transplant patients *as a group*, there is no question that they are harmful to some patients by sensitizing them. If Opelz and Terasaki's data can be confirmed, a case could be argued for not shielding patients from the immunological sequelae of blood transfusions, in the current situation. However, as success rates approach optimal levels, a procedure which unpredictably sensitizes some patients becomes unacceptable, there is little question that in the long term patients will need to be shielded from blood transfusions.

THE PROBLEM OF HYPERACUTE REJECTION

In most species, the presence in the recipient of antibodies directed against kidney graft antigens results in virtually immediate graft destruction as a result of intravascular coagulation and spasm. This is precipitated by the interaction of the antibodies with the graft vasculature and the fixation of complement. In the rat, for unknown reasons, this fortunately does not happen in most strain combinations, so that basic studies on passive enhancement can proceed without the complication of hyperacute rejection having to be considered. It is, however, a problem which must be solved before clinical application of passive enhancement is considered.

Since complement fixation seems to trigger the events of hyperacute rejection, the problem is basically to remove the ability of the antibodies to fix complement without affecting their ability to induce enhancement. There are a number of ways of preventing, or at least reducing, complement fixation by antibodies. Pepsin digestion to yield $F(ab')_2$ fragments is the most obvious, but succinylation has also been tried. In rabbits, $F(ab')_2$ fragments have been shown not to induce hyperacute rejection of kidney grafts (Holter *et al.*, 1972), and succinylation prevented antibody-mediated damage to liver grafts in baboons (Smit and Myburgh, 1974). Pepsin digested and succinylated antibodies also seem to retain their ability to induce enhancement (Myburgh and Smit, 1972; Smit and Myburgh, 1974). In the experiments of Myburgh and Smit (1972) pepsin degradation of IgG did not prevent antibody-mediated damage to liver grafts in baboons, and they suggest that factors other than complement fixation might be important. However, it should be remembered that $F(ab')_2$ fragments do fix complement, although much less than whole IgG, and this fact plus the possibility of undigested IgG being present in their preparations, could explain their results in terms of complement fixation.

There are other approaches to the problem. Host decomplementation is one possibility which has not been attempted. Another is to separate IgG from antiserum into different subclasses and to use only those subclasses with poor or absent ability to fix complement for passive enhancement. However, in mouse tumour systems, contradictory results have been obtained as to whether or not non-complement fixing IgG can induce passive enhancement. With liver grafts in baboons, Smit and Myburgh (1974) have found that a subclass of IgG with poor ability to fix complement (but which still damages grafts) induces enhancement very well.

SOME PRACTICAL POINTS IN CLINICAL APPLICATION

Possible sources of sera

Multiparous women and polytransfused patients represent the most readily available source of sera against histocompatibility antigens. However, many of these sera are probably weak, and in the absence of an *in vitro* test for enhancing potency, this source should be treated with caution. It would probably be wiser, at least in the first instance, or until a suitable *in vitro* test appears, to use sera from deliberately immunized individuals, such as relatives of patients. It should be mentioned here that the lymphocytotoxin titre of an antiserum gives little or no idea of its enhancing ability (Fabre and Morris, 1974a).

Specificity of sera

This has already been discussed to some extent in a previous section. It is likely that sera directed against the incompatible HLA antigens of the donor will be suitable, though this would involve having a large battery of different sera, given the large number of HLA antigens that have been defined. The fact that antisera show a much broader spectrum of reactivity, with respect to passive enhancement of kidney grafts than would be predicted on the basis of lymphocytotoxicity (Fabre and Morris, 1974b) and that the HLA antigens are defined on the basis of lymphocytotoxicity, suggests that it might be possible with suitable assays to define a fairly broad group of donors for which any particular antiserum will be suitable, which would simplify the logistics of serum supply.

Possible treatment schedules

Direct extrapolation from rat to man is the only guide currently available as to likely clinical dose requirements. The doses generally used in the rat are of the order of 3 ml of hyperimmune serum per animal, or about 10 ml/kg, which almost certainly is an excessive dose. The only formal dose–response studies which have been done (Fabre and Morris, 1973) found that in two different strain combinations the minimum effective dose was 50 μl per rat, or about 0·25 ml/kg. Unfortunately, these latter studies were performed with sera raised with adjuvants, and since this will not be possible clinically, the results obtained almost certainly represent an underestimate of clinical requirements. Myburgh and Smit (1972), also using sera raised with adjuvants, found that 1 ml/kg was as effective as 8 ml/kg for liver grafts in baboons. Further dose studies, in the rat and other species, are clearly needed.

The time over which the serum need be administered is well established. In the early studies of Stuart *et al.* (1968), continuing antiserum injections beyond the first week after grafting conferred no extra benefit. In another study, in a strain combination where rapid onset of severe kidney graft rejection occurred regularly towards the end of the second week in passively enhanced rats, continuing antiserum injections to the end of the second week did not influence the onset of rejection in the slightest (Fabre and Morris, 1972). Giving antiserum for several days after grafting seems to give slightly better results than a single injection at the time of grafting in some strain combinations (Fabre and Morris, 1973). Thus it seems that the optimum schedule involves treatment from the time of transplantation for 4 or 5 days.

The studies just quoted (Stuart *et al.*, 1968; Fabre and Morris, 1972) also indicate that passive enhancement is useful for preventing the *onset* of rejection but has little effect on established rejection reactions. Thus passive enhancement is unlikely to be of value for the treatment of late rejection episodes.

The possibility of immune complex nephritis

Immune complex nephritis could conceivably occur as a result of injecting antibodies against the incompatible antigens of the graft. This has not received critical attention, but it certainly does not seem to be a problem. In strain combinations where passive enhancement completely suppresses the usual rejection phenomena, the animals survive indefinitely, with excellent blood urea levels, and the grafts at around 6 months are in excellent condition. The fact that the total amount of *specific* antibody used in enhancement is likely to be very small and that the antigens released from the graft might be in large particles rather than in soluble form are both possible factors that might militate against the development of nephritis.

FUTURE PROSPECTS

The experimental work is promising, and has defined the broad framework within which passive enhancement is likely to find clinical application. There is every possibility that passive enhancement will find a place in immunosuppressive regimens either as a simple adjunct to current therapy to improve potency, or as the mainstay of therapy with non-specific agents used only in low doses and/or for short periods. In either case it will be of benefit, but in the latter case, by making immunosuppression safer, it might very much broaden the scope of transplantation as a therapeutic procedure to encompass, among other things, transplantation of the pancreas or pancreatic islets for diabetes mellitus. It would be reassuring, however, to see more results in outbred animals before considering widespread clinical application.

Induction of Specific Immunosuppression by Antigen (Active Enhancement)

INTRODUCTION

Active enhancement is a relatively complex approach to specific immunosuppression. The large number of possible variables in the approaches to active enhancement makes an experimental evaluation of the subject as a whole a much more formidable task than is the case with passive enhancement, and consequently, it is not as well defined a subject at the moment. Moreover, the results of treatment with antigen are by no means completely predictable, and the risk of causing sensitization is probably the main reason that antigen is unlikely to be used clinically in the near future. Nevertheless, it should be remembered that antigen offers a number of practical and theoretical advantages over the use of antibody and, in the long term, it might well turn out to be the method of choice for specific immunosuppression.

The advantages with the use of antigen fall into three groups. Firstly, it seems to be far more potent than antibody at inducing specific immunosuppression. It has been possible, using large doses, to induce in adult mice the life-long acceptance of skin grafts incompatible at the major histocompatibility locus, something inconceivable with the use of antibody. Secondly, if the tissues of the actual graft donor are used as the source of antigen for immunosuppression, one can be sure that all major and minor incompatibilities will be covered, without any knowledge being necessary of the actual incompatibilities involved and without any reliance having to be placed on current theories of histocompatibility. Finally, the use of antigen, whether it be from the actual graft donor or from other sources, avoids the step of having to immunize volunteers or harvest serum from multiparous women or polytransfused patients, which are distasteful yet unavoidable steps with passive enhancement.

When considering the experimental work on active enhancement there are several things which should be borne in mind. Firstly, much of the work has been done with skin grafts and while it is extremely likely that these experiments will reflect the trend of results with organ grafts, a slight but definite reservation on this point would not be completely unfounded. Secondly, because skin grafts are much more difficult to protect than organ grafts, any treatment schedule which doubles or trebles the mean survival time of skin grafts is likely to be quite potent in the context of organ grafts. Thirdly, any treatment schedule which involves *pre*treatment of the recipient in the days and weeks before grafting is of only limited clinical interest at this stage. Without major advances in organ storage, these techniques are applicable only to living donors. The only exception would be the use of broadly reactive antigen mixtures with certain pretreatment schedules (Pinto *et al.*, 1974) but such preparations have yet to be shown to be effective, and they are potentially dangerous. Finally, many experiments have used living lymphoid cells as the source of antigen. Because of the slight risk of graft-versus-host reactions, especially in patients receiving supplementary non-specific therapy, these preparations are probably unsuitable for clinical use. If suspensions of living cells are to be used clinically, they will have to be rendered free of the risk of inducing graft-versus-host reactions.

PRINCIPLE OF ACTIVE ENHANCEMENT

The principle is to treat the recipient with preparations containing the incompatible graft antigens. As will be discussed in detail later, the physical state of the antigen (i.e. whether it is given as whole cells, crude tissue extracts, solubilized cell membranes, etc.) is varied, mainly in attempts to increase the immunosuppressive potency of the preparation and to decrease its ability to sensitize. The source of antigen, for reasons of convenience, has usually been lymphoid tissue or liver. This approach, i.e. the use of tissues other than those of the graft as the antigen source for enhancement, rests on the assumption that the histocompatibility antigens of the body are widely and uniformly distributed. That this is probably more or less true is shown by the fact that lymphoid tissues and liver have frequently been used to enhance successfully kidney and skin grafts. However, it should be remembered that some antigens of the major histocompatibility system (the I region antigens) seem to be restricted to lymphoid tissue, and probably skin (Shreffler and David, 1975). Furthermore, a histocompatibility system has been described in the mouse which is restricted to skin and brain (Lance *et al.*, 1971). Thus, while in practice the use of tissues other than those of the graft is suitable for active enhancement, the assumption on which this approach is based should not be completely forgotten.

Except for the case where the tissues of the actual graft donor are used as the source of antigen, the problems of transferring active enhancement from the inbred to the clinical situation are similar to those discussed in detail with respect to passive enhancement. Thus, typing of donor and recipient for currently defined HLA antigens and treating the recipient with preparations containing the incompatible HLA antigens might leave uncovered as yet undefined antigens of the major histocompatibility system which might be important in graft rejection. Furthermore, since minor histocompatibility systems have not been defined in the human, it will not be possible to direct active enhancement against them.

The use of tissues from the actual graft donor offers considerable advantages, and, in most clinically applicable treatment schedules, it should be possible to use them without too much practical inconvenience.

POSSIBLE MECHANISMS

The mechanisms whereby a lymphocyte population distinguishes between tolerogenic and sensitizing stimuli is one of the intriguing problems of immunology. Until recently, the problem was considered in terms of how the individual lymphocyte could discriminate between the two sorts of stimuli. However, the possibility of suppressor T cells means that it can now also be considered in terms of how different stimuli activate different lymphocyte subpopulations.

Antigen can conceivably induce unresponsiveness in two broad ways, either by direct interaction with the lymphoid system, or indirectly by inducing the formation of antibodies. In certain situations in transplant systems the latter mechanism seems to operate. There is, however, no question that antigen can induce unresponsiveness without requiring the production of antibodies (e.g. Rouse and Warner, 1972). When antigen is used in conjunction with non-specific immunosuppressive agents, its function might be quite different. For instance, when antigen exposure is followed by treatment with ALS (e.g. Brent *et al.*, 1973) its function might be to induce the specifically reactive lymphocytes to recirculate and become vulnerable to the action of ALS.

The effects of antigen exposure need not necessarily be uniform, especially if crude extracts or whole cells are used. The end result of exposure could be a summation of the events which occur throughout the lymphoid system, and which might vary with local differences in exposure.

IMPORTANT VARIABLES AFFECTING THE INDUCTION OF ACTIVE ENHANCEMENT

Little is known of the basis for the different results obtained under different conditions of exposure to antigen. One can, however, attempt to construct on an empirical basis some general guidelines on conditions which favour the development of unresponsiveness. The picture that emerges is by no means a clear one. There are many contradictions, which emphasizes the complexity of the subject and our ignorance of the fundamentals involved.

Age of the recipient

The more immature the animal, the easier it is to induce unresponsiveness. The first demonstration of experimentally induced long-term unresponsiveness to grafts was made by treatment of mouse fetuses *in utero* (Billingham *et al.*, 1953). Thereafter it was shown that it was relatively easy to render mice unresponsive to skin grafts if they were treated on the day of birth, but that it became progressively more difficult with each day of life until it was quite difficult in the second week. Moreover, a treatment schedule which gave excellent unresponsiveness in 12-day-old mice resulted only in sensitization of fully mature adults (Gowland, 1965). Though these findings are of only limited clinical interest, it should be remembered that the level of immunological maturity in relation to the time of birth varies from species to species. Thus, whereas neonatal rats reject skin grafts very slowly (Medawar and Woodruff, 1958), fetal lambs do so quite promptly 40 days before birth in a 150-day gestation cycle (Schinckel and Ferguson, 1953).

Dose of antigen

In general, the higher the dose of antigen, the more likely it is to induce unresponsiveness. This has been shown on numerous occasions, especially with skin graft systems in the mouse. Moreover, Berrian and McKahn (1960) showed with skin grafts in mice that increasing antigen dose from low levels gave results progressing from no effect through sensitization to unresponsiveness. Nevertheless, there have been occasions where increasing antigen dose has given deleterious results. For example, Zimmerman et al. (1968) found that treatment of dogs with spleen extract for 2 weeks at a certain dose level gave some kidney graft prolongation, but a higher dose resulted only in sensitization. It should also be noted that in one or two difficult mouse strain combinations, even enormous doses of antigen have resulted only in sensitization to skin grafts (Gowland, 1965).

The doses of antigen required to induce consistently unresponsiveness to skin grafts in adult mice incompatible at the major histocompatibility locus are large, of the order of 3×10^8 cells or more per 25 g mouse. This corresponds, very roughly, to about 800 g of spleen per 70 kg human. With organ grafts, the doses required are fortunately much less. Numerous investigators have obtained excellent suppression of kidney graft rejection in rats with very small doses of antigen. For example, Ockner et al. (1970) required only 10^7 bone marrow cells given at optimal times pregraft.

The phenomenon of low zone tolerance, i.e. where prolonged exposure to sub-immunogenic doses of antigen results in unresponsiveness, has not been demonstrated in transplant systems.

Physical state of the antigen

As previously mentioned, antigen may be given as whole cells or as tissue extracts of varying complexity from crude whole tissue homogenates to truly solubilized cell membranes. The hope has been to increase the efficiency of inducing unresponsiveness and to decrease the risk of sensitization by altering the physical state of the antigen. There is also the consideration that tissue extracts are likely to be more clinically acceptable than suspensions of living cells, because of the risk of graft-versus-host reactions, as previously discussed.

It is often considered that soluble preparations of antigen will be more potent at inducing unresponsiveness and less likely to sensitize than crude extracts or whole cells. This proposition, however, has been examined hardly at all in transplant systems, and it probably derives much of its support from studies on the suppression of the antibody response to foreign proteins, where it is certainly true (Dresser, 1961). Recently, Little et al. (1975) treated baboons at the time of liver grafting with detergent solubilized spleen antigen and found that preparations containing single antigen molecules in solution doubled the mean survival time of grafts, whereas those with molecular aggregates had no effect. Medawar (1963) showed that antigen extracts with relatively small membrane fragments gave immuno-suppression, whereas those containing larger aggregates gave only sensitiza-tion. However, it should not be forgotten that excellent immunosuppression has been obtained on innumerable occasions with whole cells and crude extracts, and that in certain systems it is possible that soluble antigens are ineffective where crude extracts give good graft prolongation (Brent *et al.*, 1973). Moreover, the results that have been obtained with soluble prepara-tions do not seem to be superior to those where antigen in other forms, especially living cells, has been used. Nevertheless, the fact that soluble preparations have been shown to be effective, combined with the possibility that they might be less likely to sensitize, would make them the best initial choice for studies on clinically applicable regimens of active enhance-ment.

A number of methods have been used to produce so-called soluble mem-brane antigens. It should be noted in this respect that the HLA and H2 major histocompatibility antigens of man and mouse have been shown to have a hydrophobic end by which they are inserted into the lipid bilayer of the cell membrane. These molecules cannot remain in aqueous solution unless the hydrophobic end is removed (e.g. by enzymes such as papain) or stabilized by detergents. Cell disruption by sonication has frequently been used to produce supposedly soluble membrane antigens. These preparations, however, might contain tiny membrane particles as well as truly solubilized antigens (Rosenberg and McIntosh, 1968).

Timing of antigen exposure

Antigen therapy may be given at the time of grafting or at various times before and/or after grafting and either single or multiple injections may be used. The timing of antigen exposure in relation to the time of grafting is often crucial in determining the outcome of therapy. Ockner *et al.* (1970) found that a single exposure to donor bone marrow 1–2 weeks pregraft gave excellent immunosuppression, but that exposure 1 or 2 days, or 3 or more weeks, pregraft resulted in sensitization. A number of groups have obtained similar results. Timing has also been shown to be crucial for antigen therapy given after grafting. Lymphoid cells given 9 days after grafting in combination with ALS at around the time of grafting gave excellent skin graft prolongation in mice, but if the cells were given at the time of grafting or 4 days after grafting, they had no effect or were weakly sensitized (Lance and Medawar, 1969). There are, however, exceptions to the above general findings. Thus, Kim *et al.* (1972), using sonicated spleen cells as a source of antigen, found that treatment 1 day pregraft gave moderate kidney graft prolongation in rats, but that at all other time intervals it had no effect. In another system (Matalo et al., 1972) spleen cells or spleen cell membranes given at what would seem to be an optimal time (2 weeks) before heart grafts in rats resulted only in sensitization.

Frequent exposures to antigen at the rate of 2 or 3 per week have been shown on a number of occasions to be superior to single injections (e.g. Gowland, 1965). This applies to pretreatment schedules as well as to those involving postgraft antigen therapy (Lance and Medawar, 1969). Continuing pregraft therapy into the postgraft period has not been thoroughly studied. However, in a system involving a single injection of extract 16 days before skin grafting in mice, together with ALS in the first postgraft week, adding a single injection of spleen cells 12 days after grafting substantially improved results (Brent et al., 1973). Again, there are exceptions to the above findings. Kim et al. (1972) found that a single injection a day or two before kidney grafting in rats gave moderate graft prolongation, whereas multiple pregraft injections were without effect. Matalo et al. (1972) found that spleen membranes given 4 days before heart grafts in rats gave good synergism in combination with ALS around the time of grafting, but that the addition of a single injection of membranes 8 days after grafting gave results inferior to ALS alone.

Route of administration

Unresponsiveness has been induced most consistently and safely by the intravenous route. Though the intraperitoneal route has been effectively used for induction of unresponsiveness on numerous occasions, it has sometimes resulted in sensitization where, under otherwise identical conditions, the intravenous route gave unresponsiveness (e.g. Medawar, 1963). Unresponsiveness has even been induced by the subcutaneous route, but this is not usually effective.

The effect of thymectomy and splenectomy

The presence of the thymus is necessary for the maturation of newly developing T lymphocytes, so that thymectomy could conceivably play a role in preventing the rejection of grafts, especially the chronic rejection sometimes seen after the induction of active enhancement. However, thymectomy could also interfere with enhancement if suppressor T cells were important in the maintenance phase of unresponsiveness. Both Guttmann and Falk (1974) and Kilshaw et al. (1974) found that active enhancement of rat heart and mouse skin grafts respectively was slightly improved if the recipient was thymectomized prior to entering the experiment. Abbot et al. (1969) found that thymectomy markedly increased the survival of skin grafts in rats treated with ALS and antigen, but the grafts were eventually rejected.

Although thymectomy seems usually not to affect markedly the outcome of enhancement, it is interesting to note, from the point of view of mechanisms, that the tendency is for thymectomy to *improve* the results of enhancement.

The studies of Enomoto and Lucas (1973) have previously been quoted. In their experiments the spleen was essential for the induction of both active and passive enhancement of kidney grafts in rats. Though the spleen is well known to play an important role in the antibody response to certain antigens, an interference with antibody production does not seem to be the mechanism whereby splenectomy interfered with the induction of active enhancement in their experiments: the antibody response to the active enhancement schedule was completely normal, at least as measured by lymphocytotoxins. The role of the spleen in their experiments is obscure, but the general significance of their findings must await further study since, at least with the case of passive enhancement, their results could not be confirmed in a different strain combination (Fabre and Batchelor, 1975a). In the experiment of Kilshaw *et al.* (1974) splenectomy did not affect the induction of active enhancement of skin grafts.

Other possible variables

It can be seen from the foregoing discussion that the results of active enhancement are by no means uniform and predictable. The reasons for the variability in results are as yet unknown. Contributory factors could be species and strain differences in the response to active enhancement, differences in the reaction to different types of grafts, and slight differences in experimental protocol between groups studying any given approach.

THE USE OF NON-SPECIFIC IMMUNOSUPPRESSIVE AGENTS IN COMBINATION WITH ACTIVE ENHANCEMENT

It has been possible under a variety of conditions to obtain a very strong synergism between active enhancement and several of the non-specific immunosuppressive agents currently in clinical use. With kidney grafts in dogs, the use of multiple injections of donor lymphoid tissue extracts over several weeks before grafting in combination with postgraft administration of low doses of azathioprine and methylprednisolone has on occasion given remarkably good results. This is in spite of the fact that neither the tissue extracts alone nor the non-specific therapy alone had any effect at all on graft survival. One group of 14 dogs so treated had a mean survival time of 124 days (Wilson *et al.*, 1969), though in any series of experiments the best groups have usually had less striking survival times. Unfortunately, the synergism seems to be critically dependent on the dose of antigen given and the period over which it is administered within uncomfortably narrow limits, which makes clinical application difficult. Thus, in the work of Wilson et al. (1969) 3 mg of antigen over 4 weeks yielded a mean survival time of 44 days, but 5 mg over the same period had no effect at all and 3 mg over 6 weeks gave a mean survival time of only 16 days.

In skin graft systems, active enhancement has been studied most extensively with ALS, again with excellent results. In some studies (e.g. Brent et al., 1973) antigen treatment by itself has had no effect on graft survival, but if given with ALS, the results have been much better than with ALS alone. The most effective protocols have combined ALS around the time of grafting with a pregraft injection of tissue extract and a postgraft injection of spleen cells (Brent et al., 1973) or with multiple postgraft injections of lymphoid tissue (Lance and Medawar, 1969). Skin grafts incompatible at the major histocompatibility locus have survived for in excess of 100 days in the majority of treated mice. The timing and to a lesser extent the dose of antigen has been shown on many occasions to be critical for synergism to occur. Where timing or dose is inappropriate, the antigen is harmful in that the survival of the grafts is less than with ALS alone (e.g. Matalo et al., 1972; Lance and Medawar, 1969).

Other agents such as hydrocortisone (Chutnà, 1971) and methotrexate and x-irradiation (Medawar, 1963) are known to potentiate the active enhancement of skin grafts. The possibility that these non-specific agents might interfere with any active processes occurring during the induction of enhancement seems not to be a problem. However, Myburgh and Smit (1972) have noted that cyclophosphamide abolished the effectiveness of donor bone marrow when it was given in conjunction with passive enhancement for liver grafts in baboons.

THE EFFECT OF COMBINING ACTIVE AND PASSIVE ENHANCEMENT

The combined use of active and passive enhancement has been tested on only a few occasions, and in most instances it has been shown to be marginally better than either agent alone. Stuart et al. (1968) combined the use of spleen cells on the day before grafting with passive enhancement after grafting for kidney grafts in rats. Myburgh and Smit (1972) treated baboons at the time of liver grafting with donor bone marrow cells and passive enhancement. In both cases, combined therapy was better than either agent alone, but the improvement was not striking.

THE USE OF ANTIGEN–ANTIBODY COMPLEXES FORMED IN VITRO

This seems an attractive approach since passive enhancement is likely to be effective by way of antigen–antibody complexes formed between the injected antibody and antigen released from the graft. Supplying the antigen–antibody complexes already formed might be a more effective approach, though the risk of immune complex nephritis would have to be considered. However, this approach seems not to have been studied in transplant systems. One point to note is that the antigen–antibody ratio might be critical with respect to the ability of the complexes to induce unresponsiveness (Diener and Feldmann, 1970).

FUTURE PROSPECTS

Though active enhancement might eventually be the technique of choice when considering specific immunosuppression, there is clearly much work still to be done to make the results of therapy more predictable and to evaluate thoroughly promising approaches. It is worth noting that a few approaches, using active enhancement alone or in combination with short-term therapy with ALS, have given virtually life-long acceptance of skin grafts across the major histocompatibility barrier in adult mice. Thus the possibility remains open that, eventually, it might be possible to use specific immunosuppression in clinical situations requiring skin-containing grafts, e.g. directly vascularized full thickness skin flaps in plastic surgery and transplantation of digits.

The Maintenance Phase of Specific Unresponsiveness

INTRODUCTION

The mechanism whereby a foreign graft is retained more or less unmolested for the lifetime of the host, long after immunosuppressive therapy has been stopped, is an ill-understood but interesting area of study. What relationship these mechanisms have to those involved in self-tolerance, in the acceptance of the incompatible fetus during pregnancy, and in the unchecked growth of potentially immunogenic tumours is unknown, but it is likely that parallels will exist at least with tumour systems. A possibly important difference between self-tolerance and graft acceptance is that in the latter instance the foreign graft is presented to an already mature immune system.

    There is a variety of different approaches to inducing long-term graft acceptance. With the specific approach one may use passive enhancement, many different methods of active enhancement, active and passive enhancement together, or a variety of different non-specific immunosuppressive agents in combination with active or passive enhancement. Long-term graft acceptance can also be induced with the use of non-specific agents alone, and these may be given close to the time of grafting only, or continued for the life of the host, as occurs clinically. Whether or not all of these approaches lead to a final common mechanism in the maintenance phase is unknown, though one would guess that it is likely to be so.

Mechanisms of specific unresponsiveness in transplant systems are difficult to study at a basic level. Much of the fundamental work in this area has been performed in the simpler system of the antibody response to well-defined, pure and relatively simple antigens such as bovine serum albumin. Because helper T cells are involved in antibody production, these studies allow an examination of one subpopulation of T cells, though the relationship between the helper T cells and the T cells involved in graft destruction is unknown. Nevertheless, this work provides a guiding background to the more difficult subject of mechanisms in transplant systems, and for this reason some of the more interesting findings that have arisen will be discussed before going on to mechanisms of graft acceptance.

STUDIES ON THE SUPPRESSION OF THE ANTIBODY RESPONSE TO SIMPLE ANTIGENS

Some important work in this area has already been discussed in the section on induction of unresponsiveness, for example, the superiority of soluble as opposed to aggregated proteins for the induction of unresponsiveness (Dresser, 1961) and the studies suggesting that linking of surface receptors is the signal for unresponsiveness in B cells (Diener and Feldmann, 1970) but not necessarily T cells (Feldmann and Nossal, 1972). In this section I shall concentrate on recent work showing that remarkable differences exist between T and B cells in a number of facets of unresponsiveness. It should be mentioned that the unresponsive state in antibody systems is usually described as tolerance, so that this term will be used frequently in this section.

Kinetics of induction and subsequent loss of tolerance

The most interesting and extensive experiments in this area have been performed by Weigle *et al.* (1972) who studied the induction of tolerance to human gammaglobulin in thymus cells (source of helper T cells) and bone marrow cells (source of B cells). They found that the T cells were already 70% suppressed 6 hours after exposure to antigen and that at 24, 48 and 96 hours the suppression was, respectively, 85, 92 and 100%. The T cells remained completely tolerant for more than 100 days, after which responsiveness returned but very slowly. By contrast, B cells were still completely normal 7 days after antigen exposure, after which tolerance was gradually induced, and was not complete till 2–3 weeks after exposure to antigen. Complete tolerance was short-lived, and began to decay fairly rapidly from about 3 weeks, so that by 50 days after antigen exposure the B cells were once again completely normal. The tolerant state in the whole animal reflected the kinetics of T cell tolerance. Thus, for the greater part of the time that the mice were tolerant to human gammaglobulin, this was the result of tolerance in the helper T cell population only.

It is interesting to compare these data with *in vitro* studies on kinetics of tolerance induction. For example, Diener and Armstrong (1969) studied the induction of tolerance to polymerized flagellin (a thymus-independent antigen) in spleen cell populations *in vitro*. They found that the B cells were already 40–50% tolerant 15 minutes after exposure to antigen, and that thereafter tolerance induction proceeded exponentially so that it was virtually complete after a few hours.

These and other studies suggest that tolerance induction at the single cell level under conditions of optimal exposure to antigen occurs very rapidly. *In vivo*, tolerance induction takes several days to complete and has markedly different kinetics in T and B cell populations possibly because of problems of antigen distribution. Optimal exposure of a lymphocyte population might depend on unknown factors, such as lymphocyte recirculation.

These differences in kinetics in T and B cell tolerance induction *in vivo* might explain why, in some systems, passive enhancement of rat kidney grafts proceeds quite smoothly in spite of the fact that the recipients produce a normal antibody response in the first few weeks after grafting.

Dose requirements for tolerance induction

Helper T cells have been shown to require much smaller doses of antigen for tolerance induction than is the case with B cells. For instance, 2·5 mg of human gammaglobulin was found to induce tolerance to both T cells and B cells, but 100 μg tolerated only T cells (Weigle et al., 1972). Weigle (1971) has made an interesting review of the relevance of these findings to self-tolerance, and discussed data suggesting that self-tolerance might frequently involve only T cells, possibly because of the low concentration of some self-components. This might also be the case with unresponsiveness to grafts, and could explain why challenging rats bearing long-surviving kidney grafts with donor strain lymphoid tissue sometimes results in antibody production without affecting graft function (French and Batchelor, 1969).

The effect of the affinity of the surface receptors of lymphocytes

It is well established that lymphocytes with receptors of high affinity for antigen are preferentially rendered tolerant (Werblin and Siskind, 1972).

Although this statement can be made with certainty only with respect to B cells, it has been invoked in an attempt to explain why skin grafts are less readily enhanced than kidney grafts (Fabre and Morris, 1975).

Suppressor T cells

Gershon and Kondo (1971) have found that T cells must be present for tolerance induction to sheep red blood cells in mice, and they have attributed this phenomenon to 'suppressor' T cells. Whether or not the phenomenon they observed is due to a discrete T cell subpopulation with definite suppressor functions is not established, but suppressor T cells have been invoked as possible explanations for a number of phenomena, including long-term graft acceptance. It should be remembered that recipient thymectomy either slightly (Guttmann, 1974; Kilshaw et al., 1974) or markedly (Abbot et al., 1969) *increases* the effectiveness of active enhancement, which is a point against an active role being played by T cells in long-term graft acceptance.

STUDIES ON THE MAINTENANCE PHASE OF UNRESPONSIVENESS TO GRAFTS

The mechanisms involved in the maintenance phase of unresponsiveness are poorly understood and are currently the subject of much speculation. Burnet's clonal selection theory (Burnet and Fenner, 1949) postulated that self-tolerance resulted from deletion of the self-reactive clones, and the experiments performed in the 1950s on the neonatal induction of tolerance to skin grafts seemed to support this idea of clonal deletion. Those experiments are still, in fact, mostly simply interpreted on the basis of clonal deletion, though it should be remembered that the mechanisms involved in unresponsiveness induced in immature animals might be different to those where it is induced in adults. In recent years, hosts bearing tumours and grafts have been shown to possess lymphocytes reactive against the foreign tissues which they bear, together with blocking factors which will suppress those lymphocytes. As a consequence, clonal deletion has fallen into disfavour and has been supplanted by concepts involving continuous suppression of specifically reactive clones by blocking factors and/or suppressor cells. The issue, however, is not yet resolved.

Before discussing mechanisms of unresponsiveness in the maintenance phase, it is necessary first to establish that unresponsiveness does in fact persist long after the graft has been established. The possibility of graft adaptation will, therefore, be considered first, and then the evidence for and against clonal suppression and clonal deletion will be presented.

The possibility of graft adaptation

It has long been considered that a graft might in some way adapt to its host and thereby become less vulnerable to rejection. For instance, it has been postulated that the endothelium of the graft vasculature might be replaced by host endothelium, that antigen modulation (suppression of the expression of foreign antigens) might occur, or that loss of passenger leukocytes might considerably diminish the immunogenicity of the graft. It is at least conceivable that host reactivity to the graft might return but find the graft no longer susceptible to rejection. Fortunately, this question can be easily and unequivocally answered with the help of inbred strains.

If complete graft adaptation occurs, it means that an animal of strain A bearing a graft from strain B will be potentially capable of rejecting his graft, but the graft will no longer be vulnerable to rejection. In that situation if the A animal is given a fresh B graft, he will reject it, and conversely if the long-surviving B graft is retransplanted to a fresh A host, it will not be rejected. If specific unresponsiveness persists and graft adaptation has not occurred, the long-surviving A animal will not reject a fresh B graft, and the long-surviving B graft will be rejected by a fresh A host. Such experiments were first performed by Stuart et al. (1970) in a rat kidney graft system and they showed that specific unresponsiveness did indeed persist. The long-surviving hosts did not reject fresh grafts and the long-established grafts were rejected by fresh hosts. However, the rejection of the long-established grafts was significantly slower than normal, indicating that some degree of graft adaptation occurred. One can conclude from these experiments that incomplete graft adaptation does occur, but that it is irrelevant to the mechanism of long-term graft acceptance.

The possibility of clonal suppression

The most direct approach to the problem of mechanism is to attempt to demonstrate lymphocytes reactive against graft antigens in hosts bearing well-established grafts. Such a demonstration would immediately exclude clonal deletion as the mechanism of graft acceptance. There are a number of experiments which appear to do this. Firstly, due largely to the work of the Hellströms, hosts bearing well-established tumours and grafts have been shown to possess lymphocytes which will, *in vitro*, react against the foreign tissues residing in them (e.g. Stuart et al., 1971). Secondly, lymphocytes from long survivors of rat kidney grafts have been shown to have a completely normal capacity to mount graft-versus-host reactions against donor strain tissues (French et al., 1971). Thirdly, rats with long-surviving kidney grafts will reject, usually very promptly, skin grafts from the same strain as the donor kidney, without adversely affecting the survival of the kidney graft.

These data suggest that specifically reactive lymphocytes exist, but closer examination shows that they are not conclusive. If specificity has any meaning in immune reactions, it must mean that if the affinity of a lymphocyte's receptors for any particular antigen is too low, it will not be stimulated by it. It would be surprising if the affinity cut-off point were identical for all the tests to which a lymphocyte population is subjected. In the *in vitro* tests employed for detecting specifically reactive lymphocytes, the conditions for lymphocyte–target cell interaction are optimal, and it is possible that the lymphocytes detected are of only low affinity. Though they might react quite well *in vitro* they might have only a very low probability of interaction *in vivo*, where the affinity requirements might be more stringent. Thus, the lymphocytes detected by the *in vitro* tests (e.g. Stuart *et al.*, 1971) might not in fact be reactive against the graft. Secondly, there is increasing evidence that lymphocyte–lymphocyte interactions such as graft-versus-host reactions and mixed lymphocyte culture reactions are determined, at least to a large extent, by antigens restricted to lymphoid tissue (Shreffler and David, 1975) and if this is so, the graft-versus-host reaction is irrelevant as a test for lymphocytes reactive against the kidney graft. Finally, the rejection of donor strain skin grafts by long survivors of kidney grafts is difficult to explain whatever mechanism one chooses to defend—deletion or suppression. The simplest explanation is that the skin grafts are rejected by lymphocytes not reactive against the kidney, e.g. lymphocytes reactive against skin specific antigens (Lance *et al.*, 1971) or perhaps lymphocytes of lower affinity than will react with kidney. If either explanation is correct, the rejection of skin grafts is irrelevant as a test for lymphocytes reactive against the kidney graft.

If it is accepted that lymphocytes reactive against the graft exist, a mechanism must be found whereby they are prevented from destroying the graft. There is abundant evidence for the presence in long survivors of serum factors which will specifically suppress the reactive lymphocytes found by the *in vitro* tests (e.g. Stuart *et al.*, 1971). Suppressor T cells have also been postulated on the basis of the work of Gershon and Kondo (1971). There are, however, a number of points to consider. Firstly, the serum-blocking factors have usually been defined as antibodies, or antigen–antibody complexes formed with graft antigens. The work of Weigle *et al.* (1972) has shown that T cell tolerance is possible in the presence of completely normal B cells, so that the finding of antibodies or complexes in the long survivors could simply reflect a failure of unresponsiveness to extend to the B cells. Secondly, the fact that thymectomy *increases* the effectiveness of unresponsiveness argues against an active role being played by T cells in the mechanism of unresponsiveness. Finally, attempts to transfer unresponsiveness from long survivors to fresh hosts, using cells or serum, have generally been unsuccessful.

The possibility of clonal deletion

Clonal deletion has the merit of simplicity. Since in its simplest form, clonal deletion involves a complete absence of specifically reactive lymphocytes, supplying the animal with normal lymphoid tissue should replace the missing clones and lead to graft rejection. This has been done on numerous occasions in rats and mice rendered unresponsive to skin grafts by the neonatal injection of foreign tissues, and has led to the prompt rejection of long-accepted and healthy grafts. However, in rats rendered unresponsive to kidney grafts as adults, even large doses of normal or sensitized lymphocytes (Bowen et al., 1974) have completely failed to induce the host to reject his graft. Whether this difference is due to differences in the mechanism of unresponsiveness in animals rendered unresponsive as neonates and adults, or to differences in the response to skin and kidney grafts, is unknown. In any case, with the reservations previously made about blocking factors, this failure to reconstitute long survivors of kidney grafts favours clonal suppression as the mechanism of unresponsiveness in these animals.

Conclusions

It is interesting to look back at the enthusiasm which surrounded the early technical successes in experimental organ grafting. Before the problem of rejection had dampened his hopes, Carrel (1907), who had transplanted almost anything that was technically possible in dogs and cats, enthused: 'If I were a veterinary surgeon and had to treat a myxoedematous dog, I should not hesitate to transplant to its neck a thyroid gland from another dog'. He went on to say 'It is not unreasonable to believe that some transplantations, as, for instance, the transplantation of the arm a little below the elbow, may be successfully performed if an adequate technique is used' and '. . . the organs of the anthropoid apes are perhaps able to tolerate human plasma'. However, the golden age of spare parts surgery is still not upon us: seventy years later, as I hope the preceding discussion has shown, only the area covered by the first of his predictions has real hope of being realized in the near future.

References

Abbot, W. M., Monaco, A. P. and Russell, P. S. (1969). Antilymphocyte serum and cell-free antigen loading. *Transplantation*, **7**, 291

Batchelor, J. R., Fabre, J. W. and Morris, P. J. (1972). Passive enhancement of kidney grafts. Potentiation with anti-thymocyte serum. *Transplantation*, **13**, 610

Batchelor, J. R., French, M. E., Cameron, J. S., Ellis, F., Bewick, M. and Ogg, C. S. (1970). Immunological enhancement of a human kidney graft. *Lancet*, **ii**, 1007

Berrian, J. H. and McKahn, C. F. (1960). Strength of histocompatibility genes. *Ann. N.Y. Acad. Sci.*, **87**, 106

Billingham, R. E., Brent, L. and Medawar, P. B. (1953). Actively acquired tolerance of foreign cells. *Nature (London)*, **172**, 603

Bowen, J. E., Batchelor, J. R., French, M. E., Burgos, H. and Fabre, J. W. (1974). Failure of adoptive immunisation or parabiosis with hyperimmune syngeneic partners to abrogate long-term enhancement of rat kidney grafts. *Transplantation*, **18**, 322

Brent, L., Hansen, J. A., Kilshaw, P. J. and Thomas, A. V. (1973). Specific unresponsiveness to skin allografts in mice. I. Properties of tissue extracts and their synergistic effect with antilymphocyte serum. *Transplantation*, **15**, 160

Burnet, F. M. and Fenner, F. (1949). *The Production of Antibodies*. 2nd Ed. p. 76. (Melbourne: Macmillan)

Carrel, A. (1907). The surgery of blood vessels, etc. *Johns Hopkins Hosp. Bull.*, **18**, 18

Chutnà, J. (1971). The mechanism of immunological enhancement of H-2 incompatible skin grafts in mice. *Transplantation*, **12**, 28

Diener, E. and Armstrong, W. D. (1969). Immunological tolerance *in vitro*: kinetic studies at the cellular level. *J. Exp. Med.*, **129**, 521

Diener, E. and Feldmann, M. (1970). Antibody-mediated suppression of the immune response *in vitro*. II. A new approach to the phenomenon of immunological tolerance. *J. Exp. Med.*, **132**, 31

Dresser, D. W. (1961) Acquired immunological tolerance to a fraction of bovine gamma globulin. *Immunology*, **4**, 13

Enomoto, K. and Lucas, Z. J. (1973). Immunological enhancement of renal allografts in the rat. III. Role of the spleen. *Transplantation*, **15**, 8

Fabre, J. W. and Batchelor, J. R. (1975a). The role of the spleen in the rejection and enhancement of kidney grafts in rats. *Transplantation*, **20**, 219

Fabre, J. W. and Batchelor, J. R. (1975b). Prevention of blood transfusion-induced immunisation against transplantation antigens by treatment of the blood with antibody. *Transplantation*, **20**, 473

Fabre, J. W. and Morris, P. J. (1972). Experience with passive enhancement of renal allografts in a (DA × Lewis)F_1 to Lewis strain combination. *Transplantation*, **13**, 604

Fabre, J. W. and Morris, P. J. (1973). Dose–response studies in passive enhancement of rat renal allografts. *Transplantation*, **15**, 397

Fabre, J. W. and Morris, P. J. (1974a). Passive enhancement of homozygous renal allografts in the rat. *Transplantation*, **18**, 429

Fabre, J. W. and Morris, P. J. (1974b). Passive enhancement of rat renal allografts with only partial cover of the incompatible Ag-B specificities. *Transplantation*, **18**, 436

Fabre, J. W. and Morris P. J. (1975). Studies on the specific suppression of renal allograft rejection in presensitised rats. Theoretical and clinical implications. *Transplantation*, **19**, 121

Feldmann, M. and Nossal, G. J. V. (1972). Tolerance, enhancement, and the regulation of interaction between T cells, B cells, and macrophages. *Transplant. Rev.*, **13**, 3

Fine, R. N., Batchelor, J. R., French, M. E. and Shumak, K. (1973). The uptake of 125 I-labelled rat alloantibody and its loss after combination with antigen. *Transplantation*, **16,** 641

Flexner, S. and Jobling, J. W. (1906). On the promoting influence of heated tumour emulsions on tumour growth. *Proc. Soc. Exp. Biol. Med. (N. Y.)*, **4,** 156

French, M. E. and Batchelor, J. R. (1969). Immunological enhancement of rat kidney grafts. *Lancet*, **ii,** 1103

French, M. E., Batchelor, J. R. and Watts, H. G. (1971). The capacity of lymphocytes from rats bearing enhanced kidney allografts to mount graft-versus-host reactions. *Transplantation*, **12,** 45

Gershon, R. K. and Kondo, K. (1971). Infectious immunological tolerance. *Immunology*, **21,** 903

Guttmann, R. D. and Falk, R. E. (1974). The effect of recipient thymectomy on rat cardiac allograft rejection. *Transplantation*, **17,** 228

Holter, A. R., McKearn, T. J., Neu, M. R., Fitch, F. W. and Stuart, F. P. (1972). Renal transplantation in the rabbit. I. Development of a model for study of hyperacute rejection and immunological enhancement. *Transplantation*, **13,** 244

Kaliss, N., (1956). Acceptance of tumour homografts by mice injected with antiserum. II. Effect of time of injection. *Proc. Soc. Exp. Biol. Med. (N. Y.)*, **91,** 432

Kilshaw, P. J., Brent, L. and Thomas, A. V. (1974). Specific unresponsiveness to skin allografts in mice. II. The mechanism of unresponsiveness induced by tissue extracts and antilymphocyte serum. *Transplantation*, **17,** 57

Kim, J., Shaipanich, T., Sells, R. A., Maggs, P., Luki, P. and Wilson, R. E. (1972). Active enhancement of rat renal allografts with soluble splenic antigen. *Transplantation*, **13,** 322

Kinsky, R. G., Voisin, G. A. and Duc, H. T. (1972). Biological properties of transplantation immune sera. III. Relationship between transplantation (facilitation or inhibition) and serological (anaphylaxis or cytolysis) activities. *Transplantation*, **13,** 452

Lance, E. M., Boyse, E. A., Cooper, S. and Carswell, E. A. (1971). Rejection of skin allografts by radiation chimaeras: evidence for a skin specific transplantation barrier. *Transplant. Proc.*, **3,** 864

Lance, E. M. and Medawar, P. B. (1969). Quantitative studies on tissue transplantation immunity. IX. Induction of tolerance with antilymphocyte serum. *Proc. R. Soc.*, *Ser. B*, **173,** 447

Little, J., Myburgh, J. A., Austaker, J. L. and Smit, J. A. (1975). Detergent solubilisation of baboon histocompatibility antigens and their use in prolonging liver allograft survival. *Transplantation*, **19,** 53

Matalo, N. M., Reemsta, K. and de Witt, C. W. (1972). Effect of cell membranes with and without anti-lymphocyte serum on skin and heart allograft survival. *Transplantation*, **13,** 265

McKenzie, I. F. C., Koene, R. and Winn, J. H. (1971). Mechanism of skin graft enhancement in the mouse. *Transplant. Proc.*, **3,** 711

Medawar, P. B. (1963). The use of antigenic tissue extracts to weaken the immune reaction against skin homografts in mice. *Transplantation*, **1,** 21

Medawar, P. B. and Woodruff, M. F. A. (1958). The induction of tolerance by skin homografts in newborn rats. *Immunology*, **1,** 27

Myburgh, J. A. and Smit, J. A. (1972). Passive and active enhancement in baboon liver allografting. *Transplantation*, **14,** 227

Myburgh, J. A. and Smit, J. A. (1973). Enhancement and antigen suicide in the outbred primate. *Transplant. Proc.*, **5,** 597

Ockner, S. A., Guttmann, R. D. and Lindquist, R. R. (1970). Renal transplantation in the inbred rat. Modification of rejection by active immunisation with bone marrow cells. *Transplantation*, **9**, 30

Opelz, G. and Teresaki, P. I. (1974). Post kidney transplant survival in recipients with frozen blood transfusions or no transfusions. *Lancet*, **ii**, 696

Owen, R. D. (1945). Immunogenetic consequences of vascular anastomosis between bovine twins. *Science*, **102**, 400

Pinto, M., Brent, L. and Thomas, A. V. (1974). Specific unresponsiveness to skin allografts in mice. III. Synergistic effect of tissue extracts, *Bordetella pertussis*, and antilymphocyte serum. *Transplantation*, **17**, 477

Rosenberg, S. A. and McIntosh, J. R. (1968). Erythrocyte membranes: effects of sonication. *Biochim. Biophys. Acta*, **163**, 285

Rouse, B. T. and Warner, N. L. (1972). Induction of T cell tolerance in aggammaglobulinaemic chickens. *Eur. Immunol.*, **2**, 102

Schinckel, P. G. and Ferguson, K. A. (1953). Skin transplantation in foetal lambs. *Aust. J. Biol. Sci.*, **6**, 533

Shapiro, F., Martinez, C., Smith, J. M., and Good, R. A. (1961). Tolerance of skin homografts induced in adult mice by multiple injections of homologous spleen cells. *Proc. Soc. Exper. Biol. Med. (N. Y.)*, **106**, 472

Shreffler, D. C. and David, C. S. (1975). The H-2 major histocompatibility complex and the I immune response region: genetic variation, function and organisation. *Adv. Immunol.*, **20**, 125

Smit, J. A. and Myburgh, J. A. (1974). Enhancement of baboon liver allografts with noncytotoxic preparations of alloimmune IgG. *Transplantation*, **18**, 63

Staines, N. A., Guy, K. and Davies, D. A. L. (1974). Passive enhancement of mouse skin allografts. Specificity of the antiserum for major histocompatibility complex antigens. *Transplantation*, **18**, 192

Strayer, D. S., Cosenza, H., Lee, W. M. F., Rowley, D. A. and Köhler, H. (1974). Neonatal tolerance induced by antibody against antigen specific receptor. *Science*, **186**, 640

Stuart, F. P., Fitch, F. W. and Rowley, D. A. (1970). Specific suppression of renal allograft rejection by treatment with antigen and antibody. *Transplant. Proc.*, **2**, 483

Stuart, F. P., Fitch, F. W., Rowley, D. A., Biesecker, J. L., Hellström, K. E., and Hellström, I. (1971). Presence of both cell-mediated immunity and serum blocking factors in rat renal allografts enhanced by passive immunisation. *Transplantation*, **12**, 331

Stuart, F. P., Saitoh, T. and Fitch, F. W. (1968). Rejection of renal allografts: specific immunological suppression. *Science*, **160**, 1463

Tilney, N. L. and Bell, P. R. F. (1974). Studies on enhancement of cardiac and renal allografts in the rat. *Transplantation*, **18**, 31

Weigle, W. O., Chiller, J. M. and Habicht, G. S. (1972). Effect of immunological unresponsiveness on different cell populations. *Transplant. Rev.*, **8**, 3

Werblin, T. P. and Siskind, G. (1972). Effect of tolerance and immunity on antibody affinity. *Transplant. Rev.*, **8**, 104

Wilson, R. E., Maggs, P. R., Vanwyck, R., Shaipanich, T., Hol-Allen, T. J., Luki, P. and Simonian, S. J. (1971). Active enhancement of renal allografts in dog and rat by subcellular antigen. *Transplant. Proc.*, **3**, 705

Wilson, R. E., Rippen, A., Hayes, C. R., Dagher, R. K., and Busch, G. J. (1969). Prolonged renal allograft survival associated with antigen pretreatment. *Transplant. Proc.*, **1**, 290

Zimmermann, C. E., Busch, G. J., Stuart, F. P. and Wilson, R. E. (1968). Canine renal homografts after pretreatment with subcellular splenic antigen. *Surgery*, **63,** 437

Further Reading

French, M. E. and Batchelor, J. R. (1972). Enhancement of renal allografts in rats and man. *Transplant. Rev.*, **13,** 115

Gowland, G. (1965). Induction of transplantation tolerance in adult animals. *Br. Med. Bull.*, **21,** 123

Snell, G. D. (1970). Immunological enhancement. *Surg., Gynecol., Obstet.*, **130,** 1109

Uhr, J. W. and Moller, H. (1968). Regulatory effect of antibody on the immune response. *Adv. Immunol.*, **8,** 81

Weigle, W. O. (1971). Recent observations and concepts in immunological unresponsiveness and autoimmunity. *Clin. Exp. Immunol.*, **9,** 437

Weigle, W. O. (1973). Immunological unresponsiveness. *Adv. Immunol.*, **16,** 61

CHAPTER 10

Diagnosis of Allograft Rejection

R. F. M. Wood and P. R. F. Bell

In this chapter the diagnosis of renal transplant rejection is discussed in detail. Particular reference is made to the application of immunological techniques in the management of transplant patients. The diagnosis of rejection in liver and heart transplants is beyond the scope of this book but many of the immunological methods described have a wide application in all fields of transplantation.

Introduction

The rejection reaction is an inevitable consequence of transplantation in the presence of any degree of tissue incompatibility. Despite improvements in every aspect of clinical transplantation, rejection remains the greatest stumbling block to further advances. Reviews of the results of kidney transplantation show that by 2 years after operation approximately 60% of grafts have failed, the majority due to rejection. In the patient with a successful transplant, rejection and immunosuppression are finely balanced and withdrawal of immunosuppression will result in rejection. Although rejection is an immunological process, in patients with kidney, heart or liver transplants it is significant only in terms of the functional damage it causes to the graft. For example, in kidney transplants the significance of a rejection episode is reflected by the extent to which indicators of renal function, such as the serum creatinine and creatinine clearance, are affected. However, immunological techniques have an important part to play in the management of transplant patients and particularly in the early diagnosis of rejection episodes.

From a clinical standpoint, three types of rejection can be identified: hyperacute, acute and chronic. The distinction is important as only acute rejection is amenable to treatment.

HYPERACUTE REJECTION

Hyperacute rejection commences within a few minutes or hours of transplantation. It is characterized by gross swelling of the kidney and a marked reduction in blood flow, due to the accumulation of platelets and polymorphonuclear leukocytes within the vascular bed. The diagnosis is often self-evident at the time of transplantation as the organ becomes blue and flaccid. In other cases, this diagnosis is suspected when the graft becomes grossly swollen within the first 24 hours after operation. The diagnosis can be confirmed by renal biopsy.

Despite considerable research effort, attempts to reverse hyperacute rejection have been uniformly unsuccessful. The process is thought to be due to the presence of preformed cytotoxic antibodies directed against donor tissue. The incidence of hyperacute rejection has been considerably lessened by screening potential transplant recipients for the presence of cytotoxic antibodies and by performing a direct cross-match at the time of operation. In spite of these precautions, however, hyperacute rejection can still occur. Attempts have been made to improve on the detection of specific antidonor preimmunization by estimating the recovery of radioactive labelled donor platelets (Andersen et al., 1973). In an experimental study, the recovery fell from 51% in normal animals to 2% in those which subsequently developed hyperacute rejection. Sophisticated screening methods of this kind should enable the incidence of hyperacute rejection to be reduced still further.

ACUTE REJECTION

Acute rejection occurs within the first 3 or 4 months after transplantation and is thought to be mainly a cell-mediated immune phenomenon. The predominant feature of this type of rejection is invasion of the graft by large numbers of immunoblasts and lymphocytes. These cells cause a reduction in renal function by damaging vascular endothelium and attacking the specialized structures of the kidney. Investigations in experimental animals and in man have shown that reversal of acute rejection can be brought about by treatment with large doses of intravenous prednisolone or anti-lymphocyte globulin. The figures of the European Dialysis and Transplant Association for 1973 show that 40% of grafts fail within 3 months of operation. Although a proportion of these failures are due to irreversible ischaemic damage and technical problems, the vast majority are undoubtedly due to acute rejection.

Since clinical transplantation began, a large number of techniques have been used to detect acute rejection. In particular, efforts have been made to devise methods of detecting rejection before biochemical evidence of deterioration in graft function occurs. These techniques have been used on the assumption that early treatment will either abort the rejection episode or substantially reduce damage to the kidney. This assumption, however, remains unproved. The remainder of this chapter will be devoted to a discussion of the various different techniques which have been applied to the diagnosis of acute rejection.

CHRONIC REJECTION

This condition develops insidiously over a period of weeks or months and is characterized by a gradual reduction in renal function. The diagnosis is usually made by renal biopsy which characteristically shows irreversible vascular changes and interstitial fibrosis. Chronic rejection is thought to be an antibody-dependent phenomenon, and as yet there is no satisfactory treatment for the condition.

THE DIAGNOSIS OF ACUTE REJECTION

The detailed mechanisms of acute rejection have been discussed in Chapter 7. However, in order to consider the methods used to detect rejection, a summary of the important features is helpful (Figure 10.1). Sensitization of the

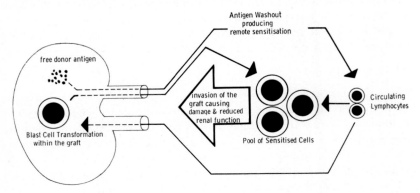

Figure 10.1 Mechanism of sensitization of recipient lymphocytes

lymphoid cell population of the recipient is an inevitable consequence of transplantation. In vascularized organs like the kidney there are two routes of sensitization. Firstly, antigenic material from the donor kidney is washed out into the recipient circulation allowing sensitization at remote sites. In addition, circulating lymphocytes are sensitized within the graft. Evidence of this initial sensitization can be found by studying cytological aspirates from the graft and the lymph draining from it. This process of sensitization undoubtedly occurs in all patients and it does not therefore inevitably result in rejection. The significant event leading to rejection is the formation of a large population of lymphoblasts specifically directed against the graft, probably stimulated by the initial pool of sensitized lymphocytes. These cells then invade the organ, damage the tubules and attack the vascular endothelium of arterioles and glomerular capillaries. In the vessels, platelets and fibrin are laid down causing a progressive reduction in renal blood flow. Fluid leaking from capillaries produces edema and hence graft swelling. The reaction affects glomerular filtration and tubular function and as a result, cells, enzymes and metabolic breakdown products are present in the urine.

The conventional methods of detecting acute rejection rely on clinical signs and a deterioration in the standard biochemical estimations of renal function. However, many other techniques have been used to diagnose rejection at an early stage and also to differentiate rejection from other causes of graft failure.

The detection of rejection will be considered under the following headings:
1. Clinical observations
2. Biochemical changes
3. Alterations in cellular and humoral immunity
4. Ancillary techniques

CLINICAL OBSERVATIONS

The following observations are of value in making the diagnosis of rejection:
1. Graft swelling and tenderness
2. Reduction in urine volume and proteinuria
3. Increase in temperature
4. Increase in blood pressure
5. Weight gain

None of these tests on their own can be taken as evidence of rejection. It usually requires an observation of two or three different variables to make this diagnosis, which in turn depends upon a good deal of clinical expertise.

Graft palpation

In about 15–20% of cases, the kidney becomes very enlarged and obviously tender in the event of a rejection episode. Other reasons for renal enlargement and tenderness, such as an abscess, a fluid collection or a leakage of urine around the kidney, should be considered. However, if the kidney is obviously enlarged and tender, it should be considered as evidence of rejection unless proved otherwise.

Urine volume and proteinuria

Urine output can be a useful and reliable indicator of rejection. Before using this measurement, however, one has to be sure that the patient has a reasonable fluid intake and is not simply dehydrated. For example, if a patient is passing about a litre of urine a day and then this drops to 500 ml and remains at that level, rejection should be suspected. A reduction in urine volume of this amount was useful in diagnosing rejection in 20% of our own patients. Proteinuria is not consistently present during rejection episodes, and is therefore probably not worth measuring routinely. In addition, patients who have not had a bilateral nephrectomy before transplantation may still be producing urine with a high protein content from their own diseased kidneys.

Temperature

As rejection is essentially an inflammatory reaction, it would be surprising if the patient did not experience an increase in temperature during these episodes. Temperatures tend to be of a relapsing variety and can easily mimic those seen with infection, and in particular with abscess formation. It is always difficult to differentiate between infection and rejection and this problem will be touched upon later under the heading of 'Differential Diagnosis'. Temperature changes alone are therefore not a sufficient indication to treat the patient for rejection. In our own experience, 60% of patients with rejection developed pyrexia and appropriate treatment often produces a dramatic fall in temperature to normal levels.

Increased blood pressure

Hypertension is seen in association with rejection in more than 50% of patients. The exact mechanism of this hypertension is not fully understood. It would be reasonable to suppose that ischaemia in the kidney during rejection would lead to stimulation of the renin/angiotensin system. In an experimental study of renal transplantation in dogs, it has been claimed that there is consistent stimulation of renin secretion during rejection (Abbrecht et al., 1968). However, consistent increases in renin levels have not always been shown to occur during rejection episodes (Blaufox et al., 1966). The explanation may lie in the observation that patients with a rejecting kidney develop a degree of sodium retention (Ogden and Holmes, 1966) which would tend to disturb the relationship between sodium balance and renin secretion.

Weight gain

An increase in weight is frequently seen during a rejection episode. Unfortunately, normal fluctuations in weight make interpretation of daily estimations difficult. However, in the presence of significant unexplained weight gain, the possibility of rejection should be considered.

BIOCHEMICAL CHANGES

The simple biochemical tests of renal function remain the mainstay of the diagnosis of rejection in patients with functioning kidneys.

Serum creatinine and creatinine clearance

In our own experience, every patient had an increase in the serum creatinine level at the time of a definite clinical rejection episode. In patients with a falling or stable serum creatinine, an increase of more than 0·2 mg/100 ml can be regarded as evidence of a rejection episode. If an improvement does not follow appropriate treatment, then this should be taken as an indication of continuing rejection and further antirejection therapy given. Changes in creatinine clearance mirror those of serum creatinine. However, creatinine clearance is not as accurate an estimation as serum creatinine, and if laboratory facilities are not available, changes in serum creatinine alone are quite adequate to handle rejection episodes.

Blood urea

Blood urea is less reliable than either serum creatinine or creatinine clearance. Although levels often change in concert with serum creatinine, it is a much cruder estimate of renal function and takes a great deal longer to return to normal after operation. In addition, fluctuations in urea can occur as a result of immunosuppression and administration of large doses of steroids. It is useful, however, as an adjunct to other tests and may be of benefit if for some reason the serum creatinine cannot be measured. However, if the serum creatinine remains stable and the blood urea increases, this should be taken as an indication to repeat the blood urea and not to treat the rejection episode.

ALTERATIONS IN CELLULAR AND HUMORAL IMMUNITY

Cellular immunity

Initial local sensitization of the lymphoid cell population of the host can be demonstrated by evidence of blast cell transformation. Blast cell activity can be studied either in the lymph draining from the transplant kidney (Pedersen and Morris, 1970) or in cytological aspirates from the graft

(Häyry *et al.*, 1972). The extent of this activity may be related to tissue incompatibility (Hamburger *et al.*, 1972). These authors found no evidence of transformation in patients where the mixed lymphocyte culture (MLC) response between donor and recipient was weak or absent. Although these techniques provide interesting research data, they cannot be considered as practical measures in the routine follow-up of transplant patients.

On the basis of the theory already mentioned in this chapter, the development of a large population of sensitized cells in the peripheral blood should give the earliest warning of impending rejection. There are a variety of immunological techniques which can be used to demonstrate this response:

    (a) Lymphoblast activity in the peripheral blood
    (b) Mixed lymphocyte culture responses
    (c) The leukocyte migration test
    (d) The rosette inhibition test
    (e) The leukocyte aggregation test
    (f) Adenylcyclase responses

(a) *Lymphoblast activity in the peripheral blood.* Lymphoblast activity can be assessed either by studying the amount of spontaneous cell division or by stimulating the cells to divide by mitogens, such as phytohaemagglutinin (see PHA-stimulation, Chapter 4). These techniques utilize the fact that the essential amino acid thymidine is incorporated into the nuclear DNA during cell division. If the thymidine is labelled with a radioactive isotope (such as ^{3}H or ^{14}C) the extent of lymphoblast activity can be estimated by the amount of radioactivity taken up by the cells.

In a follow-up study of 24 transplant recipients, spontaneous increases in lymphoblast activity were found in 14 out of 15 rejection episodes (Hersh *et al.*, 1971). The increased activity was present from 24 to 72 hours before the rejection was diagnosed on clinical grounds. Following successful treatment of the rejection episode, levels of lymphoblast activity continued to be high. This work was confirmed in a follow-up study on ten patients where the technique was again found to be of predictive value in rejection (Pagé *et al.*, 1971). In rat renal transplants the rise in thymidine incorporation occurs before clinical or histological evidence of significant rejection and is proportional to the strength of the rejection reaction, as judged by the strain combination used (Blamey *et al.*, 1973a).

However, other workers have found lymphoblast activity disappointing (Pauly *et al.*, 1973). Measuring uptake in whole blood in all nine patients studied, there was some increase in uptake in the first 15 days after operation. There were only three rejection episodes during this time and raised counts could not be related in degree or time to rejection. Lymphoblast activity in non-immunosuppressed allografted dogs was also studied with no increase in activity from the time of transplantation to death at a mean of 8 days. The authors speculate that the increased activity in their transplant patients may have been due to the effects of blood transfusion or a spill-over of myeloid cells from the marrow, due to the large initial doses of steroids. A further study, again using a whole blood technique, also found no correlation between peaks of lymphoblast activity and rejection episodes in six patients (Wu *et al.*, 1972).

Three of these authors (Hersh *et al.*, Pagé *et al.* and Pauly *et al.*) also looked at lymphoblast activity in response to PHA stimulation. In all cases the results were disappointing, and in the transplant situation spontaneous lymphoblast activity appears to be more valuable than stimulation with mitogens.

(b) *Mixed lymphocyte culture.* (See Chapter 6 for full details.) The mixed lymphocyte culture (MLC) reaction has now been shown to be a more sensitive index of tissue incompatibility than HLA typing. Studies in a group of 19 transplant recipients (Hattler and Miller, 1972) found six patients with strong MLC responses to irradiated donor cells. In these patients, the positive MLC response was maintained after transplantation and a fall noted from 1 to 4 days before evidence of clinical rejection. It is postulated that this is due to an accumulation of the sensitized cells within the graft. In a further study (Hattler *et al.*, 1973), it was found that lymphocytes separated from a rejected renal allograft retained strong MLC responses against irradiated donor cells. Although this technique may have useful applications in the future, there are two problems which restrict its value at the present time. The first is the provision of an adequate pool of donor lymphocytes for use in the test, and the second is the minimum of 3 days required for the mixed lymphocyte culture experiment to be carried out.

(c) *Leukocyte migration test* (see Chapter 6). There is now evidence to show that the leukocyte migration test is of value in the early detection of transplant rejection. The technique was originally developed as a specific measure of cellular hypersensitivity (Søborg and Bendixen, 1967). In the test, the leukocyte cell suspension is obtained from the transplant recipient. The suspension is placed in capillary tubes which are sealed and then spun down. The tubes are cut across at the cell/fluid interface and mounted in plastic wells. The wells are then filled with medium containing antigen from the transplant donor (Figure 10.2). In the presence of specific sensitization to the antigen in the well, the lymphocytes in the capillary tube produce a substance known as migration inhibition factor (MIF). This substance reduces the extent

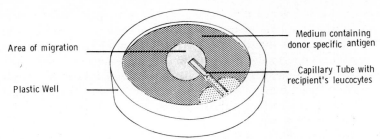

Area of migration

Plastic Well

Medium containing
donor specific antigen

Capillary Tube with
recipient's leucocytes

Figure 10.2 The leukocyte migration test

of migration of the leukocytes from the end of the capillary tube (Figure 10.3). After incubation at 37 °C for 16 hours, the migration areas can be drawn using a microscope with a camera lucida attachment. The areas are measured with a planimeter and the results expressed in terms of migration index.

$$\frac{\text{migration area with antigen}}{\text{control migration area}}.$$

In experiments on individuals sensitized by skin grafting, maximal inhibition of migration occurred where the sensitive lymphocytes were confronted with two and three HLA antigens similar to the skin graft donor (Falk et al., 1970). There was a reduced response when only one HLA similar

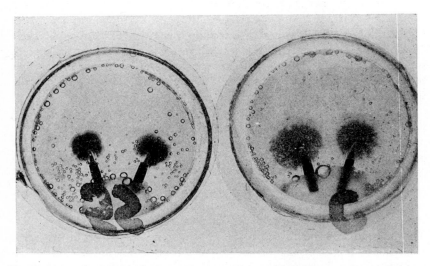

Figure 10.3 Left: Positive leukocyte migration test with inhibition of migration in response to donor antigen. Right: Normal migration of leukocytes into medium

antigen was used and slight inhibition with antigen which had none of the HLA characteristics of the donor. On the basis of this evidence, recent clinical studies have concentrated on the use of donor specific antigen. Encouraging results were reported using donor spleen extracts (Galanaud *et al.*, 1972). Using liver, spleen and lymph node antigens from cadaver donors, a study of 12 patients showed the technique to be of predictive value in eight out of ten rejection episodes (Wood *et al.*, 1973). Inhibition of migration was observed from 24 hours to 5 days before the diagnosis was made on clinical or biochemical grounds.

(d) *Rosette inhibition test*. This test was originally described as an *in vitro* method of assessing the activity of antilymphocyte globulin (ALG) (Bach and Antoine, 1968). The test depends upon the spontaneous formation of rosettes of sheep red blood cells around human lymphocytes *in vitro*. The addition of ALG to this system inhibits rosette formation. By using a range of doubling dilutions of ALG and counting rosettes per thousand lymphocytes at each dilution, a rosette inhibition curve can be drawn (Figure 10.4).

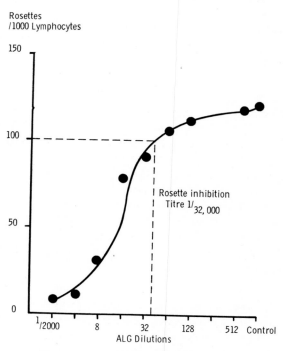

Figure 10.4 Normal rosette inhibition test

The rosette inhibition titre is taken as the point on the curve where there is a 25% reduction in numbers of rosettes compared to a controlled sample with no ALG. The test has been shown to be of predictive value in the detection of rejection (Munro *et al.*, 1971), and its use has also been described in monitoring the level of immunosuppressive therapy (Bewick *et al.*, 1972). The advantage of the rosette inhibition test over other immunological techniques is the speed with which a result can be obtained. It is possible to complete the test within 4 hours, and this gave the prospect of a rapid confirmatory test in patients who are thought to be rejecting on clinical or biochemical grounds. A further study (Wood and Gray, 1973), although confirming the presence of altered rosette inhibition titres in immunosuppressed patients, found that the test was of no value in the prediction of rejection. Spontaneous rosette formation with sheep red blood cells is now regarded as a good T cell marker. In the rosette inhibition test, the increased titres seen with immunosuppression are probably due to a metabolic effect of steroids and azathioprine on the circulating T cells, making them more readily coated with ALG. The problems with the rosette inhibition test are mainly due to the large number of variables in the technique. On theoretical grounds, one would expect an increase in T cell numbers at the time of rejection and the sophisticated techniques now available for measuring the ratio of T cells and B cells may well provide a useful means of screening transplant patients for potential rejection.

(e) *Leukocyte aggregation test.* This technique has been proposed as a more rapid method of demonstrating specific sensitivity to donor antigen than the leukocyte migration test (Kahan *et al.*, 1974). The technique has the advantage that a result can be achieved within 8 hours. Target cells derived from monolayer cultures of donor kidney or skin fibroblast cells are incubated with leukocytes from the transplant recipient. In the presence of specific sensitization, the leukocytes will aggregate around the target cells within a period of 5 hours. In a study of 23 transplant patients leukocyte aggregation *in vitro* was present several days before clinical evidence of rejection (Kahan *et al.*, 1974). After reversal of rejection, host peripheral leukocytes were unresponsive *in vitro*. However, in cases of irreversible rejection, the aggregation test remained positive.

(f) *Lymphocyte adenyl cyclase.* A recent experimental study (Wood *et al.*, 1975) has shown that raised levels of the enzyme adenyl cyclase are present in the lymphocytes of transplant recipients before biochemical evidence of rejection. Adenyl cyclase is generally regarded as being a 'second messenger' in the immune system (Watts, 1971). Antigen binding to the surface of an immunocompetent cell is thought to stimulate adenyl cyclase activity (Figure 10.5). This in turn results in the conversion of adenosine triphosphate

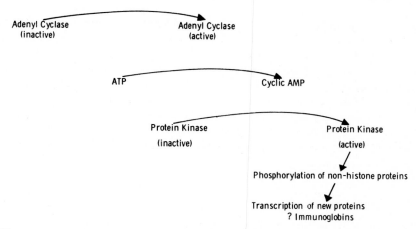

Figure 10.5 The possible mode of action of adenyl cyclase as a 'second messenger' in the immune response

to adenosine cyclic 3′-5′-monophosphate (cyclic AMP). The cyclic AMP activates protein kinases which bring about phosphorylation of non-histone proteins. This mechanism may allow the non-histone proteins to be stripped from nuclear DNA and trigger the first stage in the transcription of new proteins, which in this case are probably immunoglobulins. Adenyl cyclase may therefore play an important part in the early stages of the immune reactions leading to rejection. However, further research is obviously required to establish whether measurement of lymphocyte adenyl cyclase is of any value in the clinical situation.

Humoral immunity

(a) *Antibodies.* The increased incidence of hyperacute rejection in patients with preformed cytotoxic antibodies has already been discussed. In addition, an antivascular endothelium antibody has also been implicated in this type of rejection (Cerilli *et al.*, 1972) but other antibodies, such as the IgG antibody detected by the capillary agglutination test have been shown to have an enhancing effect with a degree of protection against early rejection crises (Stiller *et al.*, 1972). However, detection of antibodies has not been found to be of value in the early detection of conventional acute rejection.

(b) *Serum immunoglobulins.* Levels of serum IgM and IgG have both been shown to fall during rejection. Although the levels give some guide to immunosuppression and toxicity, they are of little value in predicting rejection in individual patients.

(c) *Complement.* Activation of the complement system is an important factor in rejection. Complement fixation may be involved in the antigen/antibody reactions in pre-sensitized patients and the damage to vascular endothelium in acute rejection is probably partially a complement-mediated reaction.

In postoperative patients, normal serum complement levels tend to be associated with normal renal function. Significant depression in the levels of haemolytic serum complement, factors C_3, C_4 and to a lesser extent C_1 and C_2 are seen in association with rejection (Yokoyama *et al.*, 1972). However, serial estimations of these factors show considerable fluctuation and they are of no value in the prediction of rejection (Yokoyama *et al.*, 1972).

ANCILLARY TECHNIQUES

These methods will be considered under two broad headings:

(a) *Tests on peripheral blood and urine*—These techniques are mainly concerned with identifying metabolic products formed as a result of the rejection reaction.

(b) *Techniques which investigate the graft itself*—In the main, these techniques are concerned with demonstrating reductions in renal blood flow.

Tests on peripheral blood and urine

(a) *Haematological techniques.* (1) *White cell count.* Immunosuppression tends to mask changes in both the total white cell count and the lymphocyte count that might be expected with rejection. Therefore, neither of these indices can be used as a reliable guide in diagnosing rejection.

(2) *Alterations in platelets.* Thrombocytopenia has been found to occur during hyperacute rejection and is mainly due to platelet trapping within the graft. Although platelets also have an important part to play in acute rejection, routine estimations of the platelet count are of little value in the early detection of rejection.

(b) *Enzymes.* A large number of enzymes have been studied in both serum and urine of transplant patients. These include leucine-aminopeptidase, transamidinase, glutamic-oxaloacetic transaminase, glutamic-pyruvic transaminase, aldolase, muramidase, glutaminase, carbonic anhydrase, alkaline phosphatase and lactic dehydrogenase. Although raised levels of alkaline phosphatase and lactic dehydrogenase have been shown to occur during rejection, these enzymes are common in the systemic circulation; they are therefore liable to be affected by other factors apart from rejection, and this renders them of limited value. Recent research has concentrated on the levels of the urinary lysosomal glycosidases: N-acetyl-β-D-glucosamini-dase (NAG), β-galactosidase (GAL), β-glucosidase (GLU), and β-glucuroni-dase (GON). In a study of GON levels in 38 transplant patients, raised values were present in all patients in the immediate postoperative period (Gonick et al., 1973). However, with stable renal function the levels tended to fall, and in 15 patients there were 'variable but consistent' rises with rejection. In a study of NAG levels in 19 patients, there were eight rejection episodes and NAG levels were raised in all cases (Sandman et al., 1973). A further study of urinary NAG and urinary GAL in nine patients has shown that NAG levels are of predictive value in the diagnosis of rejection (Wellwood et al., 1973).

Although the urinary lysosomal glycosidases are of considerable value in following transplant patients, they give an estimate of tubular function and therefore are totally unable to distinguish acute tubular necrosis from rejection. They are therefore only of real value in kidneys which have achieved stable function.

(c) *Examination of the urine.* (1) *Cytological examination of the urinary sediment:* This was one of the first techniques used in an attempt to predict transplantation rejection. However, there is considerable controversy in the literature over its value. A review of this subject in 1968 concludes 'it is evident that serial examinations of fixed and stained urinary sediments by an experienced observer can yield valuable information, and that the small mononuclear cells of epithelial origin correlate to some extent with rejection' (Carpenter and Austen, 1968).

Methyl green pyronine may be used to stain lymphocytes in the urinary sediment and in one study (Hrushesky et al., 1972) pyronine-positive lympho-cyturia was present in 14 out of 16 episodes of rejection. In 12 of these episodes, the test predicted rejection by at least 2 days. In a further communication from the same group (Murphy et al., 1973), the initial findings were confirmed in a 2-year follow-up of 34 transplant patients. The success of this technique depends on making a quantitative estimate of the numbers of pyroninophilic lymphocytes in the urinary sediment. This is obviously difficult to achieve with any degree of accuracy and is also subject to considerable observer error.

(2) *Measurement of urinary fibrin fibrinogen degradation products (FDP):*
FDP were first demonstrated in the urine of patients who had received
renal allografts by immunodiffusion and immunoelectrophoresis techniques
(Braun and Merrill, 1968). It was later shown that a tanned-red-cell
haemagglutination inhibition immunoassay (TRCHII) could be used to
give a sensitive and quantitative measure of urinary FDP levels following
transplantation (Clarkson *et al.*, 1970). However, this technique required
time-consuming concentration of the urine sample before testing. Interest
in FDP as a means of predicting graft rejection was considerably enhanced
by the development of a rapid latex screening test (Hulme and Pitcher, 1973)
and evidence that satisfactory results can be achieved in the TRCHII without
initial concentration of the urine (Clarkson, 1973).

In a study of 46 patients using the TRCHII assay, raised FDP excretion
was present at the time of rejection on 16 out of 18 occasions, and in nine
cases where serial information was available, raised FDP levels preceded the
diagnosis of rejection in five patients (Naish *et al.*, 1973). A further study
(Hall *et al.*, 1973) reported the follow-up of 81 human cadaver kidney
transplant patients with serial measurements of FDP using the TRCHII
method and immuno-nephelometry. In acute rejection episodes in functioning transplants, there were increased levels of FDP excretion with rejection,
which in 81% of the cases preceded the clinical diagnosis by periods of
1–7 days. Recovery from rejection was associated with a rapid fall in FDP
excretion to undetectable levels. The level of FDP excretion during a rejection episode was also related to the ultimate outcome. Irreversibly
rejecting kidneys tended to excrete much higher levels of FDP for long
periods. During the oliguric phase, kidneys which eventually functioned
well had much lower levels of FDP excretion than kidneys which eventually
turned out to be irreversibly damaged. There were occasional false-positive
results in which there was no evidence of acute clinical rejection. There
are a number of other reports in the literature of smaller series of patients
in general confirming these findings. However, both acute tubular necrosis
and vascular accidents such as renal artery and renal vein thrombosis may
complicate the correlation of the results with the onset of acute rejection.
In this country at the present time where most cadaver grafts have a relatively
long warm ischaemic time, acute tubular necrosis is present to a significant
degree after the majority of transplant operations. This tends to cause high
and often fluctuating levels of FDP in the important early days after operation. There is no doubt that in live donor transplantation and cadaver
transplantation with zero warm ischaemic time, the measurement of
urinary FDP provides a simple, non-invasive method of monitoring for
rejection.

Techniques which investigate the graft itself and are mainly concerned with showing a reduction in blood flow

(a) *Radiology.* Intravenous pyelography has little part to play in the early detection of renal transplant rejection. The only contribution it can make to the diagnosis is an estimate of the kidney size. The accuracy of this measurement is affected by a number of variables, including the size and positioning of the patient, and also the position of the kidney which may produce a degree of magnification. Arteriographic changes in experimental renal transplant rejection have been fully investigated (Dempster, 1971). The initial haemodynamic upset is a reduced perfusion of the outer cortex due to afferent vasoconstriction of varying degrees. This dramatically reduces the excretory function of the kidney, but perfusion and filtration continues in the inner cortical glomeruli. A 'crisis' of excretory function occurs when the total renal blood flow in the transplanted kidney is reduced by only 20 to 40%. At this stage, a nephrogram phase can still be observed. In the late stages of rejection, cortical flow virtually stops and with the abolition of inner cortical filtration, a nephrogram is no longer visible. In a series of 34 angiograms in 29 patients with classical acute rejection, occurring after the seventh postoperative day, the features in most cases were of a combination of stretching and irregularity of the interlobar and arcuate arteries (Pastershank *et al.*, 1973). A moderate nephrogram was present with a striated border. In the majority of cases, the arterial clearance time was prolonged. The radiological findings are very variable and asymptomatic patients with relatively normal renal function may show the classical angiographic features of rejection (Gedgaudas *et al.*, 1972).

Angiography, although having an important place in the diagnosis of renal artery stenosis or thrombosis and renal vein thrombosis, has little part to play in the diagnosis of acute rejection. The technique is invasive and therefore not without risk, and it is also for this reason that serial investigations cannot be undertaken.

(b) *Radionuclide techniques.* [131]I hippuran renography has been used for many years as a test of kidney function. The value of the technique in the detection of rejection has been considerably advanced by the advent of scintillation scanning with the gamma camera. In an experimental study in dogs, the following changes in ^{131}I hippuran occur before biochemical evidence of rejection (Hayes and Moore, 1972):

(1) A reduced renal uptake index
(2) An increased renal transit time
(3) An increased bladder entry time

(4) A reduced bladder/kidney index

(5) A reduced blood clearance index of ^{131}I hippuran

To confirm the results of this experimental series, 315 procedures were carried out on 42 postrenal transplant recipients (Hayes *et al.*, 1972). Fourteen of the patients had rejection episodes. On four occasions, impaired indices were present before rejection, and in 11 at the time of rejection. However, in seven of 11 patients, there was a transient paradoxical increase in flow before rejection, and in six of 28 cases with no evidence of rejection there were also transient falls in the bladder/kidney ratio at various times in their postoperative course.

Despite improvements in the technique of ^{131}I hippuran renography, these studies are not able to differentiate acute tubular necrosis from rejection in the anuric or oliguric patient. A further advance has been the development of a combined ^{131}I hippuran and ^{99m}Tc pertechnetate method. In the combined analysis, ^{99m}Tc pertechnetate is used to analyse abnormalities of transplant vascular perfusion while ^{131}I hippuran gives a measure of transplant function and morphology, as well as excretory progression of the tracer from the renal cortex to the pelvis and then to the bladder. In acute tubular necrosis, the ^{131}I hippuran concentration is poor and no radioactivity appears in the renal pelvis or bladder. Serial evaluations showed no change in ^{131}I hippuran concentration and clearance times remained elevated but stable. These values tend to return to normal if the kidney starts to function. However, the arterial perfusion measured by ^{99m}Tc pertechnetate remains normal at all times. In the oliguric or anuric patient, changes in ^{99m}Tc pertechnetate herald the onset of rejection. The outline of the kidney, from being well defined becomes indefinite and rather vague. This contrasts with the picture in renal artery occlusion where there is complete non-visualization of the transplant. An initial study showed the value of this technique (Weiss *et al.*, 1972) and the results were confirmed in a further study (Wibell *et al.*, 1973). ^{113m}In has been shown to be superior to ^{99m}Tc pertechnetate as the ^{113m}In is bound to transferritin and therefore remains completely within the circulation, allowing much more accurate perfusion studies to be carried out (Sampson *et al.*, 1972). The interpretation of the results can be further improved by using computer-assisted analysis.

(c) *Ultrasound*. Two different ultrasound techniques may be used to evaluate kidneys after transplantation. In the B scan, pulses of very high frequency sound are reflected from the tissues and the echoes used to build up a two-dimensional visual representation of anatomical structures. The second technique is the measurement of blood flow using Doppler ultrasound. In this technique a small fraction of the high-frequency sound is reflected back by the particles of blood to the receiving crystal. The velocity of the blood alters the frequency of the reflected sound and this frequency shift is measured by the flow meter. Frequency shift is proportional to the blood flow in a vessel of given diameter.

Results: The B scan has been shown to be useful in detecting fluid collections around the kidney and major degrees of hydronephrosis (Winterberger *et al.*, 1972). In this study, six patients had scans carried out during rejection episodes. In four of these patients the ultrasound showed significant increases in graft size.

Using Doppler ultrasound (Sampson, 1969), falls in blood flow have been shown to occur with rejection. There was a fall in blood flow through the kidney on average 7 days before treatment of rejection was started. These results have been confirmed by a further study (Dempster, 1970) which also showed that blood flow was not reduced when impaired renal function was due to either pyelonephritis or acute tubular necrosis. Both studies found that in patients where renal blood flow did not improve with antirejection therapy the patients went on to have further rejection episodes or developed chronic rejection. Doppler ultrasound is also of value in the diagnosis of vascular thrombosis in renal allografts (Marchioro *et al.*, 1969).

In a review of the subject in 1972 (Sampson *et al.*) it is concluded that ultrasound is a useful tool in the postoperative follow-up of renal transplant patients. Ultrasound has the advantage of being non-invasive, it can be repeated at frequent intervals and gives immediately available results. However, the initial alteration in renal blood flow occurs at a cortical level, and at the present time ultrasound techniques are not sufficiently developed to detect renal cortical blood flow as opposed to total renal blood flow; developments which would allow the measurement of cortical blood flow would markedly increase the sensitivity and therefore the value of the technique.

(d) ^{125}I *fibrinogen*. The injection of radioactive labelled fibrinogen has been widely used as a method for detecting deep venous thrombosis following surgical operations.

The labelled fibrinogen is incorporated into any developing thrombus and this can then be detected by monitoring the level of radioactivity over the lower limbs. The use of this method has been described for detecting rejection in renal transplant patients (Salaman, 1970). ^{125}I labelled fibrinogen is injected intravenously in a dose of 90 to 130 μCi. Uptake to the thyroid gland is blocked by giving oral potassium iodide. Subsequently, radioactivity is counted over the heart, the transplant, the bladder and the contralateral iliac fossa and the liver. In patients with acute tubular necrosis and also those with functioning transplants, the ratio of transplant counts to heart counts was less than 120%. In patients with oliguria or anuria due to rejection, the activity was always over 120%, with a range of 130 to 270%. In a series of 32 patients (Salaman, 1972a), there was only one false-positive result and no adverse side-effects were reported. The value of the technique has been confirmed by further clinical (Yeboah et al., 1973) and experimental studies (Salaman, 1972b; Blamey et al., 1973b; Howard et al., 1973).

[125]I labelled fibrinogen has a useful part to play in the follow-up of oliguric patients after transplantation. In the early days after transplantation there is really no other technique which affords the same degree of accuracy in detecting rejection. However, the technique has certain limitations:

(1) because of the relatively short half-life of ^{125}I the test period is limited to a week and satisfactory levels are really only obtainable for 5 days after injection;

(2) a full bladder, obstruction of the transplant ureter, or extravasation of urine may cause an increase in activity measured over the kidney;

(3) bleeding from the transplant or the formation of a wound haematoma may cause trapping of the radioactive labelled fibrinogen around the graft, giving falsely high readings;

(4) although the technique is relatively non-invasive, the use of human fibrinogen exposes the patient to a theoretical risk of serum hepatitis;

(5) in acute rejection episodes occurring in functioning kidneys, deposition of radioactive labelled fibrinogen is probably a rather late manifestation of rejection.

Differential Diagnosis of Rejection

The clinical picture of rejection can be mimicked by other events which require a completely different form of treatment. However, if there is any doubt the incident should initially be regarded as a rejection episode and treated accordingly. There is no place for a wait-and-see policy following renal transplantation, where 24 hours can mean the difference between survival or failure of the graft if the reaction is one of rejection.

There are two main diagnoses to consider as an alternative to rejection:

(a) The development of systemic infection
(b) Local conditions affecting the graft

SYSTEMIC INFECTION

The high doses of immunosuppression that have to be given following operation render the patient considerably more susceptible to infection. Infection with organisms that are usually of low pathogenicity (e.g. staphylococcus albus) is not uncommon and opportunistic viral and fungal infections may also occur. During rejection episodes, pyrexia frequently accompanies other signs of rejection such as reduced urine volume, hypertension and decreasing renal function. In this situation successful treatment of the rejection episode will result in a resolution of the pyrexia. However, the presence of a persistent pyrexia requires an intensive search for a source of infection. Fortunately, the application of large doses of intravenous steroids in the short term does not adversely affect the course of infection. Unless the patient's condition appears to be deteriorating, antibiotic therapy should not be started as this may encourage the establishment of fungal infections which are potentially more lethal than bacteria.

LOCAL CONDITIONS AFFECTING THE GRAFT

Acute tubular necrosis

The presence of a significant warm ischaemic interval in cadaver kidneys inevitably results in a degree of acute tubular necrosis with a delay in the onset of function. During the anuric phase, it is difficult to differentiate acute tubular necrosis from rejection. In this situation the techniques described earlier, in particular scintiscanning and ^{125}I uptake, are of value. Tubular necrosis rarely occurs once function is even partially established and any deterioration in this situation should be regarded as being due to rejection.

Renal vein thrombosis

Thrombosis of the venous drainage of the kidney is a rare event but is important as it is potentially correctable. It may occur any time in the first few days after operation. The differential diagnosis from an acute rejection episode is difficult but suspicion should be aroused if renal function diminishes and proteinuria suddenly develops in conjunction with a tender, enlarging kidney. In this situation, the episode should initially be treated as rejection by giving intravenous steroids. However, if the patient fails to respond, exploration of the graft to investigate a thrombosed renal vein should be considered.

Thrombosis of the renal artery

Unfortunately, this condition is usually not amenable to any form of treatment. Non-function of the kidney from the time of transplantation always suggests this possibility as an alternative to rejection or tubular necrosis, particularly in organs with a short warm ischaemic time. In addition, a sudden cessation in urine output following reasonable function makes the diagnosis almost certain. A ^{99m}Tc pertechnetate scan is of great value in this situation and it is usually unnecessary to resort to arteriography.

Obstruction of the ureter

Ureteric obstruction can simulate rejection as there is a fairly sudden deterioration in urine output, often with an enlarged kidney. In the first instance, the patient should be treated for rejection but if there is no improvement then the diagnosis may be made by cystoscopy and retrograde catheterization of the transplant ureter. More recently, with increasing expertise in ultrasonography, it is often possible to outline the distended renal pelvis.

Urinary leakage

The escape of urine from the bladder or ureter, due to a dehiscence of the anastomosis, the bladder incision, or necrosis of the ureter, is fortunately an uncommon event. The clue to the diagnosis is the sudden onset of severe pain and exquisite tenderness in the area of the graft. Urinary leakage usually occurs several days after the transplant operation, usually once the drain has been removed. Rejection does not usually present with such a sudden onset of symptoms, and this clinical picture requires urgent surgical exploration of the graft.

Haematoma around the kidney

Occasionally bleeding can occur following transplantation and this results in a tender mass surrounding the graft. This can be confused with rejection and if there is any doubt, the kidney must be re-explored.

Conclusions

Despite all the advances over the past ten years, the management of transplant patients remains largely empirical and intuitive. Rejection must be constantly suspected and sometimes treatment has to be started on very slim evidence. The more information that is available the better; however, the sophisticated techniques described in the latter part of this chapter cannot be used as an alternative to careful clinical examination of the patient and a reliable biochemical service.

   In clinical transplantation, it is important to select the ancillary techniques which will be of most benefit in patient management. In the immediate postoperative period if the kidney is non-functioning, the differential diagnosis usually lies between acute tubular necrosis, rejection and renal artery thrombosis. The new scintiscanning techniques offer a relatively simple method of establishing that the graft has a satisfactory blood flow. The development of an ultrasound technique for measuring renal blood flow would be a considerable advance in this area. The only certain means of knowing whether rejection is taking place in an initial anuric phase is to perform a renal biopsy or measure ^{125}I fibrinogen uptake within the graft.

In functioning kidneys there are a variety of methods of predicting the onset of rejection. The immunological technique which has been most widely used is the leukocyte migration test. When donor antigens are employed it has a very useful place in diagnosing rejection with a predictive value of from 1 to 3 days. Other immunological techniques which have been described in this chapter are less reliable, and the value of new methods such as the leukocyte aggregation test and increases in adenyl cylase activity await more detailed investigation.

The measurement of FDP and urinary enzymes, although affected by acute tubular necrosis and vascular accidents, are useful techniques in detecting rejection in kidneys with established renal function. The recent observation that transplantation with zero warm ischaemic time considerably increases the value of FDP as a means of detecting rejection may render this test of increasing importance in an era of 'heart beating' donors (Wood et al., 1974).

The value of predicting rejection in advance of biochemical and clinical criteria remains unproved. The effort is only worthwhile if it reduces the incidence of rejection and the damage caused by it. It still has to be shown that satisfactory prediction of rejection with consequent early treatment will result in an increase in graft survival and better levels of long-term renal function. Like one of the other imponderables of organ transplantation—antilymphocyte globulin—only a large-scale controlled trial will provide the answer.

References

Abbrecht, P. H., Turcotte, J. G. and Vander, A. J. (1968). Plasma erythropoietin and renin activity after canine renal allotransplantation. *J. Lab. Clin. Med.*, **71,** 766

Andersen, O. S., Tissot, R. G., Cohen, C. and Jonasson, O. (1973). Platelet survival test. An accurate prediction of hyperacute rejection of renal allografts in rabbits. *Transplantation*, **15,** 105

Bach, J. F. and Antoine, B. (1968). *In vitro* detection of immunosuppressive activity of antilymphocyte sera. *Nature (London)*, **217,** 658

Bewick, M., Ogg, C. S., Parsons, V., Snowdon, S. A. and Manuel, L. (1972). Further assessment of the rosette inhibition test in clinical organ transplantation. *Br. Med. J.*, **3,** 491

Blamey, R. W., Nicol, R. A., Baxter, T. J. and Deans, B. J. (1973a). Measurement of the immune response to a renal allograft. *Transplantation*, **16,** 1

Blamey, R. W., Renney, J. T. G., Baxter, T. J. and Deans, B. J. (1973b). The use of ^{125}I-fibrinogen in the detection of renal allograft rejection. *Transplantation*, **16,** 5

Blaufox, M. D., Birbari, A. E., Hickler, R. B. and Merrill, J. P. (1966). Peripheral plasma renin activity in renal-homotransplant recipients. *N. Engl. J. Med.*, **275,** 1165

Braun, W. E. and Merrill, J. P. (1968). Urine fibrinogen fragments in human renal allografts. *N. Engl. J. Med.*, **278**, 1366

Carpenter, C. B. and Austen, K. F. (1968). The early diagnosis of renal allograft rejection. In F. T. Rapaport and J. Dausset (eds.). *Human Transplantation*. (New York: Grune & Stratton)

Cerilli, J., Jesseph, J. E. and Miller, A. C. (1972). The significance of antivascular endothelium antibody in renal transplantation. *Surg., Gynecol., Obstet.*, **135**, 246

Clarkson, A. R., Morton, J. B. and Cash, J. D. (1970). Urinary fibrin/fibrinogen degradation products after renal homotransplantation. *Lancet*, **ii**, 1220

Clarkson, A. R. (1973). Latex-screening test for urinary FDP. *Lancet*, **i**, 109

Dempster, W. J. (1971). The nature of experimental second-set kidney transplant rejection. Nephrograms in second-set reactions and their general significance in acute renal failure. *Br. J. Exp. Pathol.*, **52**, 594

Dempster, W. J. (1970). Hypertension and acute rejection processes in allotransplanted kidneys. *Br. J. Exp. Pathol.*, **51**, 149

Falk, R. E., Thorsby, E., Möller, E. and Möller, G. (1970). *In vitro* assay of cell-mediated immunity: the inhibition of migration of sensitized human lymphocytes by HL-A antigens. *Clin. Exp. Immunol.*, **6**, 445

Galanaud, P., Crevon, M. C., Dormont, J., Mahieu, P. and Weydert, A. (1972). Leucocyte migration test and renal allograft rejection. *Transplantation*, **13**, 48

Gedgaudas, E., White, R. I., and Loken, M. K. (1972). Radiology in renal transplantation. *Radiol. Clin. N. Am.*, **10**, 529

Gonick, H. C., Kramer, H. J. and Schapiro, A. E. (1973). Urinary β-glucuronidase activity in renal disease. *Arch. Intern. Med.*, **132**, 63

Hall, C. L., Pejhan, N., Thomson, R. W., Dawson-Edwards, P., Barnes, A. D., Robinson, B. H. B., Meynell, M. J. and Blainey, J. D. (1973). Serial estimations of urinary fibrin/fibrinogen degradation products in kidney transplantation. *Br. Med. J.*, **3**, 204

Hamburger, J., Debray-Sachs, M., Dimitriu, A., Lacombe, M., Dimitriu, D. and de Grouchy, J. (1972). Lymphocyte activation in allograft recipients. *Transplant. Proc.*, **4**, 189

Hattler, B. G., Miller, J. (1972). Changes in human mixed lymphocyte culture reactivity as an indicator of kidney rejection. *Transplant. Proc.*, **4**, 655

Hattler, B. G., Rocklin, R. E., Ward, P. A. and Rickles, F. R. (1973). Functional features of lymphocytes recovered from a human renal allograft. *Cell. Immunol.*, **9**, 289

Hayes, M. and Moore, T. C. (1972). Early detection of canine renal allograft rejection by reduction in the scan bladder/kidney isotope intensity ratio. *Surgery*, **71**, 60

Hayes, M., Moore, T. C. and Taplin, G. V. (1972). Radionuclide procedures in predicting early renal transplant rejection. *Radiology*, **103**, 627

Häyry, P., Pasternack, A. and Virolainen, M. (1972). Cell proliferation within graft and in blood during renal allograft rejection. *Transplant. Proc.*, **4**, 195

Hersh, E. M., Butler ,W. T., Rossen, R. D., Morgan, R. O. and Suki, W. (1971). *In vitro* studies of the human response to organ allografts: appearance and detection of circulating activation lymphocytes. *J. Immunol.*, **107**, 571

Howard, R. J., Sutherland, D. E. R. and Najarian, J. S. (1973). Detection of renal allograft rejection with ^{125}I fibrinogen. *J. Surg. Res.*, **15**, 251

Hrushesky, W., Sampson, D. and Murphy, G. P. (1972). Lymphocyturia in human renal allograft rejection. *Arch. Surg.*, **105**, 424

Hulme, B. and Pitcher, P. M. (1973). Rapid latex-screening test for detection of fibrin/fibrinogen degradation products in urine after renal transplantation. *Lancet*, **i**, 6

Kahan, B. D., Tom, B. H., Mittal, K. K. and Bergan, J. J. (1974). Immunodiagnostic test for transplant rejection. *Lancet*, **i,** 37

Marchioro, T. L., Strandness, D. E. and Krugmire, R. B. (1969). The ultrasonic velocity detector for determining vascular patency in renal homografts. *Transplantation*, **8,** 296

Munro, A., Bewick, M., Manuel, L., Cameron, J. S., Ellis, F. G., Boulton-Jones, M. and Ogg, C. S. (1971). Clinical evaluation of a rosette inhibition test in renal allotransplantation. *Br. Med. J.*, **3,** 271

Murphy, G. P., Williams, P. D. and Merrin, C. E. (1973). Diagnostic value of lymphocyturia in renal allograft rejection in man. *Urology*, **2,** 227

Naish, P., Peters, D. K. and Shackman, R. (1973). Increased urinary fibrinogen derivatives after renal allotransplantation. *Lancet*, **i,** 1280

Ogden, D. A. and Holmes, J. H. (1966). Urinary solute excretion as an index of renal homograft rejection. *Ann. Intern. Med.*, **64,** 806

Pagé, D., Posen, G., Stewart, T. and Harris, J. (1971). Immunological detection of renal allograft rejection in man. *Transplantation*, **12,** 341

Pastershank, S. P., Chow, K. C., Baltzan, M. A., Baltzan, R. B., Cunningham, T. A. and Cross, J. W. (1973). Renal homotransplantation angiographic features in first 180 days following surgery. *J. Ass. Can. Radiol.*, **24,** 104

Pauly, J. L., Han, T., Varkarakis, M. J., Sokal, J. E., Sampson, D. and Murphy, G. P. (1973). Leukocyte [³H]thymidine uptake in short-term whole-blood cultures of human and canine renal allograft recipients. *J. Surg. Res.*, **15,** 301

Pedersen, N. C. and Morris, B. (1970). The role of the lymphatic system in the rejection of homografts: a study of lymph from renal transplants. *J. Exp. Med.*, **131,** 936

Salaman, J. R. (1970). Use of radioactive fibrinogen for detecting rejection of human renal transplants. *Br. Med. J.*, **2,** 517

Salaman, J. R. (1972a). A technique for detecting rejection episodes in human transplant recipients using radioactive fibrinogen. *Br. J. Surg.*, **59,** 138

Salaman, J. R. (1972b). Renal allograft rejection in the rat studied with ¹²⁵I fibrinogen. *Transplantation*, **14,** 74

Sampson, D., Bakshi, S. P., Bender, M. T. and Murphy, G. P. (1972). Radioisotopic evaluation of renal allografts with the digital autofluoroscope. *Transplantation*, **13,** 84

Sampson, D. (1969). Ultrasonic method for detecting rejection of human renal allotransplants. *Lancet*, **i,** 976

Sampson, D., Winterberger, A. R. and Murphy, G. P. (1972). The use of diagnostic ultrasound in renal transplantation. *Rev. Surg.*, **29,** 77

Sandman, R., Margules, R. M. and Kountz, S. L. (1973). Urinary lysosomal glycosidases after renal allotransplantation: correlation of enzyme excretion with allograft rejection and ischemia. *Clin. Chim. Acta*, **45,** 349

Søborg, M. and Bendixen, G. (1967). Human lymphocyte migration as a parameter of hypersensitivity. *Acta Med. Scand.*, **181,** 247

Stiller, C. R., Olson, L., Haystead, J. and Dossetor, J. B. (1972). The absence of early rejection crises in human renal allografts as predicted by capillary agglutinating antibodies. *Transplantation*, **14,** 521

Watts, H. G. (1971). The role of cyclic AMP in the immunocompetent cell. *Transplantation*, **12,** 229

Weiss, E. R., Blahd, W. H., Krishnamurthy, G. T. and Winston, M.A. (1972). The diagnosis of renal transplant rejection in association with acute tubular necrosis using the scintillation camera. *J. Urol.*, **107,** 917

Wellwood, J. M., Ellis, B. G., Hall, J. H., Robinson, D. R. and Thompson, A. E. (1973). Early warning of rejection? *Br. Med. J.*, **2**, 261

Wibell, L., Frödin, L., Jung, B. and Wicklund, H. (1973). Gamma-camera scintigraphy after kidney transplantation. *Scand. J. Urol. Nephrol.*, **7**, 56

Winterberger, A. R., Palma, L. D. and Murphy, G. P. (1972). Ultrasonic testing in human renal allografts. *J. Am. Med. Ass.*, **219**, 475

Wood, R. F. M., Gray, A. C., Briggs, J. D. and Bell, P. R. F. (1973). The prediction of acute rejection in human renal transplantation using the leucocyte migration test. *Transplantation*, **16**, 41

Wood, R. F. M., and Gray, A. C. (1973). Evaluation of rosette inhibition test in renal transplantation. *Br. Med. J.*, **4**, 649

Wood, R. F. M., Gray, A. C., Packer, S. G., Bell, P. R. F. and Pitcher, P. M. (1974). Urinary/fibrinogen degradation products (FDPs) as an index of rejection in canine renal transplants. *Paper presented to the British Transplantation Society, London*

Wood, R. F. M., Alston, W. C., Goudie, R., and Gray, A. C. (1975). Lymphocyte adenyl cyclase activity in canine renal transplant rejection. *Transplantation*, **19**, 188

Wu, K. T., Gordon, J., Maclean, L. D. and Guttman, R. (1972). Spontaneous thymidine incorporation by leucocytes of renal transplant recipients. *J. Surg. Res.*, **13**, 221

Yeboah, E. D., Chisholm, G. D., Short, M. D. and Petrie, A. (1973). The detection and prediction of acute rejection episodes in human renal transplants using radioactive fibrinogen. *Br. J. Urol.*, **45**, 273

Yokoyama, T., Torisu, M., Durst, A. L., Schroter, G., Groth, C. G., and Starzl, T. E. (1972). The complement system in renal homograft recipients. *Surgery*, **72**, 611

CHAPTER 11

Clinical Organ Transplantation

John R. Salaman

During the last ten years kidney transplantation has emerged as an effective form of treatment for patients with renal failure. Transplantation of the liver, heart and other organs has not been so rewarding, but some notable successes have been achieved on occasions. This chapter will consider both the practical and the immunological aspects of organ transplantation as it is practised today.

Kidney Transplantation

POTENTIAL RECIPIENTS OF KIDNEY TRANSPLANTS

It has been estimated that the number of persons under the age of 60 developing renal failure each year is about 40 per million of the population (Branch *et al.*, 1971; Pendreigh *et al.*, 1972). In the British Isles this represents over 2000 new cases a year, most of these having developed chronic glomerulonephritis or chronic pyelonephritis (Figure 11.1). Dialysis facilities are limited, and although a young adult will generally find a place on a chronic dialysis programme, a patient over the age of 45 may not. There are 42 dialysis centres in the United Kingdom, the majority of which undertake renal transplantation, or work with a nearby transplant unit. Dialysis and transplantation are intimately related and there is a frequent interchange of patients between them (Figure 11.2). In the first instance, patients are usually dialysed in hospital where they are given training so that later they will be able to continue dialysis treatment at home. At any time, however, a patient may be selected for kidney transplantation on the basis of tissue matching (Chapter 6). Should the transplant fail, it is often possible for

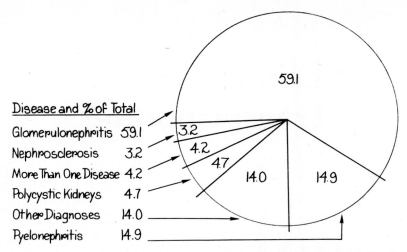

Figure 11.1 Causes of renal failure in 8 000 cases treated by renal transplantation. Data from the Tenth Report of Renal Transplant Registry—by kind permission

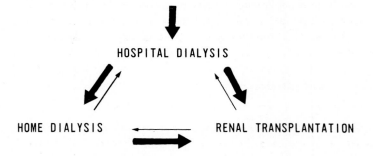

Figure 11.2 Diagram showing how patients move between dialysis and transplantation. The narrow arrows are only followed by patients with failed transplants and by those who have been unable to dialyse satisfactorily at home

previously trained patients to continue dialysis at home without over-burdening the busy hospital units.

POTENTIAL KIDNEY DONORS

Kidneys may be obtained from living or deceased individuals.

Living donors

Related living donors have provided almost half of the kidneys transplanted in the United States, whilst in Canada and Europe the emphasis has been on cadaveric donors. On the whole, kidneys from living related donors fare better than kidneys from cadavers and for this reason living donors continue to be used, despite the fact that a few may develop postoperative complications. Usually the relatives are anxious to donate a kidney and are quite willing to accept the small risk involved.

With unrelated living donors (husbands, wives or volunteers) the results have been poor and these donors are no longer used.

Cadaver donors

Kidneys from cadaver donors must be removed within one hour of death if they are to function subsequently. If this time is reduced to a few minutes, tubular damage is avoided and the kidney will then excrete urine immediately. This greatly simplifies postoperative management and improves the chance of survival.

Donors should be under 60 years of age but patients with malignant disease (other than in the central nervous system) or with infections cannot be used for fear of transferring these diseases to the recipient. Patients with pre-existing renal disease, diabetes or hypertension, are also unsuitable, which reduces the donor 'pool' to a small group of patients dying from head injuries, cerebrovascular accidents or primary cerebral tumours. These patients are often supported during their last hours by ventilation machines and vasopressor drugs. However, once it has been established that cerebral death has occurred these measures are usually withdrawn and the kidneys are removed once the heart has stopped beating. In the United Kingdom the law requires that the relatives and the hospital should both give their consent to this, and this is usually forthcoming.

It is common practice on the Continent and in North America to remove kidneys from the patients with cerebral death before the circulation fails, for in this way ischaemic damage to the kidneys can be avoided and early function of the transplant assured. There has been some reluctance by transplant surgeons in the United Kingdom to pursue this course which, it might be argued, could result in organs being removed before the patient had died. The concept of cerebral death is well recognized, however, and when the diagnosis has been made with confidence, most physicians would agree that the patient really was dead and that resuscitation should be discontinued. When this decision has been made, it would then seem reasonable to remove the kidneys in a healthy state, before the circulation had been allowed to fail completely.

Tissue Typing

This subject has been considered in Chapter 6 and will not be discussed here. Kidney transplants between identical twins are not rejected, but where genetic differences exist between donor and recipient rejection occurs, and in general the greater the genetic difference the worse the rejection. As a result most centres in Great Britain attempt to provide their patients with well-matched grafts although this is often very difficult to achieve. As there are many possible combinations of antigens it is rare to find two *unrelated* persons with the same arrangement or 'phenotype'. Nevertheless certain phenotypes are present in the population in greater numbers than might be expected by chance, which narrows the odds to some extent. All the same, a perfect match will not be found unless a pool of at least 250 potential recipients is available to choose from (Festenstein *et al.*, 1969). In Great Britain and Ireland all potential recipients have been pooled and detailed records of their tissue types are kept on a computer file at the National Organ Matching Centre at Bristol. When kidneys are removed from a cadaver donor, the Bristol Centre is informed of the tissue type, and the best-matched recipient is sought from the list of patients on the file. If a favourable match is not found, the kidneys may be offered to patients in Europe through 'Eurotransplant', 'Scandiatransplant' and other organizations. Similarly, kidneys obtained on the Continent may find their way into suitably matched recipients in the U.K. Despite national and international co-operation on this vast scale, it is only possible to match exactly for all four antigens in about 10% of the kidneys that are exchanged.

Organ Preservation

When living donor kidneys are used, the need for organ preservation does not arise. The operations on the donor and the recipient are performed synchronously and the interval between removal of the organ and its revascularization in the recipient rarely exceeds 30 minutes. Simple cooling of the kidney during this period is all that is required to ensure immediate function afterwards.

The need for preservation is much greater when cadaveric kidneys are transplanted. Quite frequently delays of up to 12–14 hours occur whilst the most suitable recipient is selected and the kidney transported to the appropriate hospital. Normothermic ischaemia for more than 2 hours causes irrecoverable damage, and if the donor has been hypotensive, even 1 hour of ischaemia may be sufficient to destroy the graft. Early cooling of the kidney is essential and simple surface cooling with ice will protect the kidney for a few hours. Better preservation may be obtained by perfusing the kidney with an electrolyte solution prior to ice storage, and a number of perfusing solutions have been tried. The two most commonly used are a Rheomacrodex/fructose–bicarbonate solution (Brunius et al., 1966) and a solution containing high concentrations of intracellular ions described by Collins et al. (1969). These simple procedures are adequate when preservation is required for less than 18 hours as is normally the case. After flushing the kidneys with Collins solution they are packed in sterile plastic bags and placed in polystyrene boxes containing ice chips. In this manner they are conveyed to the recipient hospital. If longer periods of preservation are required the viability of the kidney can be maintained only by perfusing it on a machine. Numerous preservation machines have been devised, the most successful of which circulate through the kidney a cold (10 °C) oxygenated solution of plasma or plasma derivative (Belzer and Kountz, 1970; Johnson et al., 1972).

Transplantation and Postoperative Care

The standard technique of kidney transplantation is to place the kidney in an extraperitoneal position in the left or right iliac fossa, and to anastomose the renal artery to the internal iliac artery and the renal vein to the external iliac vein. The ureter is implanted into the bladder in a manner designed to prevent ureteric reflux (Figure 11.3).

Subsequent management depends upon the state of function of the transplant. If there is a diuresis, fluid and protein restriction may be relaxed and larger doses of azathioprine given. When the kidney develops tubular necrosis, however, dietary restrictions must be continued and dialysis performed until the kidney recovers. Patients receiving immunosuppressive drugs have an increased susceptibility to infections and should be protected from potential pathogen carriers, but elaborate barrier procedures are probably unnecessary and in many units only simple precautions are taken. Patients are discharged after 2–4 weeks to be followed up in a special outpatient clinic.

Immunosuppression

This topic is dealt with in Chapter 8, and only those aspects that are pertinent to renal transplantation are covered here.

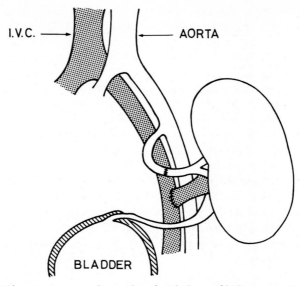

Figure 11.3 The most commonly employed technique of kidney transplantation. The renal artery is anastomosed to the internal iliac artery and the renal vein to the external iliac vein. The ureter is implanted into the bladder

PROPHYLAXIS

Immunosuppressive drugs are commenced immediately after transplantation (or in the case of living donor grafts—just before) and are continued indefinitely in an attempt to avert rejection episodes. Azathioprine is the most important drug, but is seldom given on its own. It causes leukopenia and, more rarely, liver dysfunction and must be used with great care. Over the course of months the dose may be increased gradually to a maximum of 150 mg/day.

Steroids are required in high doses in the initial postoperative period but afterwards the dosage may be gradually lowered to a maintenance level of 10–15 mg of prednisone/day. Despite the many serious side-effects of steroid therapy it is usually not possible to discontinue it altogether. One commonly employed scheme of treatment is shown in Table 11.1.

A large number of alternative treatments have been tried. Methyl prednisolone may be given intravenously in doses of 1g or more for short periods, and this drug is popular in the United States at present. Irradiation of the graft is commonly practised and has been shown to delay rejection in animal experiments (Hume and Wolf, 1967). Doses of 150 rads are given

Table 11.1 Commonly employed scheme of immunosuppression

Period	Prednisone	Azathioprine	Others
Day of transplant	150 mg	5 mg/kg	± Methyl prednisolone 1 g ± Radiotherapy 150 r ± ALG
First 3–7 days	100 mg/day	2.5 mg/kg or 1 mg/kg★	± Radiotherapy 150 r × 4 ± ALG
First 2–4 weeks	75 mg/day 40 mg/day	2.5 mg/kg or 1 mg/kg	± ALG
2nd month onwards	30 mg/day 15 mg/day	2.5 mg/kg	

★ Azathioprine reduced to 1 mg/kg if the patient develops postoperative oliguria

on the first postoperative day and then on alternate days up to a total dose of 600 rads. Antilymphocyte globulin may also be added during the first postoperative weeks. There is no doubt that this drug is effective in animal experiments, but difficulties have been encountered in preparing a globulin for human use, and although good reports have appeared (Sheil *et al.*, 1971) there have been few controlled clinical trials.

TREATMENT OF REJECTION

As soon as rejection has been diagnosed large doses of prednisone are given, either orally or intravenously as methyl prednisolone. Graft irradiation may be repeated up to a further 600 rads and actinomycin C administered intravenously on each of three successive days (Table 11.2). If these measures are unsuccessful a second course of treatment may be given, but the risks of

Table 11.2 Drugs that can be used for treatment of rejection episodes. Usually large doses of steroids are given with or without one of the other agents

Treatment	Dose
Prednisone	200 mg/day for 3 days
Methyl prednisolone	1 g 12-hourly for 3 doses
Actinomycin C	200 μg/day for 3 days
Local radiotherapy	150 r on alternative days × 4
ALG	
Heparin	

serious complications increase significantly, and if this second attempt fails, the kidney is best abandoned or removed, and the patient returned to chronic haemodialysis.

Complications of Renal Transplantation

ACUTE TUBULAR NECROSIS

This commonly follows cadaveric renal transplantation when more than 15 minutes has elapsed between death of the donor and cooling of the excised kidney. Although the majority of these kidneys recover their function satisfactorily within 3 weeks, a proportion (10–15%) do not. During the period of oliguria, haemodialysis must be continued.

REJECTION

This has been covered in Chapter 7 and only a brief account is included here. Three forms of rejection are recognized; hyperacute, acute and chronic.

Hyperacute rejection

This takes place immediately after the graft has been revascularized in the recipient. Within a few minutes the kidney changes colour from pink to a dull blue and loses all the firmness it has just regained. Despite vigorous pulsations in the renal artery very little blood flows through the graft, and pinching of the renal vein does not cause the kidney to swell. Renal biopsy reveals the presence of microthrombi consisting of platelets, fibrin, polymorphs and red cells in the arterioles and glomerular capillaries. These changes are mediated by antibodies previously present in the recipient and directed against antigens on the donor kidney. A negative cross-match test prior to transplantation should exclude the possibility of a hyperacute rejection, but the standard cytotoxicity test is not completely reliable. At present, hyperacute rejection is not irreversible and the kidney is best removed immediately.

Acute rejection

An older term was a 'rejection crisis', which in the non-immunosuppressed individual took the form of an acute toxic reaction during which the patient became febrile and oliguric. In patients receiving immunosuppressive drugs, however, the tempo of rejection is slowed considerably and the transplant recipient may be unaware that anything is amiss. Helpful indicators in diagnosing rejection are listed in Table 11.3. Several other events may occur and these include changes in the levels of the second and third components of complement, a rise in the level of lactic dehydrogenase and

Table 11.3 Clinical and biochemical features that signify a rejection episode

1. Enlargement and tenderness of the graft
2. Fever, hypertension and tachycardia
3. Decreased urine volume
4. Edema and increased weight
5. Protein and lymphocytes in the urine
6. Decreased excretion of urea, creatinine and sodium
7. Rise in blood urea and creatinine, and fall in creatinine clearance

increased excretion of alkaline phosphatase, lysozyme and fibrin degradation products in the urine. Changes in the leukocyte migration index have been described, and these may precede the rejection episode thus providing an early warning of impending trouble (Smith *et al.* 1969).

Renal biopsy can be especially helpful. Microscopically, rejection is characterized by interstitial edema and infiltration of the cortex by mononuclear cells, many of which have RNA in their cytoplasm (Figure 11.4). There is

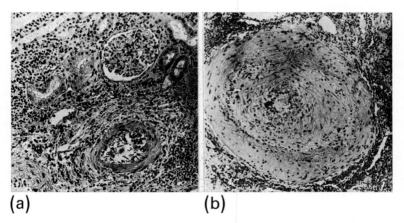

(a)   (b)

Figure 11.4 (a) The histological appearances of acute rejection. There is a perivascular and periglomerular collection of small round cells. The arteriole has leukocytes adherent to the intima. (b) Chronic rejection. The lumen of a small artery is almost totally obliterated by a thickened intima

rupture of peritubular capillaries and necrosis of tubular cells. Fibrinoid necrosis may be observed in the walls of the afferent and efferent arterioles and in severe cases may extend into the glomerular tuft. Deposits of platelets and fibrin may be seen on the intima of arterioles, although in the later stages of rejection these deposits may have become organized with resulting obliteration of the arterial lumen.

Rejection can be especially difficult to diagnose during the early post-operative period when renal function may be depressed as a result of ischaemic tubular necrosis. [131]I renography or renal scanning (after i.v. sodium pertechnetate or ^{131}I hippuran) may demonstrate the presence of a vascularized graft but these tests are of little use in differentiating rejection from tubular necrosis (Branch *et al.*, 1971). [125]I fibrinogen, however, is helpful in this respect as rejection episodes can be identified by a rise in the level of radioactivity measurable over the graft (Salaman, 1970).

In many instances rejection episodes can be reversed quite successfully using the scheme of treatment outlined above. In some cases, however, this treatment is ineffective and the kidney is destroyed. Provided that these patients have not been 'over-immunosuppressed' they will be able to return to the chronic dialysis programme without having incurred any serious complications.

Chronic rejection

This takes the form of a gradual fall in renal function commencing some months after transplantation. Proteinuria develops and the patient frequently becomes hypertensive and edematous. The histological changes are different from those seen in acute rejection, in that infiltrating lymphocytes are sparse. Thickening of the glomerular basement membrane occurs as a result of subendothelial or subepithelial collections of amorphous material containing IgM, IgG and complement. Many workers have noted a similarity between these changes and those seen in the patient's own kidneys, and it is quite possible that glomerulonephritis may recur within the graft. Vascular lesions are also very common. Initially the arterial lumen is narrowed by loose cellular tissue and this later becomes replaced by a dense fibrous matrix which may totally occlude the vessel (Figure 11.4). Chronic rejection does not readily respond to treatment; high doses of prednisone may bring about improvement but more often there is no response at all, and a decision to return the patient to chronic dialysis needs to be taken before he becomes severely debilitated.

SIDE-EFFECTS OF IMMUNOSUPPRESSIVE THERAPY

A large number of complications have been described following renal transplantation, many of which can be attributed directly or indirectly to the administration of immunosuppressive drugs (Table 11.4). Sepsis is undoubtedly the most important and is the major cause of death in most series. Although immunosuppressive drugs diminish the ability of the body to resist infections, most transplanted patients appear to cope quite satisfactorily with common ailments, although this may not be true for those patients

Table 11.4 Drug-induced complications of renal transplantation

1. Infections	New
	Latent
2. Bone disease: Osteoporosis, avascular necrosis	
3. Diabetes	
4. Cataracts	
5. Gastroduodenal ulceration	
6. Pancreatitis	
7. Liver dysfunction	
8. Malignancy	
9. Depression	
10. Hypertension	

who have received high doses of drugs to combat rejection. In these cases infections can progress rapidly and cause death within days. The liberal use of antibiotics has not improved survival because resistant strains of the more common pathogens arise, and infections with more unusual organisms can supervene. They include fungi (*Candida*, *Nocardia*, *Aspergillus*), viruses (herpes zoster, cytomegalovirus) and protozoa (*Pneumocystis*).

Occasionally a pre-existing but dormant infection may become re-activated—herpes simplex infection of the lips and pulmonary tuberculosis being examples. Infections within the transplant wound are not uncommon, and although usually benign, fatal secondary haemorrhage may occur.

Patients on long-term immunosuppression are at risk of developing malignant disease. The commonest type is a malignant lymphoma, which may arise within the brain (Schneck and Penn, 1971). The occurrence of these tumours has been ascribed to a loss of immunological surveillance so that newly formed tumour cells are no longer recognized as foreign and eradicated.

TECHNICAL PROBLEMS

These can take the form of arterial or venous thromboses or haemorrhage. The ureter may become obstructed or a urinary fistula develop. The latter condition is particularly serious as an infected urinary fistula is frequently the cause of septicaemia and death. On the whole, technical problems are fairly rare and account for only a small proportion of failures.

Results of Renal Transplantation

Although the survival rates for transplanted patients vary from centre to centre, an overall picture may be obtained from the reports of the Human Renal Transplant Registry, which are based upon the results of transplant operations carried out all over the world. The latest (11th) report (Barnes 1973) records the outcome of 12 389 renal transplant operations performed since 1961. Patient survival has always been better than transplant survival, for many of the patients have been successfully retransplanted or re-established on chronic haemodialysis following the loss of their graft. Of the transplants carried out in 1970 and 1971 those from sibling donors gave the best results, with grafts from parental donors running a close second. Grafts from cadaver donors did rather less well (Table 11.5).

Table 11.5 Patient and graft survival at two years after transplantation. Figures are from Renal Transplant Registry Eleventh Report, and apply to grafts performed during 1970 and 1971

Donor source	No. of transplants	Graft survival	Patient survival
Sibling	623	74%	83%
Parent	538	68%	81%
Cadaver	2473	47%	64%

Unfortunately these figures are little better than those obtained for previous years, and the latest figures for transplants performed during 1972 do not show any improvement. Nevertheless, certain well-experienced transplant centres, notably in the United States and Australia, have been able to produce results that are considerably better than the quoted 'world average'.

The Influence of HLA Typing on Graft Survival

When living related donor transplants are considered, a clear correlation has been found between the degree of tissue matching and the outcome after transplantation, with grafts between HLA identical sibs doing especially well (Singal et al., 1969).

It is still not clear whether tissue matching has any part to play in cadaveric renal transplantation. A few centres have noted a better outcome in well-matched cases (Oliver et al., 1972), but a large study from the United States (2172 cases) was unable to confirm this correlation (Opelz et al., 1974).

It is becoming clear that other factors besides the HLA antigens may influence the survival of cadaveric grafts. Discrepancies for the products of the MLR locus may be just as important, and, in addition, the ability to mount an immune response may be a function of yet another genetic system. Certainly those persons who fail to produce a normal antibody response when transfused with HLA incompatible blood are likely to do particularly well after kidney transplantation (Opelz et al., 1972). It is obvious that much still remains to be learnt, and until such time that these factors are better understood, cadaveric renal transplantation will remain a somewhat hit or miss procedure.

Heart Transplantation

The first successful human transplant was performed in 1967 (Barnard, 1967) and more than 230 such operations have since been carried out. The number of patients currently surviving is 33. There are no great technical difficulties to the operation which has been practised successfully in many hundreds of animal experiments. During the operation the patient is placed on cardio-pulmonary bypass, and the diseased heart is removed leaving just the remnants of the two atria with the openings of the cavae and pulmonary veins. The donor heart is anastomosed to these remnants and the aorta and pulmonary artery united with the recipient's own vessels.

The greatest obstacle to success has been rejection, and this has accounted for the majority of deaths. It may be diagnosed from changes in the electro-cardiogram such as (i) a decrease in voltage, (ii) the presence of right axis deviation, (iii) the appearance of conduction defects and arrhythmias. Other signs are weight gain, a right ventricular gallop and an elevated venous pressure. Additional evidence can be obtained from an endomyocardial biopsy. Should the heart fail, there is at present no mechanical device that can substituted for its action, in the way that dialysis may be used to save the life of a patient with a rejected kidney transplant. However, a few patients have been given second heart grafts after their first had failed. Patients that have survived a year or more have not infrequently developed coronary atheroma which has lead to a further reduction in the number of survivors. There is some evidence that this may be prevented by the use of anticoagulants and a low fat diet.

A remarkable series of 54 cases has been reported by Caves et al. (1973), where the 1- and 2-year survival rates have been 41% and 37% respectively. All these patients had been gravely ill and would have died within a few weeks had they not received a graft. Tissue matching has not influenced the outcome to any great extent, and like cadaveric kidney transplantation, heart transplantation must await new specific forms of immunosuppression before it can become a more regularly successful procedure.

Liver Transplantation

There are a number of fatal liver diseases which could, in theory, be treated by liver transplantation, including cirrhosis, biliary atresia, hepatic cell carcinoma, bile duct carcinoma and acute hepatic necrosis. However, many of these cases would be unsuitable for liver transplantation because of extra-hepatic spread of tumour or because of severe psychological disturbances as may be found in patients with cirrhosis.

The operation of liver transplantation is a prodigious exercise. The patient's own liver is often greatly enlarged and this has first to be removed, which can be a very haemorrhagic procedure especially when there is an associated coagulation defect. The new liver is placed in the space vacated by the diseased organ and its vessels anastomosed to those of the recipient. Five separate anastomoses are performed, two to the vena cava and one each to the hepatic artery, portal vein and bile duct. The immediate postoperative period can be critical as disseminated intravascular coagulation may cause further bleeding. Hypoxia, hypothermia, acidosis and hypocalcaemia may require correction, and special note has to be taken of hypo- or hyperkalaemia. Within a few hours of a successful graft, electroencephalogram recordings will show an improvement over the preoperative pattern and a previously comatosed patient may regain consciousness. The serum bilirubin usually reverts to normal within a week (Williams, 1971).

Antirejection treatment differs very little from that used for other types of transplantation. Azathioprine is normally converted by the liver into the active metabolite 6-mercaptopurine, but in the presence of liver dysfunction this may not occur, and cyclophosphamide has been suggested as an alter-native (Startzl et al., 1971). Late rejection can be a disappointing sequel. It presents as a relentless cholestatic jaundice leading finally to liver failure. Major infarction has also been encountered, and biliary fistulae may also occur. In the absence of an effective mechanical substitute, retransplantation is the only form of treatment available should the graft fail. Out of 201 liver transplants carried out since 1963 currently 15 patients are surviving.

Transplantation of Other Organs

Attempts have been made from time to time to transplant other organs to patients in extreme need. Lung transplants have been performed in cases of respiratory failure and a few of these grafts have been highly successful. However, infections and rejection have usually supervened and no case has lived longer than 10 months.

Pancreas transplantation has been carried out in an attempt to control severe diabetes. These patients have usually had an accompanying nephro-pathy and renal transplantation has been performed at the same time. The exocrine secretion of the graft is unwanted, but it may be drained into the patient's alimentary system via a segment of donor duodenum. Thirty-four such operations have been performed up to the present time. In many cases it has been possible to reduce or even withdraw the daily dose of insulin, but long survival of the graft has not been possible and only two patients are currently surviving with functioning grafts. It may become possible to transplant just the islet cells on their own, and the outcome of such research is awaited with interest.

Segments of small intestine have been transplanted successfully in dogs and it is hoped that this procedure may be feasible for patients who have had to undergo massive bowel resections. Very few clinical cases have been reported and it is too early yet to assess the results.

Future Prospects

Although rejection has been the greatest problem in transplantation it is remarkable how effectively it can be prevented in some patients with kidney or heart transplants. It is now clear that the patient's response towards his graft becomes modified in some specific way with the result that after a time only small doses of drugs are required to prevent rejection occurring. In animal experiments it has been shown that some established grafts can survive without the aid of any drugs. The exact mechanisms by which these grafts escape rejection is not known at present, but the evidence available so far would suggest that immunological enhancement has some part to play. This supposes that there are in the recipient specific antidonor antibodies that are capable of modifying the rejection process. Such antibodies have been detected in a fair proportion of patients with successful renal transplants, generally by their ability to block *in vitro* reactions between the cells of the donor and host (Quadracci et al., 1974). However, some recipients have no demonstrable blocking antibodies yet continue to do well.

Another possible explanation for the good results of transplantation is immunological tolerance. In this state the immunologically active cells that are capable of reacting to the transplant are somehow switched off or destroyed. It is possible to achieve this state in animals by injecting them with donor antigens when they are very young. So far no one has been able to make a human individual tolerant prior to transplanting a kidney. However, there is some evidence that this state of affairs may arise spontaneously afterwards, for when lymphocytes are taken from patients who have had a successful transplant for more than a year they are found to be unreactive with the antigens of the donor (Quadracci et al., 1974).

It would be very advantageous if this satisfactory state of affairs could be induced in *all* patients at the time of transplantation. Numerous experiments have been undertaken in animals to try and evolve a state of enhancement or tolerance, and some successes have been achieved. Certainly in the rat this is easily accomplished, and long-term kidney transplant survival can be obtained by injecting the recipient with donor antigens, or antidonor antibodies, or both (Stuart *et al.*, 1968). In the dog this has been much more difficult and in the monkey almost impossible. A few attempts have been made to pretreat human recipients of renal transplants by injecting donor cells (Newton and Anderson, 1973), but no striking results have been achieved. Such a regime is hazardous, as the recipient may become immunized and as a result destroy the graft all the more quickly. Passive enhancement has also been attempted. It has the attraction that the recipient cannot become immunized but requires another individual (usually a parent) to act as a source of antibody after suitable stimulation. Too few cases have been treated in this way to allow proper appraisal of the results.

It may be that better results in transplantation will follow the gen era use of one of these immunological procedures. It is more likely, however, that such complex manœuvres will remain the province of the research units and will not gain general acceptance for many years. I regard it more likely that a new safer immunosuppressive drug will be introduced in the meantime. Certainly it is strange that in the last 10 years no drug has been found to supersede azathioprine or prednisone. Since rejection remains the biggest obstacle to successful transplantation an introduction of a better immunosuppressive agent is urgently awaited.

References

Barnard, C. N. (1967). A human heart transplant. *S. Afr. Med. J.*, **41**, 1271

Barnes, A. B. (1973). The eleventh report of the Human Transplant Registry. *J. Am. Med. Ass.*, **226**, 1197

Belzer, F. O. and Kountz, S. L. (1970). Preservation and transplantation of human cadaver kidneys. *Ann. Surg.*, **172**, 394

Branch, R. A., Clark, G. W., Cochrane, A. L., Jones, J. H. and Scarborough, H. (1971). Incidence of uraemia and requirements for maintenance haemodialysis. *Br. Med. J.*, **1**, 249

Branch, R. A., Coles, G. A., Eynon, A., Jones, G. R. and Lowder, E. (1971). The use of radioactive hippuran in the management of cadaveric renal transplants. *Br. J. Radiol.*, **44**, 697

Brunius, U., Fritjofsson, A. and Gelin, L. E. (1966). Microcirculatory aspects of the preservation of kidneys for transplantation. *Bibl. Anat.*, **9**, 374

Caves, P. K., Stinson, E. B., Griepp, R. B., Rider, A. K., Dong, E. and Shumway, N. E. (1973). Results of 54 cardiac transplants. *Surgery*, **74**, 307

Collins, G. M., Bravo-Shugarman, M. and Terasaki, P. I. (1969). Kidney preservation for transplantation. *Lancet*, **ii**, 1219

Festenstein, H., Oliver, R. T. D., Hyams, A., Moorhead, J. F., Pirrie, A. J., Pegrum, G. D. and Balfour, I. C. (1969). A collaborative scheme for tissue typing and matching in renal transplantation. *Lancet*, **ii**, 389

Hume, D. M. and Wolf, J. S. (1967). Modification of renal homograft rejection by irradiation. *Transplantation*, **5,** 1175

Johnson, R. W. G., Anderson, M., Morley, A. R., Taylor, R. M. R. and Swinney, J. (1972). Twenty-four hour preservation of kidneys injured by prolonged warm ischaemia. *Transplantation*, **13,** 174

Newton, W. T. and Anderson, C. B. (1973). Planned preimmunisation of renal allograft recipients. *Surgery*, **74,** 430

Oliver, R. T. D., Sachs, J. A., Festenstein, H., Pegrum, G. D. and Moorhead, J. R. (1972). Influence of HL-A matching, antigenic strength and immune responsiveness on outcome of 349 cadaver renal grafts. *Lancet*, **ii,** 1318

Opelz, G., Mickey, M. R. and Terasaki, P. I. (1972). Identification of unresponsive kidney transplant recipients. *Lancet*, **i,** 868

Opelz, G., Mickey, M. R. and Terasaki, P. I. (1974). HL-A and kidney transplants: re-examination. *Transplantation*, **17,** 371

Pendreigh, D. M., Heasman, M. A., Howitt, L. F., Kennedy, A. C., MacDougal, A. I., MacLeod, M., Robson, J. S. and Stewart, W. K. (1972). Survey of chronic renal failure in Scotland. *Lancet*, **i,** 304

Quadracci, L. J., Tremann, J. A., Marchioro, T. L. and Striker, G. E. (1974). Serum blocking factors in human recipients of renal allografts. *Transplantation*, **17,** 361

Salaman, J. R. (1970). Use of radioactive fibrinogen for detecting rejection of human renal transplants. *Br. Med. J.*, **2,** 517

Schneck, S. A. and Penn, I. (1971). De novo brain tumours in renal transplant recipients. *Lancet*, **i,** 983

Sheil, A. G. R., Mears, D., Kelly, G. E., Rogers, J. H., Storey, B. G., Johnson, J. R., May, J., Charlesworth, J., Kalowski, S. and Stewart, J. H. (1971). Controlled clinical trial of anti-lymphocyte globulin in patients with renal allografts from cadaver donors. *Lancet*, **i,** 359

Singal, D. P., Mickey, M. R. and Terasaki, P. I. (1969). Serotyping for homotransplantation. Analysis of kidney transplants from parental versus sibling donors. *Transplantation*, **7,** 246

Smith, M. G. M., Eddleston, A. L. W. F., Dominguez, J. A., Evans, D. B., Bewick, M. and Williams, R. (1969). Changes in leucocyte migration after renal transplantation. *Br. Med. J.*, **4,** 275

Startzl, T. E., Halgrimson, C. G., Penn, I., Martineau, G., Schroter, G., Amemiya, H., Putnam, C. W. and Groth, C. G. (1971). Cyclophosphamide and human organ transplantation. *Lancet*, **ii,** 70

Stuart, F. P., Saitoh, T., Fitch, F. W. and Spargo, D. (1968). Immunological enhancement of renal allografts in the rat. *Surgery*, **64,** 17

Van Hooff, J. P., Schippers, H. M. A., Van der Steen, G. J. and Van Rood, J. J. (1972). Efficacy of HL-A matching in Eurotransplant. *Lancet*, **ii,** 1385

Williams, R. (1971). Post-operative care. In R. Y. Calne (ed.). *Clinical Organ Transplantation*. (Oxford: Blackwell Scientific Publications)

Further Reading

Bach and Good (1972). *Clinical Immunobiology*. (New York and London: Academic Press)

Calne, R. Y. (1971). *Clinical Organ Transplantation*. (Oxford and Edinburgh: Blackwell Scientific Publications)

Calne, R. Y. (1973). *Immunological Aspects of Transplantation Surgery*. (Lancaster: MTP)

Najarian and Simmons (1972) . *Transplantation*. (Philadelphia: Lea and Febiger)

CHAPTER 12

Tumour Immunology

J. E. Castro

Introduction

A dynamic interaction exists between growing cancer cells and their environment. This balance may be influenced by changes in either the tumour or host. In the tumour a rapid cell doubling time, invasiveness and a propensity to metastasize are all associated with poor prognosis. In the host genetic factors, the endocrine milieu, blood coagulation and nutritional state, as well as immunological reactions may influence tumour development and growth. Some of these features are interrelated—for example, in animals it has been shown that alterations in blood coaguability affect the incidence of metastases: increased coagulation is associated with increased metastases and anticoagulation with a decrease. But blood coagulation can be influenced by nutritional state and the hormonal milieu. In this chapter the emphasis will be on the immunological relationships of the host and his tumour.

Tumour Antigens

For a tumour to stimulate an immunological response it must possess characteristic antigens. Much of the early work on tumour antigenicity was confused because of the failure to appreciate the fact that tumours, like most other tissues, exhibit transplantation antigens. A clear understanding of the terminology that applies to tissue grafts is, therefore, germane to tumour immunology (Table 13.1). Only when syngeneic tumours are studied can consideration be given to those antigens that are characteristic of tumours. In animals this was possible after introduction of inbred mouse strains and in

Table 12.1 Terminology of tissue grafts

A syngeneic graft is a graft exchanged between individuals of identical genetic constitution: for example, grafts between identical twins or mice of the same pure line strain

An allogeneic graft is a graft exchanged between members of the same species but of different genetic constitution: for example, from one human to another or from one pure line strain of mice to a different one

A xenogeneic graft is a graft exchanged between individuals of different species: for example, from monkey to man or mouse to elephant

1953 Foley produced the first evidence for specific antigenicity of experimental tumours, findings that were soon confirmed by others (Prehn and Main, 1957; Old *et al.*, 1962).

TUMOUR-SPECIFIC TRANSPLANTATION ANTIGENS

Experiments to demonstrate tumour-specific antigens involve a demonstration that pretreatment with a syngeneic tumour will influence the growth of a subsequent challenge with the same tumour. Pretreatment may involve ligation or excision of the initial tumour after it has reached a critical size, but before dissemination (Klein *et al.*, 1960), injection of a low dose of cells which is too low to induce an overt tumour, or injection of tumour cells that have been treated chemically or physically to prevent growth and division. If pretreatment alters the growth of an inoculation of tumour cells that would normally initiate an overt tumour in a non-treated recipient, then such pretreatment has caused an immune response to the characteristic antigens of the tumour. If pretreatment alters the growth of a tumour which is different from the one used for pretreatment, then cross-reactivity between the tumours used for pretreatment and challenge is said to occur. Many of the early experiments to demonstrate tumour antigenicity used inappropriate methods and yielded negative results. Immunization was often with subcellular preparations in which tumour-associated antigens were destroyed or degraded. Frequently recipient animals were challenged with overwhelmingly large doses of tumour cells and it is now known that immunity to tumour specific antigens can protect the host against only a relatively small (10^6–10^7) number of tumour cells.

There are also *in vitro* techniques for detection of tumour antigens. Some involve the demonstration of tumour antibodies by membrane immunofluorescence, complement fixation or cytotoxicity, whilst others demonstrate lymphocyte cytotoxicity. Although antibodies to tumour antigens have been demonstrated by a variety of techniques their significance *in vivo* is poorly understood. Most attempts at passive transference of tumour immunity by sera have failed and in some circumstances enhancement of tumour growth occurs. There are many tests for measurement of cell-mediated immunity to tumours; the majority involve a cytotoxic assay that measures the ability of lymphocytes to lyse tumour cells or inhibit their growth but the relevance of such observations to the *in vivo* situation is not clear. Leukaemia cells and cultured lymphoblastic cells from patients with lymphoma, leukaemia or infective mononucleosis stimulate blastogenesis when tested against responder lymphocytes of the same donor. The blastogenic response of lymphocytes from patients with leukaemia to stimulation by leukaemia cells is of favourable clinical prognostic significance as is the presence of circulating serum factors that inhibit blastogenesis. Other tests involve the action of lymphokines, which are humoral substances elaborated by specifically sensitized lymphocytes on contact with antigen. Inhibition of macrophage migration by the products of sensitized lymphocytes is one of the best studied *in vitro* correlations of delayed hypersensitivity.

The existence of tumour-specific transplantation antigens against autochthonous methylcholanthrene-induced sarcoma has been demonstrated by transplantation techniques. Similar antigens have been demonstrated for tumours induced by other polycyclic hydrocarbons, other types of chemical carcinogens, irradiation and implanted cellophane or millipore filters. The initial view was that these induced tumours express individually distinct neoantigens whereas the antigens on virally induced tumours were cross-reacting. The immunogenicity of individual chemically induced tumours was found to vary when measured by the number of viable tumour cells a recipient could reject after a standard immunization procedure. An animal immunized with a weak antigenic tumour would reject only 10^2–10^4 tumour cells but an animal immunized with a highly antigenic tumour could reject 10^6 or 10^7 tumour cells. In every case the degree of immunity was finite and if more tumour cells were inoculated immunity was overcome. It has also been shown that immunity to tumour-specific transplantation antigens can be adoptively transferred to previously untreated syngeneic recipients by immunocompetent cells (e.g. spleen or peritoneal exudate cells) from immunized donors. However, passive transfer of antibodies produces variable results. Circulating antitumour antibodies have been detected in the serum of mice with growing tumours but only after the tumour has been excised. This may be due to the complexing of antibody to circulating tumour antigen. When the tumour is excised excess antigen is cleared and the free antibody may be measured in appropriate assays.

It is now known that chemically induced tumours express both individually characteristic tumour antigens and also cross-reacting antigens and there is increasing evidence that at least some of these cross-reacting antigens are phase specific or fetal antigens (Coggin *et al.* 1971).

VIRAL ANTIGENS

The tumour-specific transplantation antigens induced by both DNA and RNA viruses are the same for all tumours induced by a single virus, but differ from those induced by different viruses.

Tumours induced by DNA viruses (polyoma, SV 40, adenoviruses 3, 7, 12, 18 and 31, etc.) have similar immunological findings. These viruses induce neoplasms *in vivo* or *in vitro* which do not then produce infectious virus. Tumours induced by DNA virus have three neoantigens. Tumour-specific transplantation antigens, which are cell surface antigens, and T antigens which are first detected in the nucleus and persist in the malignant cell are the first two. Both these may be detected by serological methods and can be differentiated from the third group of neoantigens, the complement-fixing viral particle antigens, by physical and immunological manœuvres (Black *et al.*, 1963; Dephendi *et al.*, 1964).

Furthermore, with the exception of adenovirus 12, tumours without demonstrable infective virus do not elicit the production of viral antibodies.

RNA viruses (mouse leukaemia virus, chicken sarcoma virus, Bittner virus) differ considerably from DNA viruses, both in structure and manner of replication. Unlike the DNA viruses there is continued production of infectious RNA viruses in most neoplasms induced by them. It is, therefore, difficult to distinguish between tumour-specific antigens and viral antigens.

FETAL ANTIGENS

The inappropriate expression of normal tissue antigens has been found in a variety of animal tumours. Examples of these phase-specific antigens are thymus–leukaemia antigen, Gix antigen and fetal antigens. The TL antigen can be detected serologically on normal thymus cells from some mouse strains (TL positive) but not others (TL negative). Leukaemias developing in TL negative mice frequently carry the TL antigen and it is probable that there is a repressed structural gene coding for TL determinant which is only derepressed by the malignant process. The Gix antigen is similar and occurs in the serum of rats immunized with a syngeneic virally induced tumour. It has specificity for the thymocytes of certain mouse strains.

Baldwin, Glaves and Pimm (1971) have shown by immunofluorescence that chemically induced tumours have fetal antigens on their surface. Integral to appreciating the significance of these fetal antigens is a demonstration that adult syngeneic animals are capable of mounting an immune response against them.

Cytotoxic tests *in vitro* have demonstrated that lymphocytes from tumour bearers are sensitized against fetal antigens. When fetal tissues are implanted in mice made deficient in cell-mediated immunity (Castro *et al.*, 1974) it was observed that they grow considerably larger than in normal, immunologically competent adults. There is also a marked difference in the variety of histological types of tissues found in these implants as in the normal mice identifiable tissues were limited and a lymphocyte infiltrate was found at the junction of the fetal implant with host tissues. This may be contrasted with the appearance of fetal implants in immunologically depressed mice where few histological types of tissues could be identified and no infiltrate could be seen at the junction of the graft and recipient tissue. This finding, together with the observation that pretreatment with fetal tissues would modify the growth of a second fetal tissue implant, suggests that early syngeneic fetal tissues may provoke a transplantation reaction in normal mice. Parmiani and Della Porta (1973) have examined the effects of immunization with fetal tissues in a different way. They pretreated adult mice with syngeneic-adult tissues, sarcoma, fetus or with allogeneic adult tissues and observed the effects of these treatments on litter size, premature birth and viability of progeny. There was a significant reduction in the frequency of pregnancies and in the litter sizes after sarcoma or fetal tissues but not after treatments with adult tissues. It is suggested that these effects result from the induction of a specific immune cytotoxic action of embryo cells after sensitization to fetal antigens by pretreatment with embryonic or tumour tissues.

The relationship between fetal and tumour antigens has been examined in a variety of ways (Stonehill and Benditch, 1968). In 1916, Schöne (1906) showed a relationship between immunization with fetal tissues and growth of tumours. More recent workers, using genetically defined mice, have confirmed the relationship between fetal and tumour antigens. Most have found that pretreatment with fetal tissues protects against subsequent tumour challenge (Coggin *et al.*, 1971), but some have found that tumour growth is enhanced and others have found no significant effects. The reasons for these contradictory results are not known.

It has recently been shown that embryo-immune rats are capable of limiting metastatic growth of tumours. This may result because intravenous inoculation of tumour cells may facilitate direct contact with cytotoxic effector mechanisms or, in addition, tumour cells may be unable to lodge in the lungs due to mechanisms other than those of an immunological nature.

It would appear that tumours may contain several antigens capable of stimulating an immune response (Table 13.2). The relationship between tumours, specific transplantation antigens and fetal antigens is not clear.

Table 13.2 Tumour antigens

Transplantation antigen
Tumour-specific antigens
Viral antigens
Fetal antigens

Whether tumour-specific antigens are dependent on new genetic information resulting from mutation or viral infection or whether they represent a derepressed fetal gene has yet to be established. A brief exposure to an oncogenic agent might produce derepression within a cellular genome. The derepressed gene groups may code for synthesis of antigenic substances recognized experimentally as tumour-specific transplantation antigens. Most experimental work suggests that tumour-specific transplantation antigens and fetal antigens are not the same, for pretreatment with the former is far more efficient at causing tumour elimination than treatment with fetal antigens.

Human Tumour Antigens

It is obviously not possible to demonstrate tumour-specific antigens in human tumours by transplantation techniques. Methods rely upon the demonstration of cell-mediated immunity or humoral immune responses against tumour cells or tumour cell extracts. Using the techniques of immunofluorescence and *in vitro* cytotoxicity or cytostasis, antibodies have been demonstrated against Burkitt's lymphoma, neuroblastoma, malignant melanoma, osteosarcoma and many other tumours including cancer of the bladder, renal cell cancer, testicular tumours, Wilm's tumour, gliomas, meningiomas, leukaemias and carcinomas of the breast, lung, endometrium and ovary.

Patients with Burkitt's lymphoma were the first to demonstrate tumour-associated antigens and the geographical distribution of the tumours suggested that it might result from infection spread by an arthropod vector. Cross-reactivity of antigens between different patients with Burkitt's tumour and isolation of a DNA virus (Epstein Barr or EB virus) from cultured cell lines of Burkitt's tumour support this view. However, many tumours contain viruses which may be contaminants (passenger viruses) and it is, therefore, not possible to show definitely that EB virus is the aetiological agent of Burkitt's lymphoma. EB virus is either identical or very similar to the virus responsible for infectious mononucleosis. Four antigens have been demonstrated in cells from Burkitt's tumour. Viral capsid antigens are located in the cytoplasm, they have no correlation with the clinical course of the disease and can be found in normal sera. Membrane antigens are located on the cell surface of living cells and they do correlate with clinical progress, titres being high when patients are in remission and low when the disease recurs. Another group of antigens can be found on the surface of acetone-fixed Burkitt's cells and in sera from patients with Burkitt's tumour, naso-pharyngeal cancer and infectious mononucleosis and precipitating antigens found in sera of patients with active disease. In addition cell-mediated im-mune responses have been demonstrated by delayed cutaneous hypersensi-tivity reactions to extracts of autologous tumour cells and by lymphocyte-mediated cytotoxic reactions of cells from tumour-bearing patients.

The clinical course of neuroblastoma sometimes suggests that immuno-logical mechanisms may be important in its control, for regression of meta-stases has been reported after excision of the primary tumour and clinical cure may follow even incomplete tumour excision. It was the first human tumour in which antigens were demonstrated by lymphocyte-mediated cytotoxicity. The possibility that viral infection during pregnancy may be an important aetiological factor in neuroblastoma is suggested by the finding of cross-reactivity between neuroblastomas and demonstration of lymphocyte cytotoxicity by cells from the mothers of children with neuroblastoma.

Many techniques have been used to show antibodies against melanoma cells and cross-reactivity has frequently been shown. A possible relationship be-tween the antigen of osteogenic sarcoma and an infectious agent was sug-gested by the high incidence of antibodies to tumour antigens in sera from relatives and close friends of patients with the disease. Furthermore, C-type virus particles, similar to avian and murine sarcoma viruses, have been isolated from cell lines of a human liposarcoma and cell-free extracts of sarcomas induced a sarcoma-specific antigen in normal human embryonic fibroblasts in culture. High levels of antibody indicate a good prognosis but it is not clear whether the decreased level of antibodies allows the develop-ment of metastases or whether increasing tumour load neutralizes antibodies by forming antigen–antibody complexes.

Generally human tumours contain common antigens shared by most, if not all, tumours of the same histological type. Cross-reactivity between tumours of different histological types is not usually found. This antigenic specificity is similar to that found in experimental tumours and it is suggestive evidence for a viral aetiology of most human tumours. Some human tumours have been shown to contain individually unique as well as common antigens which is similar to the situation observed in murine mammary carcinomas induced by the mouse mammary tumour virus.

Immunosurveillance

The mechanisms whereby the host mounts a response against the antigens expressed by the tumour is known as immunosurveillance. Immunosurveillance as a mechanism for control of cancer was suggested by Green in 1954 and elaborated by Burnet (1970) thus, 'A major function of the immunological mechanism is to recognize and eliminate foreign patterns of behaviour arising in the body by somatic mutation or some other equivalent process'. This concept suggests that a mutant cell, which is potentially responsible for overt tumour development, has at least one antigen with a biochemical sequence different from that normally found in the host. An immunological response is, therefore, mounted against this antigen and, if there is sufficient of it, a clone of immunologically competent cells appears and eliminates the abnormal mutants.

There is general agreement that some form of surveillance occurs continuously but the points of debate are whether or not the surveillance mechanism requires immunological rejection rather than elimination by non-immunological mechanisms and whether it has specificity. There is evidence both for and against these contentions. For example, the effect on tumour induction and growth of manœuvres that suppress cell-mediated immunity have been studied. Nehlsen (1971) gave a group of mice long-term rabbit antimouse antithymocyte serum (ATS). She found the incidence of tumours after this treatment was not increased but when mice given ATS were exposed to an oncogenic virus (polyoma) the incidence of tumour was very high compared with appropriate controls. There are some exceptions to the association of increased tumour incidence with immunosuppression. A decreased incidence of tumours induced by mammary tumour virus has been observed following neonatal thymectomy. In addition, the low incidence of papillomas induced by the Shope papilloma virus was not increased by immunosuppression. Balner and Dersjant (1969) have reported similar results, for mice given ATS alone developed no more tumours than the control untreated mice whereas those given ATS and a chemical carcinogen developed more tumours and at an earlier time than mice given carcinogen alone. Generally it has been difficult to facilitate the induction of tumours by chemical carcinogens after immunosuppression but this may be related to the immunosuppressive effects of the oncogenic drugs themselves.

The finding that mice deprived of cell-mediated immunity and exposed to an oncogenic agent develop more tumours is evidence in favour of immunosurveillance. However, the observation that immunosuppressed mice do not have more tumours than untreated mice is evidence against the theory.

In human patients taking immunosuppressive drugs after renal transplantation there is an increased incidence of tumours. Penn (1975) reported an overall corrected incidence of 5·6% compared with an incidence of 0·058% for a normal age-matched population. The distribution of the histological types of these tumours is markedly different from that found in the normal population, for nearly 50% of tumours were mesenchymal in origin and many of these were reticulum cell sarcomas. This abnormal distribution of tumours suggests that the mechanisms operating in immunosuppressed patients may be different from that involved in oncogenesis in the normal population. The finding may be partially explained by the suggestion that some of the agents used for immunosuppression are themselves oncogenic, that immunosuppressed patients are subject to opportunist viral infections (some of which may be oncogenic) or that the antigen drive of allogeneic transplanted organs may contribute to the development of tumours, particularly lymphomas or reticulum cell sarcomas.

The importance of host resistance to tumours has been demonstrated in other ways. Stimulation of immune reactivity by specific immunization or non-specific immunopotentiation causes a decreased incidence of tumours and prolongation of their induction time after infection with some oncogenic viruses. However, attempts to prevent chemical carcinogenesis by immunological means have failed. Complimentary evidence for the importance of host resistance comes from the relationship between congenital or acquired immunodeficiency disease and tumour development (Good and Finstead, 1969).

There is an increased incidence of both lymphoreticular and solid tumours in these diseases but particularly those like ataxia-telangectasia or the Wiskott–Aldrich syndrome which affect cell-mediated immunity (Fialkow, 1967). There is also an increased incidence of tumours at the extremes of life and a relative decrease in immunity has been documented among ageing animals and humans.

Circumstantial evidence for the importance of immunity against human tumours comes from the occasional cases of spontaneous regression of primary tumours that occur and from those rare cases where regression of metastases occurs after excision of the primary tumour (Everson and Cole, 1966). The difference between the reported incidence of clinical tumours and the higher incidence found unexpectedly during postmortem suggests that people are developing tumours that regress. The frequent infiltration of tumours by lymphocytes and demonstration of immunological reactivity by *in vitro* tests is further evidence of an immunological response against human tumours.

If surveillance is not due to immunological mechanisms, what are the alternatives? One suggestion by Hellström (1966) is that tumour destruction is due to allogeneic inhibition. This is a consequence of the observation, in mice, that cytotoxicity to tumour cells can be effected by allogeneic lymphocytes immunized against normal or tumour cells of the mouse in which the tumour arose. Furthermore, if normal allogeneic cells were used tumour cytotoxicity did not occur, but the situation was reversed when the same allogeneic and tumour cells were brought into close apposition (for example, by phytohaemagglutinin). In contrast, syngeneic cells even in apposition were not cytotoxic. It may be that several types of surveillance against tumours are operational and only one is mediated through the immune system.

Escape from Surveillance

That tumours develop in animals and man and grow progressively and kill the host is an all too common observation in clinical practice. If immunological surveillance exists there must be escape mechanisms by which tumours evade the control of immune responses. There are several suggested mechanisms of escape (Table 13.3).

Table 13.3 Escape from surveillance

1. Tumour antigenicity
2. Immunoresistance
3. Sneaking through
4. Vascularization
5. Genetic factors
6. Immunosuppressants
7. Anergy
8. Blocking factors

TUMOUR ANTIGENICITY

It is pertinent to ask whether surveillance operates selectively against some tumours or whether it is relevant to all tumours and also to question its importance *in vivo*. Tumours which arise spontaneously seem to be considerably less antigenic than induced ones; tumour immunologists tend to concentrate on antigenic or biologically unsuccessful tumours whereas tumour growth under natural conditions favours less antigenic or non-antigenic tumours. Furthermore, very few animal tumours metastasize.

Immunosurveillance may be highly efficient in destroying antigenic tumours but may be ineffective against other tumours. Evidence for the effectiveness of surveillance *in vivo* is limited. However, Lappé (1968) found that when mouse skin was treated with 3-methylcholanthrene and grafted on to syngeneic mice the outcome was affected by treatment of the recipient. Irradiation decreased the latent period whereas non-specific stimulation with BCG lengthened the latent period and increased the number of spontaneous regressions of these skin papillomas.

IMMUNORESISTANCE

When antigenic autochthonous tumours are exposed to immunological reactions that do not entirely eliminate them, immunoresistance may develop. This diminished sensitivity to rejection may develop in the same way that bacteria develop resistance to chemotherapeutic agents, selective pressures favouring those cells expressing less antibody-binding sites on their surfaces. It has indeed been shown by binding tests that immunoresistant cells do, in fact, show a decrease in the number of relevant antibody-binding sites for each cell rather than a complete antigenic loss. Other phenotypic changes that resemble immunoresistance may develop—for example, when faced with a persistent immunological reaction the surface of the tumour cell is altered or modulated so that it is no longer expressing a configuration which will be recognized by the sensitized lymphoid cells (Boyse and Old, 1969). This was first detected in the case of the TL antigen in mice, but it has not yet been confirmed for human tumours. Another mechanism for immuno-resistance is that the target molecules on the surface of tumour cells may be continuously shed into the surrounding extracellular fluid. The cell surface will then be comparatively immunoresistant and the locality flooded with excess antigen. Tumours that shed antigen most rapidly are presumably those of low immunogenicity which metastasize most rapidly.

SNEAKING THROUGH

The concept of tumours sneaking through is based on the observations of Old *et al.* (1962). They found that medium-sized inocula of antigenic tumour cells would grow progressively. The large dose of tumour cells overwhelms the immune mechanism but a small number of cells can grow to an ir-reversible tumour colony before an immune reaction is mounted. This may be a very important mechanism in the natural establishment of tumours and it may be that vascularization is the time when the nascent tumour colony becomes invulnerable to immune attack.

VASCULARIZATION

It has been suggested by Folkmann that tumour growth occurs in two phases; the first is an avascular one whereby nutrients and waste are exchanged by simple diffusion and during this stage growth of tumours is slow. Whilst the tumour colony is still small, proliferation from the host vascular system begins and most tumours are vascularized after reaching 1–2 mm diameter. Tumour vascularization occurs by an ingrowth of host vascular channels into the tumour and once established rapid growth of the tumour occurs. In an established tumour it is mainly the vascular endothelium that is exposed to immunological attack by the host defences, but because vascularization results from ingrowth of host cells it is recognized as 'self'.

GENETIC FACTORS

The successful escape of tumours from surveillance can also result from changes in the host. In animals the response to various antigens has been shown to vary in different animal populations which are then designated high or low responders; a similar response may be true for tumour antigens. The mechanisms which effect the altered response to antigens are not clear but evidence from studies with Marek's disease in chickens, which results from horizontal infection with a herpes virus, suggests that some factors may operate through cell-mediated immunity. The clinical manifestation of the infection may be a highly malignant disease, a benign lymphoproliferative condition or no disease at all. In susceptible animals thymectomy does not increase the high incidence of malignant disease but it does increase the incidence in normally resistant chicks.

IMMUNOSUPPRESSION AND ANERGY

Exogenous administration of immunosuppressants can also diminish the host immune response and the effects of this on tumour incidence has already been discussed. However, patients with tumours show a non-specific depression of immune responses or anergy. Whilst the occurrence of both cellular and humoral immunosuppression in tumour-bearing patients has some prognostic significance the mechanisms causing this immunosuppression are not clearly understood. Tumour extracts, circulating serum factors and tumour-induced ascites will cause immunological depression *in vitro* and *in vivo* and the immunosuppression is greatest when the serum or ascites are from patients showing anergy. It has also been suggested that suppressor cells may contribute to anergy. However, the central question in immunosuppression and cancer is whether subjects who develop cancer are intrinsically immunosuppressed or whether the growing tumour itself, either directly or indirectly, induces a state of immunosuppression. There is evidence for both possibilities: the finding of depressed immunological reactivity in patients with very early and *in situ* cancer suggests inherent immunosuppression in patients developing cancer, whilst the correlation between the stage of the disease and frequency of anergy suggests factors associated with the tumour-inducing immunosuppression.

BLOCKING FACTORS

Successful adaptation of tumours may be due to systemic factors which block the usual interaction of host defences and tumour cells, therefore protecting the tumour from destruction. Several serum factors have been incriminated in this inhibitory activity; blocking antibodies (Hellström *et al.*, 1971), antigen–antibody complexes (Baldwin and Embleton, 1971) and excess soluble antigen (Currie and Basham, 1972) have all been invoked.

Stimulation of Tumour Growth by the Immune Response

Recently Prehn (1972) has suggested that stimulation of the immune response may encourage tumours to develop. Although specific immune reactivity may sometimes be adequate to control a neoplasm, lesser degrees of immune reactivity may promote growth of latent tumours. If the response to tumours is biphasic in this way a similar reaction would be expected with other immunological reactions. A possible example has been reported in respect of the parasite *Plasmodium berghei* infection in mice. It has been found that antilymphocyte serum decreases the number of parasites and prolongs the life of infected hosts but only in situations where there is little natural resistance. In mouse strains with more immunity antilymphocyte serum shortens life from this same infection. These data are similar to the situation with mouse mammary tumours (Prehn, 1971): C_3H mouse mammary tumour produced by milk agent is quite immunogenic when grown in C_3H mice which lack the virus, but grown in a subline which contains virus it has very little immunogenicity. Attempts at immunization against the tumour implants in virus-containing mice sometimes caused enhanced tumour growth and irradiation or neonatal thymectomy may decrease the growth of tumour transplants. In the C_3H mice, in which the tumours are more immunogenic, reduction of immune capacity by thymectomy or irradiation increases tumour growth. The results could, however, be explained by alteration in the balance between blocking factors and cellular immunity. There are other data that support the immune stimulation theory. When thymectomized, x-irradiated mice were injected with various numbers of spleen cells from specifically immunized mice but mixed with a constant number of target cells, different results were obtained dependent on the proportions of the cell populations. Small numbers of immune spleen cells caused acceleration of tumour growth when compared with controls of non-immune spleen cells or spleen cells from animals immunized against different non-cross-reacting tumours. Large numbers of specifically immune spleen cells, however, produced inhibition of tumour growth. Such data suggest that early in the course of disease, or in situations where the immune reaction to tumour is weak, stimulation of tumour growth may occur whereas inhibition occurs at other times. The *in vitro* experiments of Jeejeebhoy (1974) gave similar results. At early stages of tumour development when lesions were not palpable the cellular antitumour immune responses of mice were found to be capable of specifically stimulating tumour growth *in vitro*. However, when the tumours enlarged and were palpable, it was found that the stimulatory pattern seen early in the development had changed to an inhibitory one.

Effector Mechanisms of Tumour Destruction

Tumour immunity is frequently assumed to be a variant of that found in transplantation and, therefore, mediated by the same mechanisms. The data to support this assumption are minimal; the immunological mechanisms of tumour cell destruction are not known and there is disagreement about the relative roles of the separate components of the immunological apparatus in this process. It has not been possible to implicate any one cytotoxic mechanism in the immune elimination of tumours and different mechanisms seen to be dominant in varying situations.

THYMUS-DEPENDENT CELLS

The importance of T lymphocytes is clear, for specifically sensitized T lymphocytes are able to destroy tumour cells in an *in vitro* assay and *in vivo*. They can transfer immunity to non-immune animals and infusion of syngeneic or allogeneic immune lymphocytes into tumour-bearing animals sometimes has therapeutic effects. T cell cytotoxic cells recognize target cell antigens and T cell killing *in vitro* is paralleled by protection *in vivo*, for sensitized T cells can be transferred to mice made deficient of T cells by irradiation and this transfer confers protection.

There is also considerable evidence for cytotoxic cells other than T lymphocytes (Woodruff et al., 1973). For example, neonatally thymectomized rats are able to generate cytotoxic lymphocytes against Rous sarcoma antigens in the colony inhibition assay. Experiments based on studies with differential radio-resistance and kinetics of cytotoxicity suggest there are several types of effector cells.

THYMUS-INDEPENDENT CELLS

One cytotoxic mechanism is effected by thymus-independent cells, now designated K cells, which have no direct affinity for target cell antigen but are triggered to kill by antigen bound to the target cells (MacLennon, 1972). K cells develop independently of the thymus, they are not actively adherent to glass and they are not phagocytic. Several types of cells may be active in the assay, B cells, polymorphonuclear cells and null cells (Greenberg *et al.*, 1973).

ANTIBODIES

The antibody involved in killing with the thymus-independent cells is lymphocyte-dependent antibody (LDA) and is found only in the IgG fraction, and cytotoxicity is independent of complement. Because antibodies must have an intact Fc fragment it has been suggested that the Fc fragment of an IgG molecule attaches to the target cell (Larsson and Perlmann, 1972). Even in the presence of adequate numbers of antibody-producing cells, antibody production is dependent upon sufficient numbers of T helper cells. Although transfer of antibody alone will confer protection *in vivo* it is not clear whether this is due to collaboration with effector cells and the significance *in vivo* of killing by thymus-independent lymphocytes in concert with lymphocyte-dependent cytotoxic antibody has yet to be established.

A second type of serum that promotes cytotoxicity has been termed 'unblocking' serum by Hellström *et al.* (1975). This is thought to represent the interaction of free antibody with blocking complexes. They found that serum from patients who were disease free or 'cured' seldom contained blocking activity. When such serum samples were mixed with those from patients with progressive disease, which normally had blocking activity, this action was abrogated. Unblocking activity *in vitro* has been correlated with tumour regression *in vivo* (Bansal and Sjögren, 1972). The exact mechanism of unblocking is not known but there are several possible explanations. One is that cytotoxic antibody in the presence of complement causes direct lysis of tumour cells. It is more likely that unblocking serum is antitumour antibody which saturates the available antigen sites of the soluble antigen–antibody complexes and prevents interaction with immune lymphocytes. If this is the case it suggests that blocking is not due to antibody alone. The final possibility is that unblocking activity is equivalent to antibody-dependent cellular cytotoxicity. Tumour cells can be rapidly destroyed by antibodies alone in the presence of complement in *in vitro* systems. Lymphoma and leukaemia cells are very sensitive to such attack whereas sarcoma cells are resistant. The role of this cytotoxic mechanism is far from clear and even *in vitro* the culture conditions of the test are all important. In general, tumour-specific cytotoxic antibodies cannot be detected in tumour-bearing animals but in the very immunogenic lymphomas induced by the oncorna viruses antibodies can be detected in the earlier stages of tumour growth

(Currie, 1973) but in chemically induced sarcomas they can never be found whilst the tumour is *in situ*. In some patients with human tumours complement-dependent cytotoxic antibodies can be found in the early phases of tumour growth but disappear with extension of the disease.

Apart from a cytotoxic effect antibodies may have functions other than cytotoxicity that may be beneficial to the host. Inhibition of tumour cell growth is one action but it is often difficult to distinguish this from a slow lytic effect and its *in vivo* significance is not clear. Inhibition of tumour cell motility by antibody is another phenomenon easily demonstrated *in vitro* and if the effects are also found *in vivo* they could be important in limiting the local and metastatic spread of tumours (Currie and Sime, 1973).

PHAGOCYTIC CELLS

There are two categories of phagocytic cells, namely the polymorphonuclear phagocytes (granulocytes) and the mononuclear phagocytes. In various aspects these cell lines resemble each other. Both originate primarily from the bone marrow, enter the bloodstream and circulate for 1–3 days before randomly leaving the circulation to become fixed macrophages (Roser, 1970). Their subsequent terminology depends upon the site at which they settle— Kupffer cells in the liver, fixed splenic histiocytes, pulmonary alveolar macrophages, epithelioid cells and so forth. There are, however, differences between the two cell lines, particularly regarding cellular kinetics, the number of ancestor cells in the bone marrow and the characteristics of the proliferation and differentiation of the cells. They also differ in the time spent in the circulation and tissues. Other differences concern their capacity to phagocytize and pinocytize, to kill ingested micro-organisms and to ingest intracellular materials.

The actual role of phagocytes in tumour destruction is not clear but resistance of animals to tumours parallels reticuloendothelial phagocytic activity. During growth of transplanted, syngeneic tumours there is an increased production and function of macrophages which result from changes in cellular factors rather than opsonins. Although stimulation of reticuloendothelial function protects against some tumours the biological mechanisms underlying these observations is not clear.

The evidence suggests that phagocytic cells exert a critical role in initiating and maintaining immune reactions (Feldman and Palmer, 1971. In particular, there is a wealth of experimental work to show that localization of antigens, including tumour antigens, on the phagocytic cells is an essential part of the primary immune response. Of necessity this invokes the concept of phagocytic cells interacting with antigen-reactive lymphoid cells in such a way that exposure or transfer of antigen or other messenger material takes place. Both

in vitro and *in vivo* the relationship between phagocytic cells and lymphocytes is such that there is ample opportunity for such transfer to occur. *In
vitro* lymphocytes cluster around macrophages and eventually become firmly
attached to them by means of a single cytoplasmic process or 'foot ap-
pendage'. Subsequently lymphocytes transform into blast cells. *In vivo*
electron microscopic studies show the presence of clusters of lymphocytes
around macrophages in the medullary cords of lymph nodes and red pulp of
the spleen. There are also infrequent areas of distinct communication between
the cytoplasm of phagocytic cells and adjacent lymphocytes.

Apart from processing antigen for lymphoid cells, phagocytic cells may be
a significant effector mechanism in tumour destruction (Evans and Alexander,
1972). If monolayer cultures of phagocytic cells are established from cells
taken from mice with growing lymphomas they will specifically inhibit the
in vitro replication of the appropriate cultured lymphoma cells. In a syngeneic system, such as this, the effects of confrontation between immune
macrophages and target tumour cells are detected only by an inhibition of
cell growth, whereas in an allogeneic system tumour cell lysis can occur.

The 'arming' of normal phagocytic cells by exposing them to immune
lymphoid cells can produce specifically cytostatic phagocytic cells. The
nature of this arming process has been partially elucidated and it is due to
a soluble supernatant factor which is produced by the lymphoid cells and
affects the phagocytic cells. When an armed phagocyte encounters an
appropriate specific target cell it becomes 'angry', as evidenced by its
vacuolation and hyperactivity. Furthermore, the cytostatic activity of such a
cell becomes non-specific for it causes cytostasis of a variety of unrelated
tumour cells *in vitro*. Similarly activated phagocytic cells can be produced by
the *in vitro* treatment of normal peritoneal exudate cells with low doses of
endotoxin, and also in animals infected with intracellular parasites like
Toxoplasma gondii. Although the cytostatic effects of activated phagocytic
cells is immunologically non-specific, they are only effective against malignant cells; benign cells are not affected.

The relationship of phagocytic cell cytotoxicity *in vitro* to the tumour
protection observed *in vivo* is complex for the interaction of these cells with
other lymphoid cell types makes it difficult to establish their importance in
tumour destruction. However, it has been shown that there is contamination
with large numbers of phagocytic cells in many solid rodent tumours. In
some, and particularly those of higher immunogenicity, up to 50% of the
cells constituting the tumours are phagocytes, and this is the equivalent of ten
billion in a growing tumour. When tumour, free from phagocytic cells, is
inoculated into normal animals it is rapidly infiltrated by phagocytes until the
cellular proportions approximate those in the normal tumour.

This influx of phagocytes may affect phagocytosis at other sites. Many studies have shown alteration and phagocytic activity during progression of malignant disease in animal and in man. In mice with Friend virus leukaemia there is a marked and progressive rise in phagocytosis and an increase in liver and spleen weights as the condition develops but in the terminal phase phagocytosis decreases. In mice with spontaneous mammary neoplasms and solid tumours induced by methylcholanthrene phagocyosis is slightly increased, at least in the early phase of tumour growth. It has been shown, however, that the failure of delayed cutaneous hypersensitivity seen in tumour-bearing animals can be corrected by the addition of normal macrophages to the test inoculation of antigen and it has been suggested that the failure of such delayed hypersensitivity responses seen in patients with cancer is not a primary defect of lymphocytes but it is a consequence of excessive consumption of phagocytes by growing antigenic tumours.

In humans radio-labelled heat-aggregated human serum albumen is cleared more rapidly from patients with advanced Hodgkin's disease than in animals. However, other studies have shown no significant difference in phagocytic activity between controls and patients with localized solid tumours, but when dissemination occurs phagocytic activity is inhibited (Magarey, 1972).

Phagocytic cells have other functions that may be important for the control of tumours. They have been shown to be essential for the response of lymphoid cells to the mitogen phytohaemagglutinin. Furthermore, in many tumour situations the normal interactions of cytotoxic lymphocytes and target tumour cells are inhibited by circulating blocking factors. The nature of such blocking factors is not clear; antibody, antigen or antigen–antibody complexes have been invoked and these different agents may be important at different points in the immune response. Phagocytes, by removal of excess antigen or complexes from the circulation, may play an important part in restoring a balance between cellular immunity and blocking.

PHAGOCYTIC CELLS AND TUMOUR METASTASES

Many variables affect the distribution of metastases including mechanical circulating factors and the local chemical environment. Phagocytic cells may also be important. In both animals and man extensive proliferation of phagocytes in the sinuses of the local drainage lymph nodes is regarded as a favourable prognostic sign. When hamsters are grafted with a tumour which metastasizes widely, there is no phagocyte response in the drainage lymph nodes. When a similar tumour which only rarely metastasizes is used, there is marked hyperplasia in the regional lymph nodes and cells from the tumour are phagocytosed in the nodes.

Similar changes have been observed in patients with cancer. Proliferation of phagocytic cells in the draining lymph nodes is associated with good prognosis especially if associated with infiltration of the primary tumour by mononuclear cells. However, these observations are still matters for debate because proliferation of the phagocytic cells may be non-specific as it has been observed in the absence of malignant tumours and it is also particularly noticeable when tumour necrosis is seen.

References

Baldwin, R. W., Glaves, D. and Pimm, M. V. (1971). Tumour-associated antigens as expressions of chemically induced neoplasia and their involvement in tumour host interaction. *Prog. Immunol.*, **1** 907

Baldwin, R. W. and Embleton, M. J. (1971). Demonstration by colony inhibition methods of cellular and humoral immune reactions to tumour specific antigens associated with aminoazo-dye-induced rat hepatomas. *Int. J. Cancer*, **7**, 17

Balner, H. and Dersjant, H. (1969). Increased oncogenic effect of methylcholanthrene after treatment with antilymphocyte serum. *Nature (London)*, **224**, 376

Bansal, S. C. and Sjögren, H. O. (1972). Counteractions of the blocking cell-mediated tumour immunity by inoculation of unblocking sera and splenectomy and immuno-therapeutic effects of primary polyoma tumours in rats. *Int. J. Cancer*, **9**, 490

Black, P., Rowe, W. P., Turner, H. C. and Heubner, R. J. (1963). A specific complement-fixing antigen present in SV 40 tumour and transformed cells. *Proc. Nat. Acad. Sci.*, **50**, 1148

Boyse, E. A. and Old, L. J. (1969). Some aspects of normal and abnormal cell surface genetics. *Ann. Rev. Genet.*, **3**, 270

Burnet, F. M. (1970). *Immunological Surveillance*. (Oxford: Pergamon Press)

Castro, J. E., Hunt, R., Lance, E. M. and Medawar, P. B. (1974). Implications of the fetal antigen theory for fetal transplantation. *Cancer Res.*, **34**, 2055

Coggin, J. H., Ambrose, K. R. and Anderson, N. G. (1971). Immunization against tumours with fetal antigens. *Proceedings of the 1st Conference and Workshop on Embryonic and Fetal Antigens in Cancer*. Oak Ridge National Laboratory, Oak Ridge, Tennessee May 24–26, 1971, pp. 185–202. USEAC Report Conference 710527. Springfield V United States Department of Commerce, 1971

Currie, G. A. and Basham, C. (1972). Cell-mediated inhibition of the immunological reactions of the patient to his own tumour: a possible role for circulating antigen. *Br. J. Cancer*, **26**, 427

Currie, G. A. (1973). Effect of active immunization with irradiated tumour cells on specific serum inhibitors of cell-mediated immunity in patients with disseminated cancer. *Br. J. Cancer*, **28**, 25

Currie, G. A. and Sime, G. C. (1973). Syngeneic immune serum specifically inhibits the motility of tumour cells. *Nature (New Biology)* **241**, 284

Dephendi, V., Ephrussi, B. and Koprowski, H. (1964). Expression of polyoma-induced cellular antigen(s) in hybrid cells. *Nature (London)*, **203**, 495

Evans, R. and Alexander, P. (1972). Mechanisms of immunologically specific killing of tumour cells by macrophages. *Nature (London)*, **236**, 168

Everson, T. C. and Cole, W. (1966). *Spontaneous Regression of Cancer*. (Philadelphia: W. B. Saunders)

Feldman, M. and Palmer, J. (1971). The requirements for macrophages in the secondary immune response to antigens of small and large size *in vitro*. *Immunology*, **21**, 685

Fialkow, P. J. (1967). Immunologic oncogenesis. *Blood*, **30**, 338

Foley, E. J. (1953). Antigen properties of methylcholanthrene-induced tumours in mice of strain of origin. *Cancer Res.*, **13**, 835

Folkmann, J. (1974). Tumour angiogenesis. In G. Klein and S. Weinhause (eds.), *Advances in Cancer Research*, Vol. 19, 331

Good, R. A. and Finstead, F. (1969). Essential relationship between the lymphoid system of immunity and malignancy. *J. Cancer Inst. Monograph*, **3**, 41

Green, H. N. (1954). An immunological concept of cancer: a preliminary report. *Br. Med. J.*, **2**, 1374

Greenberg, A. H., Hudson, E., Shen, E. and Roitt, I. M. (1973). Antibody-dependent cell-mediated cytotoxicity due to a 'null' lymphoid cell. *Nature (New Biology)*, **242**, 111

Hellström, I. E., Hellström, K. E., Pierce, G. D. and Young, J. P. (1966). Cellular and humoral immunity to different types of human neoplasms. *Nature (London)*, **220**, 1352

Hellström, I. E., Hellström, K. E., Sjögren, H. O. *et al.* (1971). Serum factors in tumour-free patients cancelling the blocking of cell-mediated tumour immunity. *Int. J. Cancer*, **8**, 185

Jeejeebhoy, H. F. (1974). Stimulation of tumour growth by the immune response. *Int. J. Cancer*, **13**, 665

Klein, G., Sjögren, H. E., Klein, E. and Hellström, K. E. (1960). Demonstration of resistance against methylcholanthrene-induced sarcomas in the primary autochthonous host. *Cancer Res.*, **20**, 1561

Lappé, M. A. (1968). Evidence for the antigenicity of papillomas induced by 3-methylcholanthrene. *J. Natl. Cancer Inst.*, **40**, 823

Larsson, A. and Perlmann, P. (1972). Study of Fab and F(ab)1 from rabbit IgG for capacity to induce lymphocyte mediated target cell destruction *in vitro*. *Int. Arch. Allergy Appl. Immunol.*, **43**, 80

MacLennon, I. C. M. (1972). Antibody in the induction and inhibition of lymphocyte cytotoxicity. *Transpl. Rev.*, **13**, 67

Magarey, C. J. (1972). The control of cancer spread by the reticuloendothelial system. *Ann. R. Coll. Surg. Engl.* **52**, 238

Nehlsen, S. L. (1971). Prolonged administration of anti-thymocyte serum in mice. I. Observations on cellular and humoral immunity. *Clin. Exp. Biol.*, **9**, 63

Old, L. J., Boyse, E. A., Clarke, D. A. and Carswell, E. A. (1962). Antigenic properties of chemically induced tumours. *Ann. N.Y. Acad. Sci.*, **101**, 80

Old, L. J., Boyse, E. A., Oettgen, H. F., De Harven, E., Geering, G., Williamson, B. and Clifford, P. Precipitating antibody in human serum to an antigen present in Burkitt's lymphoma cells. *Proc. Nat. Acad. Sci.*, *U.S.A.*, **56**, 1699

Parmiani, G. and Della Porta, G. (1973). Effects of antitumour immunity on pregnancy in the mouse. *Nature (New Biology)*, **241**, 26

Penn, I. (1975). Cancer in immunosuppressed patients. *Transplant. Proc.*, **7**, No. 1, Supplement 1, 553

Prehn, R. T. and Main, J. M. (1957). Immunity to methylcholanthrene-induced sarcomas. *J. Nat. Cancer Inst.*, **18**, 769

Prehn, R. T. (1971). Perspectives in oncogenesis: does immunity stimulate or inhibit neoplasia? *J. Reticuloendothelial Soc.*, **10**, 1

Prehn, R. T. (1972). The immune reaction as a stimulator of tumour growth. *Science*,
   176, 170
Roser, B. (1970). The migration of lymphocytes *in vivo*: In R. van Furth (ed.). *Mononuclear
   Phagocytes*, p. 166 (Oxford: Blackwell Scientific Publications)
Schöne, G. (1906). Tumour immunity in mice. *Munchener medizin. Wochenschr.*, **43**, 2517
Stonehill, E. H. and Benditch, A. (1968). Retrogenic expression: the reappearance of
   embryonal antigens in cancer cells. *Nature (New Biology)*, **228**, 370
Woodruff, M. F. A., Dunbar, N. and Ghaffar, A. (1973). The growth of tumours in
   T cell-deprived mice and their response to treatment with *Corynebacterium parvum*.
   Proc. R. Soc. Lond. Ser. B, **1**, **184**, 97

Further Reading

Amos, B. (1971). *Progress in Immunology*. (New York and London: Academic Press)
Bach, F. H. and Good, R. A. (1974). *Clinical Immunobiology*. Vol. 2. (New York and
   London: Academic Press)
Bloom, B. R. and Glade, P. R. (1971). *In vitro Methods in Cell Mediated Immunity*. (New
   York: Academic Press)
Burkitt, D. P. and Wright, D. H. (1970). *Burkitt's Lymphoma*. (Edinburgh: Livingstone)
Burnet, F. M. (1969). *Cellular Immunology*. (London: Cambridge University Press)
Burnet, F. M. (1970) *Immunological Surveillance*. (Oxford: Pergamon Press)
Currie, G. A. (1974). *Cancer and the Immune Response*. (London: Edward Arnold)
van Furth, R. (1970). *Mononuclear Phagocytes*. (Oxford: Blackwell Scientific Publications)
Pilch Y., Myers, G. H., Sparks F. C. and Golub, S. H. (1975). *Prospects for the Immuno-
   therapy of Cancer*, Part 1. (Chicago: Year Book Medical Publishers Inc.)
Smith, R. T. and Landy, M. (1970). *Immune Surveillance*. (New York and London:
   Academic Press)

CHAPTER 13

Approaches to the Immunological Treatment of Tumours

J. E. Castro

Introduction

Most cancers at the present time are treated by surgical operation, radiotherapy or chemotherapeutic drugs. With surgery there is increased risk of mortality, morbidity and complications. This approach lacks selectivity and only affects tumour cells at the site of treatment. Radiation therapy is a regional treatment, is injurious to normal tissues and also causes complications, deformity and functional impairment. Chemotherapeutics affect normal tissues as well as tumour cells and therefore have considerable side-effects. Both radiation and chemotherapy act by first order kinetics and usually fail to eradicate the disease totally; however, their effects are systemic and suitable for the treatment of disseminated tumours.

Theoretically, an immunological approach to the treatment of cancer has several factors to commend it. Ideally there should be immunological specificity which would affect only cancer cells and would, therefore, be free from significant toxicity. Provided the tumour has the appropriate antigens, all the malignant cells would respond and the systemic nature of the treatment should mean that metastases were also dealt with.

So far, these theoretical advantages have not been fulfilled. It may be that the immune response is inadequate to cope with the tumour: alternatively, the best methods for manipulation of opposing functions of the immune response have yet to be discovered. From a biological standpoint, factors which allow the immunological escape of tumours may nullify immune responses and other forms of non-immunological treatment may be required to alter them. Because most human tumours are antigenic, the basic aim of immunotherapy is to make existing immunity more effective in the control of growth and the ultimate goal is the immunological destruction of tumours by the potentiation or depression of separate arms of the immune response to different degrees and at will. This has yet to be achieved although several approaches have been tried. The purpose of this chapter is to outline some of the different immunological methods aimed at the control of cancer.

Immunotherapy may be specific (designed to cope with a particular tumour) or non-specific (where the overall immunological reactivity of the host will be changed) and treatments may be combined. Many aspects of specific immunotherapy are applicable in non-specific circumstances depending upon whether treatment is directed towards a specific or a cross-reacting antigen, which is found in several tumours.

Immunoprophylaxis and Immunotherapy

It is important to distinguish between these two entities. Immunoprophylaxis is the induction of resistance to tumour prior to its development or grafting and immunotherapy is the treatment of established tumours and/or their metastases. Immunoprophylaxis has been encouraging whereas the results of immunotherapy in laboratory animals and humans have been disappointing.

IMMUNOPROPHYLAXIS

Immunoprophylaxis has had startling effects on bacterial and viral infections. Similar results for the treatment of tumours might be accomplished in the following ways:

(1) Immunization against the aetiological agents of cancer. At present the causes for the majority of human cancers are not clearly defined, although there is increasing evidence that some tumours may be virally induced; even if this theory is correct it is still not clear whether transmission is vertical or horizontal.

(2) Immunization against tumour antigen acquired at the time of malignant transformation. Many tumours have type-specific antigens and, therefore, a polyvalent vaccine may be required; as yet these antigens have not been isolated in a sufficiently purified form. Vaccines for cross-reacting antigens may be directed against the aetiological agent in the case of virally-induced tumours. However, other cross-reacting antigens (particularly embryonic ones) may be suitable targets for attack, but in animal models variable results have been recorded (see p. 337).

(3) Increase of immune surveillance by non-specific immunopotentiating adjuvants (see p. 336).

Immunoprophylaxis and immunotherapy merge imperceptibly when immunological treatments are used as an adjunct to conventional methods, such as surgery, radiotherapy or chemotherapy, to prevent recurrent disease. We have used the metastasizing Lewis lung tumour for some of our own experiments in mice. Cells are released into the circulation from the primary tumour 6 days after implantation and metastases are easily visible at 21 days. Macroscopic pulmonary metastases are not observed 10 days after tumour inoculation; however, if the primary tumour is excised on day 10 metastases are always found by day 21. This model was used to simulate the clinical condition where the primary tumour is removed surgically but the patient dies from metastases. If immunoprophylaxis, in the form of *Corynebacterium parvum* (*C. parvum*) (see p. 369) was given a few days before excision of the primary tumour this considerably reduced the number of metastases, when compared with animals treated by operation alone. Some mice treated by a combination of operation and *C. parvum* were permanently cured of tumour (Sadler and Castro, 1976).

Whilst most animal studies involve immunoprophylaxis, in humans this has not so far been practised in the true sense. However, in Chicago, Rosenthal *et al.* (1972) reported a retrospective analysis of the leukaemia death rate in an infant population (aged 0–6 years) which received BCG compared with a similar population that had not received the vaccine. During the years 1964–1969 there was one death from leukaemia in 54414 infants who were vaccinated from 1–6 months, a rate of 0.31/100000/year. In contrast, there were 21 deaths from leukaemia in 172986 infants who did not receive BCG, a rate of 2.02/100000/year. The retrospective nature of this study (with the inherent problems of selection) is a reason for criticism. Similar results have been reported from Canada but other investigations have not confirmed the Chicago findings (Comstock, 1971; Kinlen and Pike, 1971).

IMMUNOTHERAPY

Immunotherapy results have been disappointing. This may be due to the limitations of the immune response or to its weakness. It is rare for immunotherapy to cause large tumour masses to disappear; presumably this is because those mechanisms which have allowed the escape of tumour cells through the normal surveillance systems are still operational. Such therapy is effective primarily in the treatment of certain specific tumours or when there is minimal residual disease.

No distinction will be made between immunoprophylaxis and immunotherapy in the rest of this discussion. Consideration will be given to possible approaches and combinations of treatment by immunological methods. These may be (a) specifically designed to cope with a particular tumour or (b) non-specific, i.e. when the overall immunological reactivity of the host will be changed. Many aspects of specific immunotherapy can be applied for non-specific purposes dependent on whether treatment is directed either towards a specific tumour antigen or a cross-reacting antigen.

Specific Immunotherapy

This can be passive, adoptive or active.

PASSIVE SPECIFIC IMMUNOTHERAPY

Tumour antisera may be raised in syngeneic, allogeneic or even xenogeneic recipients followed by specific absorption. When antibodies are used, selective production of cytotoxic (as opposed to enhancing) sera is an unsolved problem which is vital both to tumour and transplantation biologists. Several features are important in the preferential stimulation of antibodies having a particular biological function—for example, the dose of antigen used to raise antibody, its route of administration to the animal in which antibody is being raised, and the time interval between priming and harvesting. In the recipient, the dosage and route of antibody administration are also important in obtaining a particular biological reaction. Attempts physically to separate cytotoxic from enhancing immunoglobulins have been unsuccessful.

However, there are sporadic but convincing reports that serum therapy can provide a beneficial response. After immunization of CBA mice with C57Bl leukaemia, the immune serum from the CBA mice protected C57Bl mice against subsequent challenge with tumour and also retarded growth of cancer cells injected 2 days before serotherapy. Immune serum incubated with tumour cells or administered a few days before or after a small number of malignant cells retards the growth of most lymphoid, and occasionally non-lymphoid, tumours. Serum therapy is rarely effective against challenge with a large number of cells or clinically detectable tumours.

Despite these difficulties, cytotoxic antibodies may be of use in the treatment of human cancers. Carefully timed serum samples could be taken from a patient at intervals after surgical removal of a tumour and the cytotoxicity of the serum could be determined *in vitro*. Those samples showing cytotoxicity might be used *in vivo* to treat residual or recurrent tumours. Alternatively, allogeneic serum from patients with immunologically similar tumours could be used and even xenogeneic sera specifically absorbed might be useful.

In contrast, xenogeneic sera against tumour-specific transplantation antigens may have an effect upon tumour growth. We have used a rabbit anti-mouse Meth. A tumour serum which was shown to have cytotoxic activity against Meth. A cells *in vitro*. When intravenous antiserum was given followed by intraperitoneal administration of the ascitic Meth. A tumour, causing it to grow in ascitic form, there was good protective effect. This decreased with prolongation of the interval between tumour and antibody administration. There was, however, still good protection when the interval was 2 weeks between injection of intraperitoneal tumour and intravenous antibody. When intravenous antiserum was given and the ascitic tumour was injected subcutaneously, so that it grew in solid form, different results were obtained; if antiserum and tumour were given simultaneously good protection was achieved, but with prolongation of the tumour–antibody interval the protective effects of antiserum were less, and when the interval was 2 weeks there was no antitumour action.

The failure of antiserum to destroy or inhibit established solid tumours could be caused by ineffective antibody distribution because it is necessary for the antibody and tumour cells to make contact. This could be facilitated by combining cytotoxic antibodies with pharmaceutical agents which would improve their penetration or, alternatively, by infusion or regional perfusion of the tumour. The combination of antibody administration and other immunological manipulations might facilitate tumour inhibition or destruction.

An alternative use of antitumour antibodies is as vehicles for transporting antitumour agents to the surface of the cancer so that a high concentration of these reaches the tumour site: at the same time the generalized systemic side effects of such agents are minimized. Preliminary results reported by those using melanoma antibody linked with chlorambucil are encouraging (Ghose and Nigam, 1972).

Recently there has been renewed interest in the utilization of immune sera for immunotherapy of cancer. This has been stimulated by studies of the 'unblocking' activities of certain sera (Sjögren, 1973), by the discovery of lymphocyte-dependent antibodies which appear to arm cells and by investigations into sera which activate macrophages. Experiments have been reported using serum with known unblocking activity injected in a dose large enough to reverse the blocking effect of the tumour-bearing animal's own serum. Unblocking serum was given from the day of inoculation of a syngeneic polyoma tumour and those animals which never showed blocking activity in their sera developed tumours within 7–10 days, but these had completely regressed 2 weeks later. The same process did not occur in animals whose sera was shown to have blocking activity despite treatment with unblocking serum. The observation that the tumours first appeared and subsequently regressed in the cured rats implies that the administered serum caused the host's developing cell-mediated immunity to be more effective. It is unlikely that it had a direct cytotoxic effect on the tumour cells. Other experiments showed that splenectomy combined with administration of unblocking sera caused arrest or regression of growth of polyoma tumours in rats. In another study Hersey (1973) has shown that slight therapeutic effects can be achieved by giving xenogeneic sera, known to contain lymphocyte-dependent antibodies, to rats with lymphomas. The mechanisms of this action are not clear and no effect was seen with allogeneic or syngeneic sera.

Many tumours, however, are not readily susceptible to the cytotoxic effects of antisera *in vitro* and it might be that blocking factors rather than toxic agents could be administered: this would then result in tumour enhancement rather than regression. Such an effect has been repeatedly demonstrated in allogeneic tumour systems and can be deliberately induced with sera known to have blocking activity *in vitro*. This fear of enhancing tumour growth, coupled with the inability to distinguish clearly between cytotoxic and blocking sera *in vitro*, has inhibited the development of passive immunotherapy.

ADOPTIVE SPECIFIC IMMUNOTHERAPY

Tumour-bearing animals lose both specific antitumour immunity and general immune competence during tumour growth. The adoptive transfer of immunocompetent cells has frequently been tried as a method of immunoprophylaxis or immunotherapy against cancer. Either syngeneic, allogeneic or xenogeneic lymphoid cells from specifically immunized donors can be transferred to tumour-bearing recipients. In neonatally thymectomized mice infected with polyoma the transfer of sensitized lymphocytes destroys small foci of tumours and prevents development of new tumours. However, adoptive immunotherapy is usually ineffective if instituted after clinical manifestation of a tumour.

Although adoptive specific immunotherapy may be suitable for inbred strains of animals, in humans the recipient appears rapidly to reject the allogeneic cellular inoculation or the immunocompetent cells may cause a graft-versus-host (GVH) reaction (see Chapter 7) against the immunodepressed patient.

When viable immune syngeneic lymphocytes are incubated with tumour cells, or administered systemically soon after inoculation of the malignant cells, they inhibit tumour implants. Similarly, when immune lymphocytes are given to animals incubating an oncogenic virus, but before the development of an overt cancer, this will suppress tumour growth. For inhibition to occur in these systems large numbers of sensitized cells must be transferred and they must be harvested at precise times after immunization.

Adoptive immunotherapy has been used in combination with chemotherapy for treatment of an established systemically disseminated viral leukaemia. Mice given either chemotherapy or this type of immunotherapy alone always died with tumour but, when the two were combined, survival was not uncommon. Success may have resulted because chemotherapy decreased the tumour bulk and thus the immunotherapy was more effective. Alternatively, the capacity of the recipient to reject allogeneic lymphocytes could have been inhibited by chemotherapeutic agents.

To control GVH, potential donor lymphoid cells might be sensitized *in vitro* to those of normal allogeneic patients. Responding donor lymphoid cells could be inactivated by 5-BUdR or radioactive isotopes thus stimulating others capable of causing GVH reaction without affecting the antitumour clones. The remaining cells could then be infused with massive doses of irradiation or chemotherapeutic drugs. An alternative approach to reducing GVH effects of adoptive transfer is by sensitizing autochthonous lymphocytes to tumour cells *in vitro* before infusion. This approach presumes inhibitory factors *in vivo* which interfere with effective sensitization of autochthonous cells.

Non-immune lymphoid cells can be converted to specific immunoreactivity by incubation with RNA mouse extracts (Fishman, 1961), and similar findings have been described for the transference of skin allograft immunity. The system is exemplified by the following experiments: guinea-pigs were immunized to murine tumour-specific transplantation antigens. This immunity was then transferred to previously untreated mice by injection of syngeneic lymphoid cells which had been preincubated with RNA extracted from the sensitized guinea-pigs' lymphoid cells. RNA from guinea-pigs injected with normal mouse tissues did not protect against tumours and the effect appeared specific for particular tumour types used to sensitize the guinea-pigs. Similar results have been obtained with *in vitro* tumour assay systems where appropriate RNA converts normal lymphoid cells into killer cells.

The mechanisms involved in the transfer of immunoreactivity by RNA are not fully understood. One type of immunologically active RNA contains antigen fragments and it may behave as a super antigen. The other type is free from antigen and may be informational RNA which can be incorporated into the lymphoid cells and evoke a specific immune response. Both types may exist in the same immune RNA extract. It has recently been shown that immune RNA is localized within the cytoplasm of lymphoid cells. Nuclear and cytoplasmic RNA have been extracted individually from the cells of sensitized spleens. It was shown that nuclear RNA was devoid of immunological activity but that this was present in the cytoplasmic RNA.

Several other subcellular products may be of value for immunotherapy. They are the biochemicals associated with states of delayed hypersensitivity—collectively called lymphokines. At present they have been incompletely characterized and they may prove to be identical or at least related to each other. The most widely studied substance is transfer factor. This is a dialysable, non-antigenic non-immunoglobulin of 10000 molecular weight resident in circulating leukocytes. Parenteral administration of transfer factor *in vivo* converts non-sensitive recipient circulating lymphocytes to a responsive state against specific antigens, including those of tumours (Lawrence, 1972). The goal in using transfer factor is to provide the patient with a means of instructing a clone of his own lymphocytes to recognize and reject the tumour. Four potential sources of antitumour transfer factor have been suggested. It could be obtained from (a) normal donors, (b) patients in remission from tumours which share a common antigen with the recipient's tumour, (c) patients deliberately immunized to allogeneic tumour antigens, or (d) a tumour bearer. Unfortunately, transfer factor is at present only detectable in human systems (and possibly other primates); it is difficult to assay and cell populations which respond to it may not be present in the recipient. So far, references to its use for treating human tumours have been limited to anecdotal case reports, particularly of patients with malignant melanoma, and although some success has been claimed its specificity has recently been questioned; suggestions have been made that it may be acting as a non-specific potentiator of immune responses.

ACTIVE SPECIFIC IMMUNOTHERAPY

Tumour antigens are generally weak immunogens so that the resulting immunity is either ineffective or incomplete. Antigens can be rendered more immunogenic by changing the dose or route of administration and also by alteration of the cells in the following ways:

(1) Physical treatments
(2) Viral incorporation
(3) Chemical modification
(4) Surface changes by enzymes
(5) Coupling with immunogens

Physical treatments

A common method to render animals immune is to inoculate them with tumour cells that cannot grow. These cells irradiated *in vitro* with x-rays, γ-rays or ultraviolet rays before injection can immunize the recipients against subsequent viable tumour cells, but there is evidence that immunogenicity may be lost above a certain level of irradiation and treated cells have not been shown to have any immunotherapeutic effect in animals bearing advanced tumours. It is not clear whether irradiation actually increases immunogenicity or if its effect is related to the high dosage of tumour cells that can be given after such treatments.

Tumour cells have also been altered by freezing, thawing, lyophilization, high pressure and mechanical homogenization. Subcellular fractions and various cellular extracts have been used, but comparative studies suggest that there is no significant improvement in the protective effects obtained after these more complicated manœuvres.

Virus incorporation

The incorporation of virus into malignant cells is another approach to increasing tumour immunogenicity. It has been observed that mice which recover from transplantation of tumours after viral oncolysis are immune when challenged with uninfected tumour cells. It is possible that the virus used in oncolysis may act as a carrier for haptenic determinants of tumour cells: evidence for this has been provided by the observation that antiviral antibody added in excess to a virus oncolysate inhibits the antitumour response. Antigens may become incorporated into the virus envelope but this explanation for adjuvanticity of viruses, although the easiest to investigate, is not the only possible mechanism for it could result from increased immunogenicity of host cell debris. Antigens from these cells become attached to the viral proteins and the resulting molecules could carry antigenic determinants which are characteristic of the cell in addition to the possible carrier–hapten type. Other less specific interactions are conceivable: effects of neurominidase in uncovering new antigenic sites after the removal of sialic acid are well established (*vide infra*) and nucleic acids have adjuvant effects. Local immunostimulation, perhaps by attraction of specialized cells to critical sites, is also possible; some bacteria have been shown to act in this way and it is probably also true for most viruses. Certainly, the conjugation of tumour cells with hapten could theoretically increase antigenicity either by increasing helper cell effect or by providing new targets for immunological attack. This approach appears promising but its place in the treatment of established tumours has yet to be shown.

Chemical modification

Extensive investigations have been carried out to modify the tumour with reagents specific to molecular components on the cell surface. Sanderson and Frost (1974) have demonstrated the use of gluteraldehyde-treated cells for the induction of immunity to Meth. A tumour in syngeneic murine hosts. Gluteraldehyde solution contains polymeric alpha and beta saturated aldehydes. These react rapidly with protein amino groups in mild conditions and crosslink the protein molecules. The modification is irreversible and does not disorder the crystalline structure and for these reasons gluteraldehyde is used as a fixative for electron microscopy and x-ray diffraction. Non-immunized control mice challenged with 10^5 tumour cells survived for approximately 20 days whereas mice immunized with gluteraldehyde-treated cells were completely protected against this challenge but not against 10^6 tumour cells. In contrast, mice immunized with the same number of irradiated cells showed less protection. These results applied when the interval between gluteraldehyde-treated cells and tumour challenge was 2 weeks but, when mice were left for 27 days between immunization and challenge, only partial protection was obtained indicating that immunity decreased at that time. Two factors might operate in producing this effect: firstly, gluteraldehyde may be preserving the tumour antigenicity and, secondly, the chemical modification of the proteins may produce an enhanced cellular immunity at the expense of humoral response.

One advantage of chemical modification of the cell surface is that both antigenically strong and weak haptens on the cell surface can be selected. It is possible to vaccinate against several tumour lines using malignant cells treated with sulphhydryl-blocking agents like iodoacetate, iodoacetamide, N-ethylmaleimide and p-hydroxymercuribenzoate. Although p-hydroxymercuribenzoate is a good hapten it is ineffective in increasing tumour cell immunogenicity whereas the three other agents do, an observation which suggests that blocking the sulphhydryl group is not the only mechanism involved in increasing immunogenicity. Although cells treated with iodoacetamide are effective for immunoprophylaxis no effect on established tumours has been shown. Vaccination by tumour cells treated with periodate (to alter hydroxyl groups) and dinitrophenol or formaldehyde (to alter amino groups) are less effective for immunoprophylaxis. Treatment of immunogens by acetoacetylation can change the predominant immunological reaction from a humoral to a cellular response.

Surface changes by enzymes

Several enzymes, like trypsin, pepsin, bromolin-collagenase and chymotrypsin have been used to modify the immunogenicity of tumour cells. *Vibrio cholera neuraminidase* (VCN) has been studied in the greatest detail and has been shown to affect the growth of established solid tumours.

It is believed that sialic acid and other glycoproteins normally cover the tumour cell and so prevent detection of surface antigens (Currie and Bagshawe, 1968). VCN removes sialic acid and so exposes these antigenic sites. It has also been shown that cancer cells treated with VCN are less effective in establishing tumours than untreated cells. Furthermore VCN increases the immunogenicity of a variety of strong and weak transplantation antigens both *in vitro* and *in vivo*. There is no increase in the ability of VCN-treated cells to absorb anti-H2 antibody in the case of strong histocompatibility antigens and neither is there unmasking of new histocompatibility sites to match the increased immunogenicity (Simmons and Rios, 1972).

It has been demonstrated that small, but well-established, methylcholanthrene-induced sarcomas would regress after inoculation of the mice with tumour cells treated with VCN *in vitro*. There were no effects on the various control groups of mice treated with heat-inactivated VCN, or active VCN in combination with excess sialic acid or *N*-neuroamino lactose (which acts by substrate inhibition). Several types of tumour have been affected in this way but their inhibition was immunospecific and occurred only if the inoculated cancer cells and the growing tumour were of the same type. Similar therapeutic results have been reported after intratumour injection of VCN, but repeated inoculations over a long period of time are necessary. The effects of these were also immunospecific, for regression of tumours of a similar type occurred at distant sites whereas those of different types were unaffected. More recent investigations of the effect of VCN on spontaneous mammary tumours in mice have been disappointing for, despite a good effect on established growth, there was a high incidence of new tumours of identical histological type in uninjected mammary glands. This observation is probably explained by VCN increasing the immunogenicity of the 'private' tumour-specific transplantation antigens but not affecting the immunogenicity of the cross-reacting viral antigens of the mammary tumour virus; it is not known whether VCN actually depresses the immunogenicity of the viral antigen.

The increased immunogenicity of weak antigens by VCN is a matter of interest. It has been suggested that sialic acid normally prevents tumour antigen from making contact with antigen-handling cells or interferes with this reaction in some other way. As VCN removes sialic acid it may counteract these effects and by this action uncover neoantigens. Another action of VCN is to reduce the negative charge on the cell surface. This increases cellular contact and facilitates interaction between tumour cells and the host defences. Treatment of cells with VCN facilitates opsonization and phagocytosis and they are easily lysed by complement.

Coupling with immunogens

When tumour cells are conjugated with hapten the process may increase immunogenicity either by increasing helper cell effect or by providing new targets for immunological attack.

An example of this is the coupling of rabbit gammaglobulin to tumour cells using bisdiazotized benzidine. When the cells, treated in this way, were given to mice having spontaneous mammary adenocarcinomas tumour growth was markedly depressed but regression did not occur.

Non-specific Immunotherapy

MECHANISM OF ACTION OF ADJUVANTS

A substance which increases response to an antigen is an adjuvant. Some knowledge of the mechanisms which regulate the immune response is necessary in order to understand the mode of action of adjuvants and their application to non-specific immunotherapy. There appear to be ways in which regulation may occur either from within by a self-contained self-regulating system or from without. The first theory suggests that immunological processes are self-controlled, regulated by inputs and outputs which have a negative or positive feedback mechanism. The alternative is that the system is controlled by influences from without which depend upon a system of promoting or inhibiting hormones which have feedback controls.

Although much remains to be learned about the factors which influence the adjuvant activity, there are several ways, recently reviewed by Allison (1973), which might explain their mode of action. They may be effective either by alteration of the antigen itself or by influencing the immunological reaction to it. The former may alter the release of antigen. Slowing can frequently be achieved by injections in a water in oil emulsion and under certain circumstances alum can slow the release of antigen. However, the response to some soluble antigens can be increased by injecting the adjuvant at a different site from the antigen and this suggests that the depot effect of adjuvants is only one contributory factor to its mode of action.

Some antigens can be denatured or made particulate by emulsification or absorption on to alum, bentonite or other particles. Denatured or particulate proteins become associated with macrophage membranes or other non-immunocompetent cells so that antigen is presented to lymphocytes in a highly immunogenic form.

Adjuvants may also effect the cellular response to an antigen but the fundamental mechanisms involved in adjuvanticity and the selective stimulation of separate arms of the immune response are not clear. One possibility is to affect the sequestration of lymphocytes in lymphoid organs (lymphocyte trapping); adjuvants of very varied types cause trapping. They differ from antigens in at least two ways. Firstly, the duration of trapping induced by adjuvants is much longer than after antigens and, secondly, immunogenicity of the adjuvant is not essential to produce trapping. Administration of substances which affect macrophages causes subsequent trapping. This latter observation and the discovery that the transfer of peritoneal cells is best for adoptive transfer of trapping suggest that macrophages are essential to this mechanism.

There is other evidence that macrophages are important for increasing the response to an antigen. For example, when macrophages containing adjuvant and antigen are transferred to syngeneic mice antibody formation is increased. In contrast, addition of adjuvant to lymphocytes used to reconstitute immune responses in irradiated recipients does not affect the amount of antibody formed.

Adjuvants may affect other immunologically competent cells. With some like *Bordatella pertussis*, beryllium, Freund's complete adjuvant or vitamin A, thymus-derived lymphocytes are required for antibody formation. In contrast, *E. coli* lipopolysaccharides can stimulate B lymphocytes directly with only indirect effects on T lymphocytes. Antigens and adjuvants such as poly A-poly U have synergistic stimulatory effects on T lymphocytes *in vitro* and Freund's complete adjuvant increases the number of effector cells which participate in antibody-dependent cell-mediated cytotoxicity.

APPROACHES TO NON-SPECIFIC IMMUNOTHERAPY

A prerequisite for the non-specific manipulation of the immune response is a comprehension of those aspects of the immunological mechanisms that are advantageous to tumour destruction. At present, such mechanisms are not understood and there is disagreement as to the relative roles in this process of the separate components of the immunological apparatus. It has not been possible to implicate any one cytotoxic mechanism in immune elimination of tumours since they vary in different circumstances.

Recent investigations show at least two cellular cytotoxic mechanisms. One involves thymus-processed cytotoxic cells which recognise target antigens and the other is caused by a thymus-independent effector cell which has no direct affinity with target antigen; these are triggered to kill by antibody bound to the target. On other occasions, antibodies or macrophages may be important in tumour destruction. Most attempts at the immunological control of cancer have been dominated by the concept that stimulation of cellular mechanisms is beneficial, whilst humoral immunity should be depressed since it is likely to produce antibodies which promote tumour growth. This simplistic view, however, takes no account of the role of cytotoxic antibodies or of macrophages in tumour destruction.

With present knowledge four methods for stimulation of host responses are available which might retard tumour growth:

(1) Increased or improved localization of cytotoxic antibody
(2) Suppression of blocking factors
(3) More effective macrophage activity
(4) Improved cell-mediated immunity

Increased or improved localization of cytotoxic antibody

In the non-specific use of cytotoxic sera, cross-reacting antigens must be used to raise the antisera. Antigens on virus-induced tumours are cross-reacting, showing viral specificity. Therefore, antibodies raised against the viral genome might be useful for tumours of different histological types which are induced by the same oncogenic virus. There is, however, increasing evidence that chemically induced tumours express cross-reacting antigens and at least some of these are phase-specific or fetal antigens. Despite the frequent observations that pretreatment with fetal tissues will alter the growth of subsequent tumour inoculum, we have, as yet, been unable to influence tumour growth by administration of xenogeneic anti-fetal antibody but this could reflect the weak immunogenicity of fetal antigens.

Suppression of blocking factors

Serum blocking factors, which interfere with the normal interaction of cytotoxic and tumour cells, have been described both in laboratory animals and in humans. Their occurrence and disappearance after conventional treatments seem to correlate with the clinical course of tumours but their exact nature is not clear. Antibody, antigen excess and antibody–antigen complexes have been invoked and these agents may be important either at various points in the immune response or in different circumstances.

Theoretically there are more approaches to the removal of blocking factors than to stimulation of antibody formation of a particular biological class. By removing blocking factors, the normal antitumour mechanisms may be able to eliminate tumour cells. Selective suppression of those cells which are responsible for antibody production has been claimed after the use of cyclophosphamide (Turk and Poulter, 1972) and in animals antisera have seen raised against antibody-producing cells (Raff, Nase and Mitchison, 1971). In practice, however, use of these antisera is disappointing. Once blocking factors are present, they may be removed by immunoabsorption or by plasmaphoresis. Antigen–antibody complexes, if they are important, could be dissociated with the added benefit that the liberated antibody might itself be cytotoxic.

More effective macrophage activity

'*There is at bottom only one genuinely scientific treatment of all diseases and that is to stimulate the phagocytes . . . They devour the disease; and the patient recovers —unless of course he's too far gone.*' (George Bernard Shaw)

There is little doubt that phagocytic cells are involved in establishing the host's response to his own tumour, for immunity can be transferred by the injection of syngeneic phagocytic cells or by lymphocytes from animals immunized against the specific tumour. Indeed, cells of peritoneal exudate are more effective than those of lymph node for causing growth suppression of some tumour types.

Many factors cause inhibition of phagocytic function both in animal and in man and such is the case with severe stress, irradiation and cytotoxic drugs. There is an impression that surgical operation may be associated with accelerated growth of tumour metastases: in certain circumstances cytotoxic drugs and irradiation can increase the growth and spread of experimental tumours. These findings can be explained in part by the depression of phagocytosis which may be produced by these agents.

One approach to therapy is to stimulate those parts of the host's defence which are known to protect against cancer. There is considerable evidence that agents which stimulate phagocytosis have powerful antitumour effects. A variety of substances act in this way, i.e. BCG, poly I-poly C, Zymosan, diethylstilbestrol and diethylstilbestrol dimethyl ether (which has only one-twentieth the estrogenic effect of diethylstilbestrol). But so far, as regards antitumour activity and stimulation of phagocytosis, none of these agents is as promising as active strains of *C. parvum*.

C. parvum is a powerful stimulant of phagocytic activity and, given either intravenously or intraperitoneally, it will increase spleen or liver size. Histological examination of these organs shows the enlargement to be due to increased phagocytes and their function is markedly enhanced.

Concomitant with these changes, resistance to tumours develops and we have shown that pretreatment with *C. parvum* decreases the death rate of Balb C mice inoculated intraperitoneally with Meth. A ascitic tumour, of CBA mice given S37 ascitic tumour and of C3H/He mice given Ehrlich's ascitic tumour.

It is interesting that intravenous *C. parvum* does not affect the death rate from solid Meth. A tumour. However, a study carried out to investigate the effects of *C. parvum* on the growth of the primary Lewis lung tumour showed that some inhibition of tumour growth was obtained after intravenous or intraperitoneal administration of *C. parvum* but that subcutaneous inoculation of the vaccine had no effect. These data would suggest that *C. parvum* is more effective when tumour cells are dissociated as opposed to growing as a solid vascularized tumour.

We have shown that the protective effect of intraperitoneal *C. parvum* on ascitic Meth. A tumour is maximal with low tumour dose and the duration of its effect is between 25 and 50 days. Splenectomy did not affect the antitumour activity and, despite the recent studies which suggest that large doses of BCG given orally retain some of the antitumour effects seen after injection, we were unable to observe any immunological effects of oral *C. parvum*, despite massive doses of the vaccine. In particular, oral *C. parvum* did not significantly increase spleen weight or stimulate formation of antibodies against *C. parvum* itself and, furthermore, it had no effect upon the growth of tumours which are inhibited by intravenous administration of the vaccine.

Improved cell-mediated immunity

Despite the demonstration of antitumour activity without any increase in cell-mediated immunity after *C. parvum* (Castro, 1974), there is no doubt about the importance of cell-mediated immunity in some tumour situations.

Most immunological adjuvants act on several components of the immune system. However, it has recently been shown that *Bordatella pertussis* organisms, which were known to affect macrophages, have an orientation towards both T and B lymphocytes whereas lipopolysaccharides, from *S. typhi*, chiefly affect B lymphocytes. Selective stimulation of cell-mediated immunity has been claimed for lentinan, a polysaccharide extracted from the edible Japanese mushroom (*Lentinus edodes*) (Dresser and Phillips, 1973). The effects of lentinan on normal mice seem to be variable, for we have found that it affects neither skin allograft survival nor thymus or lymph node weights. We have been unable to demonstrate its protective effect in Balb C mice given Meth. A tumour (whether the inoculation was intraperitoneal or subcutaneous), in CBA mice given S37 ascites sarcoma or in C3H/He mice given Ehrlich's ascitic tumour. It would seem that the previously reported antitumour effects of lentinan are limited only to specific tumours in particular strains of mice.

The development of a transient GVH *in vivo* exerts a striking influence on immune responses to a variety of antigens, including those of tumours. This is termed the allogeneic effect. Many workers have attempted to utilize the GVH reaction as an immunotherapeutic tool but the effects appear to be transient, although it may have an antileukaemic effect. During the induction and expression of the GVH in mice it has been reported that two separate cytotoxic reactions are detectable. One represents the specific sensitization of donor cells to recipient antigens leading to lysis; the other is the non-specific cytodestruction of unrelated tumour cells by host spleen cells. To eliminate the clone of cells initiating GVH reactions, without affecting antitumour clones, it has been suggested that potential donor lymphoid cells could be sensitized *in vitro* to normal allogeneic patient cells; the responding clones would then be inactivated with physical agents or chemicals like 5-BUdR. The remaining clones should be those directed against the tumour and they could be infused into patients treated with irradiation or chemo-therapeutic drugs.

Combined Specific and Non-specific Immunotherapy

A combination of specific and non-specific therapy has been the most com-mon approach to immunotherapy in clinical practice (Mathé, 1971). The rationale for the treatment is that non-specific adjuvants will generally boost the immune response including any reaction to specific antigens.

Local immunotherapy is applied directly to the tumour (Klein, 1969). Several workers have treated superficial skin cancer and premalignant lesions with DNCB or a related chemical. After sensitizing the patient to these com-pounds the local lesion is treated. Whether or not immunological mechanisms are involved is a matter for debate. Such treatments offer little advantage over conventional methods.

In some cases the agents used for non-specific immunopotentiation, like BCG and *C. parvum*, have been injected into the growing tumour. The mechanism of regression following intralesional immunotherapy with BCG is obscure; it probably has no direct antitumour effect since it does not cause regression in tuberculin-negative patients, which suggests that it results from delayed hypersensitivity occurring within the tumour nodule. Occasionally, specific response to cancer occurs, for uninjected nodules may regress ac-companied by an increase in titres of antitumour antibodies.

Certainly, the immunological mechanism differs according to whether the immunopotentiating agents are used either systemically or locally. If the former method is used for administration of *C. parvum* it is unlikely that cell-mediated immunity is involved for its effects against tumours have been maintained despite adult thymectomy or treatment with ALS, manœuvres which inhibit cell-mediated immunity. In contrast, the effect of intralesional *C. parvum* on tumours is dependent upon the presence of T lymphocytes.

Conclusions

Far more needs to be known about the biological effects of agents that affect host response to tumours. Then, with a clearer understanding, there might be a more rational approach to immunotherapy. For the moment it is as well to remember the words of William Heberden: *'New medicines, and new methods of cure, always work miracles for a while . . .'.*

References

Allison, A. C. (1973). Effects of adjuvants on different cell types and their interactions in immune responses. In G. E. W. Wolstenholme and J. Knight (eds.) *Immunopotentiation*. (Amsterdam, London, New York: Associated Scientific Publishers)

Castro, J. E. (1974). Antitumour effects of *C. parvum*. *Eur. J. Cancer*, **10**, 115

Comstock, G. W. (1971). Leukaemia and BCG. *Lancet*, **2**, 1062

Currie, G. A. and Bagshawe, K. D. (1968). The role of sialic acid in antigenic expressions. *Br. J. Cancer*, **22**, 843

Dresser, D. W. and Phillips, J. M. (1973). The cellular targets for the action of adjuvants: T-adjuvants, B-adjuvants. In G. E. W. Wolstenholme and J. Knight (eds.) *Immunopotentiation*. (Amsterdam, London, New York: Associated Scientific Publishers)

Fishman, M. (1961). Antibody formation *in vitro*. *J. Exp. Med.*, **114**, 837

Ghose, T. and Nigam, S. P. (1972). Antibody as a carrier of chlorambucil. *Cancer*, **20**, 1398

Hersey, P. (1973). New look at antiserum therapy of leukaemia. *Nature (New Biology)*, **244**, 22

Kinlen, L. J. and Pike, M. C. (1971). BCG vaccination and leukaemia. *Lancet*, **2**, 398

Klein, E. (1969). Hypersensitivity reactions at tumour sites. *Cancer Res.*, **27**, 2351

Lawrence, H. S. (1972). Immunotherapy with transfer factor. *N. Engl. J. Med.*, **287**, 1092

Mathé, G. (1971). Active immunotherapy. *Adv. Cancer Res.*, **14**, 1

Raff, M. C., Nase, S. and Mitchison, N. A. (1971). Mouse specific bone marrow-derived lymphocyte antigen as a marker for thymus-independent lymphocytes. *Nature (London)*, **230**, 50

Rosenthal, S. R., Grispan, R. G. and Thorne, M. G. *et al.* (1972). BCG vaccination and leukaemia mortality. *J. Am. Med. Ass.*, **222**, 1543

Sadler, T. E. and Castro, J. E. (1976). Treatment of a metastasizing murine tumour with *Corynebacterium parvum*. *Br. J. Cancer* (**63**, 292)

Sanderson, C. J. and Frost, P. (1974). The induction of tumour immunity in mice using gluteraldehyde-treated tumour cells. *Nature (London)*, **248**, 690

Simmons, R. L. and Rios, A. (1972). Immunospecific regression of methylcholanthrene fibrosarcoma using neuraminidase. *Surgery*, **71**, 556

Sjögren, H. O. (1973). Blocking and unblocking of cell-mediated tumour immunity. In H. Busch (ed.), *Methods in Cancer Research*. (New York: Academic Press)

Turk, J. L. and Poulter, L. W. (1972). Selective depletion of lymphoid tissue by cyclophosphamide. *Clin. Exp. Immunol.*, **10**, 285

Further Reading

Smith, R. T. (1971). Potentials for immunologic intervention in cancer. In B. Amos (ed.) *Progress in Immunology*. (New York and London: Academic Press)

Lindermann, J. and Klein, P. A. (1976). *Immunological Aspects of Viral Oncogenesis*. (New York: Springer-Verlag)

Halpern, B. (1975). *Corynebacterium parvum: Applications in Experimental and Clinical Oncology*. (New York and London: Plenum Press)

Bach, F. H. and Good, R. A. (eds.) (1974). *Clinical Immunobiology*. Vol. 2. (New York and London: Academic Press)

Prager, M. D. and Baechtel, F. S. (1973). Methods for modification of cancer cells to enhance their antigenicity. In H. Busch (ed.), *Methods in Cancer Research*. (New York: Academic Press)

Currie, G. A. (1974). *Cancer and the Immune Response*. (London: Edward Arnold)

Braun, W. and Ungar, J. (eds.) (1973). *'Non specific' Factors Influencing Host Resistance*. (Basel: S. Karger)

Pilch, Y., Myers, G. H., Sparks, F. C. and Golub, S. H. (1975). Prospects for the immunotherapy of cancer. In *Current Problems in Surgery*. (Chicago: Year Book Medical Publishers, Inc.)

Wolstenholme, G. E. W. and Knight, J. (eds.) (1973). *Immunopotentiation*. (Amsterdam: Associated Scientific Publishers)

Katz, D. H. (1972). The allogeneic effect on immune response. *Transplant. Rev.*, **12**, 141

CHAPTER 14

Immunotherapy of Human Tumours

G. Currie

Introduction

The cancer problem is the problem of disseminated disease. Primary tumours and complications due to local invasion can, with a few notable exceptions, be controlled by surgery or irradiation. It is improbable that improvements in technique for the local management of primary tumours will have any major impact on the overall survival of patients with most forms of cancer. Current orthodoxy suggests that only when methods for the earlier diagnosis of primary tumours become available may significant increases in survival be anticipated from the use of local treatment alone. However, in many tumours there is now increasing evidence that the development of foci of metastatic disease may precede the detection of the primary tumour by months or even years. In diseases such as carcinomas of the breast and bronchus, detection of a primary tumour should perhaps be best regarded as a local manifestation of a systemic disease.

The failure of contemporary treatment methods to control metastatic disease reflects their lack of selectivity, the capacity to distinguish between normal and malignant cells. It is in this context that immunotherapy becomes such an attractive concept and therein lies a danger. Much of the enthusiasm for immunotherapy, both past and present, seems to stem less from experimental evidence than from aesthetic motives, from the innate attraction of the idea. While a nice idea can provide a suitable impetus for basic research it can hardly be used as the rationale for the treatment of patients. To flirt with a nice idea because it is attractive is a laudable activity; to be seduced by it is foolhardy.

Immunotherapy for the treatment of cancer patients has a long and undistinguished history. This is hardly surprising since there is as yet no rational basis for the use of most of the techniques that have been employed. A place for immunotherapy in the treatment of cancer must depend upon an understanding of the role, if any, of immune responses in the biology of tumour development, growth and dissemination and how such responses can be manipulated.

Perhaps the earliest reported series of patients treated with a form of immunotherapy is that described by Hericourt and Richet (1895). In the first 10 years of this century immunotherapy dominated the literature as the favoured method of treating cancer patients despite the total absence of any recorded success. This early phase and the intermittent vogues enjoyed by immunotherapy since then have been comprehensively reviewed by Southam (1961) and by Currie (1972). It is distressing to note the similarities between this early work and the current immunotherapy boom, such similarities being most noticeable in the results obtained. It must be emphasized that most of the earlier studies and many of the contemporary ones have involved the treatment of patients with advanced disease and often after the failure of conventional treatment methods. Furthermore, it has often been used alone and its failure so far may, one hopes, reflect an overall strategic misuse of immunotherapy rather than any inherent defects in the underlying concepts.

Latent Metastases—a Target for Immunotherapy

What is the role of specific antitumour immune responses in host resistance? Some clues can be obtained by examining the effects of immunosuppression on the growth of syngeneic rodent tumours. Surprisingly there is little consistent evidence about the effects of immunosuppression on the growth of primary tumours. Most studies have revealed minimal effects on the growth rate of such tumours and seem to indicate the relatively feeble effect of immune responses on the growth of an organized mass of tumour cells. However, there is now abundant and convincing evidence that a variety of immunosuppressive procedures can evoke the appearance of metastatic disease in animals bearing tumours that do not normally metastasize. In other words a tumour which, when growing in an intact animal can be cured by simple surgical excision will, when implanted into an immunologically crippled host become incurable by surgical means. Although the primary tumour can be successfully removed the compromised host will die with metastatic disease. Whole-body irradiation can promote such appearance of metastatic disease in a variety of animal models (Carnaud et al., 1974; Vaage et al., 1974; Globerson and Feldman, 1964).

Antilymphocyte serum treatment can also accelerate metastases as seen in studies of a hamster lymphoma (Gershon and Carter, 1970) and chronic drainage of the thoracic duct in sarcoma-bearing rats will provoke extensive metastatic disease (Proctor, Rudenstam and Alexander, 1973). These observations indicate that specific immunological responses to tumour cells may have considerable significance for the biological behaviour of tumours. It is in the development of metastatic disease that considerations of tumour immunity should have their greatest impact on clinical practice. In rats bearing surgically curable fibrosarcomas, amputation of a tumour-bearing limb leads to prolonged disease-free survival. However, if such animals are subsequently immunosuppressed, they develop overt metastases (S. Eccles—personal communication, 1975). The failure of these tumours to develop overt metastases when grown in normal animals suggests that immunological responses may be involved in determining the success or failure of treatment of a primary tumour. Such observations lead one to speculate that in patients undergoing surgical treatment of a primary tumour, clinically undetectable metastatic disease is already present and that the eventual outcome depends upon the capacity of the host's immune responses to suppress these latent metastatic foci. There is, however, a flaw in this argument. In experimental animals surgical excision of a growing primary tumour can evoke specific immunity to challenge with cells from the same tumour line and this immunity lasts for several weeks. These same animals will also develop overt metastases when subsequently immunosuppressed. This observation implies that the dormant foci of metastatic tumour are not destroyed despite being lodged in an 'immune' environment for several weeks. Such an observation seems to suggest that the immunological destruction of latent metastases may require substantially more knowledge than is currently available about both antitumour immune responses and the susceptibility of the latent foci.

Before dealing with the particular modes of immunological attack which are being explored at the moment, it is perhaps worth speculating as to the nature of these latent foci of metastatic disease, for they should perhaps represent the main target for immunotherapeutic attack.

The most striking feature of latent metastatic disease and the one that perplexes biologists and clinicians alike is 'dormancy'. From clinical experience with diseases like breast carcinoma it is clear that metastatic disease can remain clinically undetectable for many years. The biological basis of dormant metastatic disease is not understood. It seems improbable that such cells are mitotically dormant sitting in an organ for many years in say, G_0. A more plausible explanation for such clinically undetectable 'dormant' tumour would be some sort of dynamic equilibrium between cell proliferation and cell losses occurring in a steady-state tissue mass. Although there is as yet no convincing demonstration of an appropriate structural basis for dormancy, current research has provided a possible mechanism. Most experimental manipulations of tumour cells involve the use of single cell suspensions or monolayer cultures, both geometric forms which can have little relevance to the *in vivo* growth of tumour cells in three dimensions. Folkman and Hochberg (1973) have emphasized the fact that the growth of malignant cells in a two-dimensional form such as monolayer culture is not self-limiting, i.e. cells will proliferate as long as fresh medium and vacant substratum are available. When forced to grow in three dimensions (as spheroids) tumour cells will not grow beyond a critical cell number and the mass will not exceed a critical diameter. These authors have cultured such structures for long periods (several months) and have shown that they rapidly reach a maximum mean diameter beyond which no further expansion occurs. This they called the 'dormant diameter'. Such a dormant spheroid can contain up to 10^5 living tumour cells. Cell proliferation occurs in the outer rim of the structure and cell losses into a necrotic centre account for its failure to expand. Hidden in an organ such as the liver or lung such 'dormant' spheroids would not be detectable using currently available methods. The self-regulating property of such spheroids is probably dictated by the relationship of surface area to cell number and the consequent limitations imposed upon diffusion of gases, nutrients and metabolites into and out of the structures. In order to exceed its dormant diameter and develop into a clinically detectable tumour a spheroid will have to acquire a blood supply. Such a blood supply apparently develops in response to a tumour cell product known as tumour angiogenic factor (TAF). Vascularization of dormant spheroids may represent a crucial step in the development of overt metastatic disease. Before vascularization occurs such spheroids, if they represent the biological basis of dormancy, could present a serious clinical problem. The limitations of access which dictate their dormant state may similarly apply to access of chemotherapeutic agents, antibodies and cytotoxic cells. The therapeutic efficiency of irradiation may also be limited by the presence of a hypoxic central zone.

Optimism about the potential role of immunotherapy in situations of minimal tumour burden, in the prevention of metastases, must be tempered by the recognition of the biological complexity of the problem of tumour dormancy. Other methods for the disruption of latent metastatic foci may well be required before immunological manipulations can exert a clinically beneficial effect.

Immunological Escape

The existence of tumour-specific transplantation antigens (TSTA) on many experimental rodent tumours can be readily demonstrated by simple transplantation experiments in suitably inbred animals. Furthermore, in an animal bearing an established tumour, specific immunological reactions to the TSTA can be detected by both *in vivo* and *in vitro* methods. Although such evidence is less clear-cut in the case of human tumours, currently available results certainly lend weight to the notion that tumours are antigenic (i.e. they possess on their surfaces structural determinants which are recognizably 'not-self') and that the host reacts to them in an immunologically specific manner. Woodruff (1964), recognizing the paradoxical nature of this situation, has coined the term 'immunological escape' to describe those mechanisms, whatever they may be, which permit the development, growth and dissemination of a malignant cell clone in the face of a potentially cytocidal immune response.

There are a great many possible explanations for the escape of tumours from host restraint (see Chapter 12) and the precise contribution of any or all of them is quite unknown at present. However, there are experimental observations which seem relevant to the clinical situation and which may give important clues about the nature of the escape phenomenon. Concomitant immunity was first described by Bashford in 1908. He demonstrated the resistance of a tumour-bearing animal to challenge with cells from the same tumour implanted at a distant site and his findings have been amply confirmed in recent years. Indeed, animal models now exist which indicate that the development of metastatic disease is associated with the failure of concomitant immunity. An examination of this situation indicates that animals in whom concomitant immunity has failed still possess lymphocytes which show specifically cytotoxic effects on cultured tumour cells. The failure of concomitant immunity is apparently associated with the appearance of factors in the serum which can abrogate these cytotoxic effects. Such inhibitory or 'blocking' factors are now frequently invoked as a major contributory factor in the escape of tumours. Current results suggest that these factors comprise soluble tumour-specific antigens released from the tumour cells in a non-immunogenic form and that, either free in the extracellular fluid or bound to antibody as soluble immune complexes, such antigenic determinants may abrogate specific immunological effector mechanisms. Furthermore, as suggested by Currie and Alexander (1974) the spontaneous liberation of soluble cell membrane components may be an integral feature of the malignant cell and there may exist a quantitative relationship between the rate of liberation of soluble TSTA and the overall malignancy of the cell (i.e. capacity to metastasize and antigenicity). In this way the tumour cell itself may have a built-in escape mechanism and the ability to generate a smokescreen by which it can evade destruction by the host.

Immunological escape is central to any considerations about immunotherapy since if a tumour cell can evade host immune responses it may similarly escape from a form of therapy which employs a similar form of attack. Indeed there is a case for regarding immunological escape as the major conceptual target for immunotherapy.

How can we convert rather nebulous ideas about manipulating the immune response of cancer patients into some sort of practical reality? It is apparent that a well-established rational basis is required before clinical immunotherapy can become anything more than a haphazard clinical adventure, a shot-in-the-dark, hope-for-the-best activity.

Animal Model Systems

How well does immunotherapy work in experimental animals? Model systems in which immunological treatment can be shown to be effective may be so far removed from their clinical analogues as to be totally irrelevant. There is still no satisfactory animal model comprising a spontaneously metastasizing tumour in which excision of the primary tumour followed by immunotherapy (of any sort) can be curative, and it is surely this sort of model that is needed.

Most animal models have been selected for their suitability for the detection of tumour-specific immune reactions and unfortunately those in which such reactions are easiest to demonstrate are the least like clinical cancer. An example of this situation are the Moloney virus-induced sarcomas. Such tumours are in histological terms granulomas, their content of identifiable malignant cells is extremely low and they not surprisingly undergo spontaneous regression. Successful immunotherapeutic ablation of a tumour which regresses anyway or can be simply cured by surgery or chemotherapy is hardly a therapeutic triumph but unfortunately constitutes the bulk of experimental evidence for the effectiveness of immunotherapy. It seems clear that the first and arguably the major requirement for further progress is the development of *realistic* animal models.

Assays of Tumour Immunity

Apart from the numerous theoretical problems that must be resolved there are many practical obstacles to overcome before clinical studies can be performed. Supposing a treatment method becomes available, let us say a vaccine, and the proposal is to treat a group of patients. The clinicians involved would obviously start asking a lot of questions. Is it toxic? What dose should be given? By what route? How often? It is improbable that precise answers to such questions would be obtained by mere trial and error without divine intervention. A brief examination of basic pharmacological practice shows that such questions when asked of a new drug are answered by recourse to assay systems for measuring drug levels and their effects in small groups of intensively investigated patients. Is such an approach feasible for immunological treatments? Can we develop an immunopharmacology? So far there are no really satisfactory assay systems for examining the immune response of a patient *vis-à-vis* his or her own tumour. Many different *in vitro* phenomena are currently being examined in order to develop such tests (see Chapter 4) and it would be premature to recommend any single approach. However, an examination of the effects of any so-called immunotherapy on measurable variables of host resistance should allow the answers to the above questions to be obtained and thereby allow the application of a given form of immunotherapy to larger clinical series.

In our present state of understanding there are only a limited number of number of possible manœuvres one can perform in order to bring the immune response to bear on a tumour and so far the results obtained from such manœuvres are disappointing.

Intralesional Immunotherapy

Klein (1968) has drawn attention to the fact that the development of an acute inflammatory reaction within or around a tumour and induced by a delayed cutaneous hypersensitivity reaction to an exogenous sensitizing agent will cause regression of the affected lesion. Starting with basal cell carcinomas of the skin he demonstrated that the application of dinitrochlorobenzene (DNCB) can cause complete regression of the tumour. This concept has been widely adopted and many different agents have been applied to or injected into many tumour types. BCG (Morton *et al.* 1970) and vaccinia virus (Hunter-Craig *et al.*, 1970) when injected into cutaneous nodules of melanoma can frequently cause regression of the injected lesions. Occasionally regression of uninjected lesions has been described but this is a relatively rare phenomenon and its occurrence cannot be used as a justification for the general use of such intralesional agents. Two main questionmarks hang over this sort of treatment: (a) What evidence is there that it constitutes 'immunotherapy' as opposed to 'inflammation therapy'? and (b) What is the clinical usefulness of such a procedure? The fact that a vigorous inflammatory reaction with the inevitable tissue damage which occurs is inimical to tumour growth is hardly surprising but there are very few clinical situations in which the treatment of metastases by this local means can be justified. There is as yet no evidence that intralesional BCG is of any greater value than surgery or diathermy. The major clinical benefit to be obtained from the use of this treatment in the management of cutaneous metastases is likely to be seen in the psyche of the clinician rather than the disease of the patient.

The induction of a catastrophic inflammatory reaction within a tumour by the injection of say BCG may prove to be of value in the treatment of primary tumours. Evidence from animal models indicates that such a procedure can inhibit the development of subsequent regional node metastases. There is as yet no consistent clinical evidence on this point but the animal data certainly give every reason to be optimistic.

Serotherapy (Specific Passive Immunotherapy)

In 1895 Hericourt and Richet employed antitumour antisera in the treatment of 50 cancer patients. While it is unclear from the description as to whether there was any objective clinical benefit this approach has been used extensively.

If an antiserum can be raised which binds specifically to the surface of the patients' tumour cells but not normal cells then this could be of considerable value. While such an antiserum should, by co-operation with either K cells or complement, lyse the tumour cells, it could also be used as a carrier for radioactive isotopes or chemotherapeutic agents. In experimental models there is evidence that the combination of antibody and cytotoxic drugs can be more effective than either component of the cocktail used alone. However, the major obstacle to this approach is the availability of a truly tumour-specific antibody. Conventional immunization of another species and subsequent absorption of the serum on donor normal tissues constitutes the commonest technical approach to the development of antitumour antisera and it so frequently fails. There is little or no evidence so far that in xenogeneic systems specific antibodies can be raised which are directed at tumour-specific transplantation antigens, i.e. those antigens against which the host reacts.

In model systems syngeneic immune sera have been used with some effect. Bansal and Sjögren (1971) have shown that in rats bearing polyoma-induced tumours the injection of 'immune 'serum led to the disappearance of circulating blocking factors which were occasionally associated with regression of the tumours. However, it is clear that the indiscriminate injection of a variety of poorly characterized antisera is unlikely to provide a useful result and confirmation of this scepticism is readily available in the literature describing passive immunotherapy as practised so far.

Adoptive Immunotherapy

The use of lymphoid cells and their products for the immunotherapy of cancer is a relatively new development. The basic premise for its use is that patients may have defective cell-mediated responses to their tumours and that the defect can be corrected by the infusion of sensitized cells. Unfortunately, there is no evidence for this view. Furthermore, evidence to the contrary suggests that the cellular apparatus in cancer patients is essentially intact but may be inhibited by serum factors (see Chapter 12). The infusion of sensitized cells into a patient whose extracellular fluid is flooded by factors whose major effect is the inhibition of cellular immunity would hardly seem to be a rational occupation. However, this does not deter clinicians from trying it anyway. A major potential hazard to be anticipated from the infusion of massive numbers of allogeneic lymphoid cells would be acute allogeneic disease and graft-versus-host disease, both lethal (or potentially so) complications resulting from the infused cells reacting against the host. This could be overcome by the use of irradiated cells or extracts from them. Although there is at present no real rational basis for adoptive immunotherapy many studies are being performed and described in the literature.

LYMPHOCYTES

The largest series (so far) of cases treated by adoptive lymphocyte therapy is that described by Nadler and Moore (1969). Their method was to cross-immunize pairs of patients with tumour cells and subsequently to cross-infuse peripheral blood lymphocytes. The use of pairs of patients in this way is irrational as the immunization step would ensure that the subsequent lymphocyte infusion was rapidly destroyed by immune mechanisms. The results obtained from this extensive study have failed to justify its widespread application, there being little evidence of objective tumour regression. Andrews and his colleagues (1967) immunized donors with tumour and then cannulated their thoracic ducts to obtain lymphocytes in vast numbers. No therapeutic effects were obtained in patients with either leukaemia or malignant melanoma and there was a suspicion that graft-versus-host disease may have occurred.

TRANSFER FACTOR (see chapter 12)

As long ago as 1955 Lawrence claimed that specific cell-mediated immunity could be adoptively transferred from previously sensitized donors to unsensitized recipients by the administration of extracts of peripheral blood lymphocytes. He called this extract 'transfer factor'. Unfortunately at present there is considerable controversy concerning the biological activity of transfer factor and its possible uses. Perhaps the most confusing aspect is the general inability to confirm the observations in experimental animal models. Most concern centres around the specificity of transfer factor. Many of its effects could be attributed to either the inclusion of antigen in the preparation or the fact that transfer factor may be a non-specific agent capable of causing a general heightening in immunological reactivity as one might anticipate from an immunological hormone such as thymosin. If transfer factor is a specific information-carrying molecule then it is a molecule unique in biology in view of its extremely low molecular weight. Furthermore, it is alleged to adoptively transfer cell-mediated responses only. Sceptics, the author of this chapter included, tend to question the specific nature of the transfer phenomenon. However a non-specific hormone-like effect could be of considerable clinical value.

Unfortunately most clinical data obtained from its use consist of anecdotes or small uncontrolled series of cases and it is obvious that detailed controlled studies will be needed to evaluate transfer factor both for the ability to change cell-mediated reactivity and to induce improvement in the clinical status of the patients. Clinical benefit has been claimed from the use of transfer factor in the treatment of chronic mucocutaneous candidiasis, chronic coccidioidomycosis and pulmonary tuberculosis but no controlled studies have yet been reported. Similar anecdotal reports have appeared claiming responses in cancer patients given transfer factor derived from various sources, usually from patients 'cured' of the same diseases. Such reports have described its use in patients with malignant melanoma, breast carcinoma, nasopharyngeal carcinoma, acute leukaemia and one patient with a sarcoma. However, none of these reports provide satisfactory evidence that the transfer factor given had any objective effect on the patients' malignant diseases in view of the fact that most of the patients were also treated with conventional methods either previously or concurrently and that the responses were not dramatic.

The criticisms of adoptive cellular immunotherapy mentioned above apply equally well to any putative subcellular transfer method. Unfortunately assay systems for evaluating tumour-specific immunological responses are at present too unreliable and unsophisticated to allow assessment of the effects of agents such as transfer factor on tumour-directed immunological reactivity and this sort of information will be necessary for the rational application of agents like transfer factor.

IMMUNE RNA

Alexander and Delorme (1971) have shown that a subcellular extract from suitably sensitized lymphoid cells would show significant antitumour activity *in vivo*. Furthermore, this effect was immunologically specific. This information-carrying extract contained mainly RNA with some contaminating DNA and protein. Most of the evidence suggests that the active principle in such an extract is RNA and subsequent studies by other workers have shown that such specific RNA preparations act directly on lymphoid cells conferring upon them specifically cytotoxic activity. Although at present there is no totally unequivocal proof of the existence of immunologically specific information-transfer RNA such an approach obviously deserves closer investigation and validation and will undoubtedly be the subject of clinical studies in the not-too-distant future.

Specific Active Immunotherapy

The earliest documented patients treated with a tumour cell vaccine were those described by von Leyden and Blumenthal (1902). No evidence of objective regression was recorded. In the subsequent years very many trials were performed, most of them involving the inoculation of autologous or allogeneic tumour cell macerates into patients with extensive disease. Coca, Dorrance and Lebredo (1912) treated 79 patients; 39 were given autologous tumour cells and 48 were given allogeneic cells (several being given both types). Of the 79 so treated 5, all receiving the allogeneic cell vaccine, demonstrated objective regression. On closer inspection regression could be attributed to the immunotherapy in only one case and that regression was short-lived. This important early study set the pattern for subsequent investigations (and results). Its authors concluded that 'active immunization against malignant tumours in man is impracticable'. Over the last 75 years many clinical studies of active immunotherapy have been described and the results have shown a striking if unrewarding similarity. Despite its track record this form of treatment is still under investigation. It must be emphasized that until recently specific active immunotherapy has been used almost exclusively in patients with disseminated disease and it has been used alone as the only form of treatment. Its failure when used in this way does not rule out the possibility that it may prove to be of value when combined with other cytoreductive treatments. Furthermore, until we know how to prepare and use such cell vaccines (by using *in vitro* tests for antitumour immune responses) it is unlikely that much progress will be made in this direction.

Active immunization has been tested recently as an adjunct to surgery and radiotherapy in the treatment of glioblastoma multiforme (Bloom *et al.*, 1973). There was not the slightest evidence of benefit.

The injection of crude tumour cell preparations is obviously an unsophisticated approach to active immunization. Currently, considerable effort is being expended to develop stable preparations with enhanced immunogenicity. Among such approaches are the use of helper determinants to increase the immunizing potential of the cells. For example, tumour cells can be chemically coupled to xenogeneic proteins or can be fused with normal xenogeneic cells using viruses to give heterokaryons. It is still unclear whether or not such preparations are more effective than irradiated tumour cells in inducing immunological responses in the host. Furthermore we still do not know what contribution specific immunological responses make to the host's resistance and in consequence the potential value of specific immunization procedures must remain in question.

Immunostimulation (Non-specific Active Immunotherapy)

Many substances are known to induce intense stimulation of the reticuloendothelial system (RES) and this stimulation is often associated with non-specific accentuation of immunological reactions to unrelated antigens. These substances are mostly derived from micro-organisms such as yeasts and bacteria although polysaccharides from bamboo leaves, wheatstraw, bagasse and edible mushrooms are also alleged to show such activity. One of the most active and widely studied 'immunostimulants' (or systemic adjuvants) is Bacillus Calmette-Guerin (BCG). The resistance of mice to a variety of heterologous infections can be increased by prior treatment with BCG. Similar pretreatment of female $C_{57}Bl$ mice with BCG will accelerate their subsequent rejection of a syngeneic graft of male skin. Old, Clarke and Benacerraf (1959) have shown that resistance to challenge with transplantable allogeneic tumours was heightened by similar BCG treatment. Subsequently, Weiss, Bonhag and De Ome (1961) showed that both intact and fractionated mycobacteria when injected into mice can induce protection against syngeneic chemically induced fibrosarcomas. Another agent currently receiving close scrutiny is *Corynebacterium parvum*. Described by Halpern and his colleagues (1963) as a potent stimulant of RES activity, this diphtheroid organism is a powerful systemic adjuvant for both cell-mediated and humoral immune responses. A heat-killed suspension of *Corynebacterium parvum* can induce protection against a variety of experimental syngeneic tumours and, unusual amongst the RES stimulants, it has been shown to inhibit the growth of tumours when given systemically after inoculation of the tumour cell challenge.

The inoculation of BCG into sites other than the tumour itself, being intended to produce non-specific elevation of immunological responsiveness to tumour antigens, constitutes the currently favoured though perhaps least logical mode of immunotherapy of cancer in man. Evidence for the anti-tumour activity of BCG is almost entirely derived from experiments involving pretreatment of animals with BCG. As immunotherapy, in the treatment of established experimental tumours, it is remarkably ineffective. Nevertheless, many clinical trials have been performed. In many series the investigators have not unnaturally assumed that the BCG should be employed for the eradication of minimal residual disease and have therefore used it as an adjunct to other forms of treatment such as surgery or chemotherapy. For instance, in acute lymphoblastic leukaemia in childhood, two randomized controlled trials have failed to demonstrate any therapeutic effect (M.R.C. 1971, Heyn et al., 1973). In Burkitt's lymphoma, a controlled trial by Ziegler and Magrath (1973) has similarly failed to show any evidence of benefit. Nemato, Rosner and Dao (1975) have tested BCG as an adjunct to cyclophosphamide in a randomized controlled trial in patients with metastatic breast cancer. Objective response rate and duration of response were quite unaffected by treatment with BCG. There are also a great many uncontrolled or poorly controlled studies of BCG treatment of disseminated cancer but these similarly provide little evidence for a therapeutic effect of BCG.

Have there been any successes? In acute myeloblastic leukaemia immunotherapy with irradiated leukaemic blast cells and BCG does appear to prolong the survival time of those patients achieving haematological remission (Powles et al., 1973). Vogler and Chan (1974) have obtained similar results by using a short course of BCG alone as the immunotherapy. Although the BCG treatment seems to prolong the survival of patients with this disease there is no evidence that this is in any sense immunotherapy. In a retrospectively controlled study of patients with disseminated malignant melanoma Gutterman and his colleagues (1974) have shown that local scarification with BCG will increase the response rate of tumour within the BCG drainage area to treatment with systemic chemotherapy using dimethyl-triazeno-imidazole carboxamide (DTIC). There was, however, no significant effect on distant metastases and this result may have to be regarded as another manifestation of the local effects of BCG.

From this brief examination of the available evidence it is difficult to endorse the current enthusiasm for the almost indiscriminate use of BCG in the treatment of cancer patients. However, there is as yet no reason to discard this approach. Once again we do not know how best to use such agents. Considerations of dosage and route of administration have been based on convenience rather than immunology. The use of BCG and agents such as *C. parvum* may yet play an important role in the overall attack on tumour cells. Both agents, as well as heightening specific immunity, also lead to increased host resistance which is not strictly speaking immunological (i.e. it shows little or no tumour specificity) and may well be mediated by macrophages without the intervention of any form of specific antitumour immunity. Indeed, in animals treated with *C. parvum*, about the only agent in this group capable of influencing the growth of an established tumour, there is a notable absence of T cell reactivity, once thought to represent the major effector mechanism operating in tumour immunity. In such animals the most striking finding is the presence of activated macrophages which probably make the most significant contribution to resistance to tumour growth. Although when used alone systemic *C. parvum* does not cure experimental tumours (it causes a degree of growth inhibition only), when suitably combined with chemotherapeutic cytoreduction, complete and lasting regressions can be obtained (Currie and Bagshawe, 1970).

Immunotherapy Combined with Other Treatments

SURGERY

In experimental rodent tumours the simplest and most effective means of inducing specific antitumour immunity is to excise an established tumour. If immunity is, as we currently believe, a significant factor in host resistance to tumour growth, then the best form of immunotherapy seems to be surgery. Another important feature of most animal model systems is the strict dose-dependence of tumour immunity: in such animals a potent immune response is capable of destroying a very limited number of tumour cells, frequently less than 10^6 cells *in toto*. The destruction of such cells, however, does not obey the usual kinetic rules of chemotherapeutic kill and is not exponential. Consequently it is generally agreed that immunological mechanisms may play their most vital role in situations of minimal residual disease following, say, surgical excision of a tumour mass. The major impact of such a notion on surgical practice is the recognition that ablation of tumour mass is crucial and therefore as much tumour as is surgically accessible should be removed.

One area of intense speculation currently dominating the literature is the surgical approach to regional lymph nodes. Perhaps the most important consideration in the management of such nodes should be the practice of medicine rather than the impact of rather nebulous but fashionable ideas about immunity. There can be, in the light of present knowledge (as opposed to speculation), no justification for not treating involved lymph nodes.

Disease where it exists should be treated either by surgery, radiotherapy or chemotherapy. Similarly there is at present no evidence to justify the removal of uninvolved nodes. With the sophisticated methods of investigation currently available such as lymphography, decisions as to whether lymph nodes should be removed ought to be dictated by whether or not they contain metastatic disease. This is, however, the counsel of perfection and many situations it is not always clear whether nodes are involved. However, in the absence of unequivocal knowledge on this subject the performance of drastic and often mutilating operations is hard to justify unless they can be shown to induce a significant prolongation of survival. Partial resolution of these arguments is becoming available as current studies of the management of carcinoma of the breast are completed.

From studies of animal model systems it can be seen that the regional lymph nodes draining a tumour contain large numbers of immunologically active cells; in fact, the major site of circulating antibody production and the generation of cytotoxic cells appears to be these nodes. However, with increasing growth of a primary tumour these nodes become paralysed, failing to release sensitized effector cells and losing their complement of specifically cytotoxic lymphocytes. Following tumour excision the nodes rapidly regain these functions, unless they contain metastases. As well as having immunological functions it must be remembered that regional lymph nodes also act as an efficient filter for the removal of cells from the extracellular fluid compartment draining through them. The destruction of such cells in the regional nodes does undoubtedly have an immunological component but it is likely that immunologically non-specific destruction mechanisms also operate in them. Current investigations in both animals and man are being performed to determine whether the application of non-specific stimulants such as BCG and *C. parvum* can be applied to the drainage area at the time of tumour excision and whether the stimulation of the regional nodes induced by these agents can diminish the incidence of nodal metastases.

IRRADIATION AND CHEMOTHERAPY

Irradiation treatment and cytotoxic chemotherapy are undoubtedly immunosuppressive. Some authors have suggested that both treatment modalities should be avoided or minimized because of the risks of immunosuppression. This is a totally fallacious argument. In the presence of a tumour mass it is most unlikely that the immune response is playing an important role in limiting its growth. Only when the tumour burden has been drastically reduced is there any reason to believe that immunity to the tumour is going to play a significant role. To avoid using treatments which are known to reduce tumour mass because of a series of totally theoretical considerations is foolhardy. It is much more important to kill tumour cells than to spare the immune response. If it were possible to achieve drastic cytoreduction without immunosuppression then such a regime would be preferable. Without such methods being available, however, it seems to be much more important to kill large numbers of tumour cells than to spare an already feeble and ineffective immune response from temporary abrogation. Furthermore, even the most severe immunosuppression induced by vigorous chemotherapy is usually rapidly reversible. The use of modern chemotherapy, especially when given in intermittent high doses has surprisingly little overall impact on immunological reactivity. At present although it seems advisable to use irradiation and cytotoxic drugs in a manner which is least immunosuppressive, theoretical considerations about the role of immunity in host resistance should not override the practical aspects of trying to ablate tumours as effectively as possible. Furthermore once the tumour burden has been drastically reduced immunotherapeutic manipulations may then be expected to contribute their feeble but specific effects to eradicate residual tumour cells. This has been the thinking behind most recent attempts to use immunotherapy and there are promising fragments of evidence slowly accumulating. For instance immunization with allogeneic irradiated leukaemia blast cells plus BCG has been shown to prolong the survival in those patients with acute myeloblastic leukaemia achieving haematological remission after vigorous chemotherapy (Powles et al., 1973). In disseminated malignant melanoma the effects of DTIC, currently the most favoured form of chemotherapy for this particularly intractable disease, are alleged to have been improved by the concurrent administration of BCG (Gutterman et al., 1974) or irradiated melanoma cells plus BCG (Currie and McElwain, 1975).

Serendipity often plays an important role in the development of new treatment methods. Chance does not seem to have favoured those working on the immunotherapy of tumours but whether this is due to the lack of prepared minds working in this field is open to discussion. The general lack of success of immunotherapy so far must dictate caution in both the design of experiments and the interpretation of data. Recently acquired information, however, does provide a reason for optimism. Our increasing knowledge of the immunological mechanisms operating in the tumour-bearing individual gives every reason to hope that such mechanisms may eventually be manipulated for clinical benefit. It is also clear that to achieve such a result will require considerably more knowledge about the immunological interactions of host and tumour than is currently available.

References

Alexander, P and Delorme, E. J. (1971). The use of irradiated immune lymphoid cells for immunotherapy of primary tumors in rats. *Israel J. Med. Sci.*, **7**, 239

Andrews, G. A., Congdon, C. C. *et al.* (1967). Preliminary trials of clinical immunotherapy. *Cancer Res.*, **27**, 2535

Bansal, S. C. and Sjögren, H. O. (1971). 'Unblocking' serum activity *in vitro* in the polyoma system may correlate with antitumour effects of antiserum *in vivo*. *Nature New Biol.*, **233**, 76

Bashford, E. F. (1908). Contributions to the study of the development of sarcoma under experimental conditions. In *3rd Scientific Report. Imperial Cancer Research Fund.* (London: Taylor and Francis)

Bloom, H. J. G., Peckham, M. J., Richardson, A. E., Alexander, P. and Payne, P. M. (1973). Glioblastoma multiforme: a controlled trial to assess the value of specific active immunotherapy in patients treated by radical surgery and radiotherapy. *Br. J. Cancer*, **27**, 253

Carnaud, C., Hoch, B. and Trainin, N. (1974). Influence of immunologic competence of the host on metastases induced by the 3LL Lewis tumor in mice. *J. Natl. Cancer Inst.*, **52**, 395

Coca, A. F., Dorrance, G. M. and Lebredo, M. G. (1912). 'Vaccination' in cancer. A report of the results of the vaccination therapy as applied in seventy-nine cases of human cancer. *Z. Immun. Exp. Therap.*, **13**, 543

Currie, G. A. and Bagshawe, K. D. (1970). Active immunotherapy with *Corynebacterium parvum* and chemotherapy in murine fibrosarcomas. *Br. Med. J.*, **1**, 541

Currie, G. A. (1972). Eighty years of immunotherapy: a review of immunological methods used for the treatment of human cancer. *Br. J. Cancer*, **26**, 141

Currie, G. A. and Alexander, P. (1974). Spontaneous shedding of TSTA by viable sarcoma cells; its possible role in facilitating metastatic spread. *Br. J. Cancer*, **29**, 72

Currie, G. A. and McElwain, T. J. (1975). Active immunotherapy as an adjunct to chemotherapy in the treatment of disseminated malignant melanoma: a pilot study. *Br. J. Cancer*, **31**, 143

Dubos, R. J. (1957). Effects of cellular constituents of mycobacteria on the resistance of mice to heterologous infections. I. Protective effects. *J. Exp. Med.*, **106**, 703

Folkman, J. and Hochberg, M. (1973). Self-regulation of growth in three dimensions. *J. Exp. Med.*, **138**, 745

Gershon, R. and Carter, R. L. (1970). Facilitation of metastatic growth by antilymphocyte serum. *Nature (London)*, **226**, 368

Globerson, A. and Feldman, M. (1964). Antigenic specificity of benzo(a)pyrene-induced sarcomas. *J. Natl. Cancer Inst.*, **32**, 1229

Gutterman, J. U., Mavligit, G., Gottlieb, J. A. *et al.* (1974). Chemoimmunotherapy of disseminated malignant melanoma with DTIC and BCG. *N. Engl. J. Med.*, **291**, 592

Halpern, B. N. *et al.* (1963). Stimulation de l'activité phagocytaire du système reticuloendothelial provoquée par *Corynebacterium parvum*. *J. Reticulo-endothelial Soc.*, **1**, 77

Hericourt, J. and Richet, C. (1895). Physiologie pathologique de la Serotherapie dans le traitement du cancer. *C.R. Hebd. Séances Acad. Sci.*, **121**, 567

Heyn, R., Borges, W., Joo, P. *et al.* (1973). BCG in the treatment of acute lymphocytic leukemia (ALL). *Proc. Am. Ass. Cancer Res.*, **14**, 45

Hunter-Craig, I., Newton, K. A., Westbury, G. and Lacey, B. W. (1970). Use of vaccinia virus in the treatment of metastatic malignant melanoma. *Br. Med. J.*, **2**, 512

Klein, E. (1968). Tumors of the skin X. Immunotherapy of cutaneous and mucosal neoplasms. *N.Y. J. Med.*, **68,** 900

Lawrence, H. S. (1955). The transfer in humans of delayed skin sensitivity to streptococca M substance and to tuberculin with disrupted leucocytes. *J. Clin. Invest.*, **34,** 219

M.R.C. (1971). Treatment of acute lymphoblastic leukaemia: comparison of immunotherapy (BCG), intermittent methotrexate, and no therapy after a five-month intensive cytotoxic regimen (Concord Trial). Preliminary Report to the Medical Research Council by the Leukaemia Committee and the Working Party on leukaemia in childhood. *Br. Med. J.*, **4,** 189

Morton, D., Eilber, F. R. and Malmgren, R. A. (1970). Immunological factors which influence response to immunotherapy in malignant melanoma. *Surgery*, **68,** 158

Nadler, S. H. and Moore, G. E. (1969). Immunotherapy of malignant disease. *Arch. Surg.*, **99,** 376

Nemato, T., Rosner, D. and Dao, T. (1975). In Proceedings of the XIth International Cancer Congress. (In press)

Powles, R. L., Crowther, D., Bateman, C. J. T. et al. (1973). Immunotherapy for acute myelogenous leukaemia. *Br. J. Cancer*, **28,** 365

Proctor, J. W., Rudenstam, C. M. and Alexander, P. (1973). A factor preventing the development of lung metastases in rats with sarcomas. *Nature (London)*, **242,** 29

Southam, C. M. (1961). Applications of immunology to clinical cancer: past attempts and future possibilities. *Cancer Res.*, **21,** 1302

Vaage, J., Doroshaw, J. A. and Dubois, T. T. (1974). Radiation-induced changes in established tumor immunity. *Cancer Res.*, **34,** 129

Vogler, W. R. and Chan, Y-K. (1974). Prolonging remission in myeloblastic leukaemia by Tice-strain bacillus Calmette-Guerin. *Lancet*, **ii,** 128

von Leyden, V. E. and Blumenthal, F. (1902). Vorlaufige Mitteilungen uber einige Ergebnisse der Krebsforschung auf der 1 medizinische Klinik. *Deutsche Med. Wochenschr.*, **28,** 637

Weiss, D. W., Bonhag, R. S. and De Ome, K.B. (1961). Protective activity of fractions of tubercle bacilli against isologous tumours in mice. *Nature (London)*, **190,** 889

Woodruff, M. F. A. (1964). Immunological aspects of cancer. *Lancet*, **ii,** 265

Ziegler, J. L. and Magrath, I. T. (1973). BCG immunotherapy in Burkitt's lymphoma: preliminary results of a randomized clinical trial. *Natl. Cancer Inst. Monogr.*, **39,** 199

Further Reading

Alexander, P. (1968). Immunotherapy of cancer. *Proc. Exp. Tumor Res.*, **10,** 22

Currie, G. A. (1974). *Cancer and the Immune Response.* (London: Edward Arnold)

Klein, G. (1966). Tumour antigens. *Ann. Rev. Microbiol.*, **20,** 223

Mitchison, N. A. (1970). Immunologic approach to cancer. *Transplant. Proc.*, **2,** 92

Smith, R. T. (1972). Possibilities and problems of immunologic intervention in cancer. *N. Engl. J. Med.*, **287,** 439

Index